INTERFERON AND INTERFERON INDUCERS

MODERN PHARMACOLOGY-TOXICOLOGY

A Series of Monographs and Textbooks

COORDINATING EDITOR   ASSOCIATE EDITOR

William F. Bousquet   *Roger F. Palmer*

Division of Biological Research   University of Miami
Searle Laboratories, G. D. Searle & Co.   School of Medicine
Chicago, Illinois   Miami, Florida

Additional Volumes in Preparation

INTERFERON AND INTERFERON INDUCERS

Clinical Applications

Edited by Dale A. Stringfellow

Experimental Biology Research
The Upjohn Company
Kalamazoo, Michigan

MARCEL DEKKER, INC.   New York and Basel

Library of Congress Cataloging in Publication Data

Main entry under title:

Interferon and interferon inducers, clinical applica-
    tions.

    (Modern pharmacology-toxicology ; v. 17)
    Includes indexes.
    1. Interferons. 2. Interferon inducers.
3. Interferons--Therapeutic use. 4. Interferon
inducers--Therapeutic use. I. Stringfellow, Dale A.,
[date]   [DNLM: 1. Interferon. 2. Interferon
inducers. W1 M0167T v. 17 / QW 800 I59]
QR187.5.I5718   616.07'95   80-13726
ISBN 0-8247-6931-7

MARCEL DEKKER, INC.
270 Madison Avenue, New York, New York 10016

Current printing (last digit):
10 9 8 7 6 5 4 3 2 1

PRINTED IN THE UNITED STATES OF AMERICA

To my daughters:

Jennifer, Wendy, and Ashley

PREFACE

During the past two decades interferon research has steadily increased and intensified. At first, the discovery of interferon was of interest to only a handful of virologists involved in the phenomenon of viral interference. As more became known about this unique group of molecules, interest in their potential use in treating viral infections increased, bringing new investigators into the field. Interest then seemed to wane due to the difficulties in utilizing interferon or its inducers for treating human viral diseases. In the past few years, however, a new era of interferon research has developed. The role of interferon in cellular control processes has expanded beyond modulation of antiviral resistance to include immune regulation and cancer chemotherapy. These developments have rekindled awareness of interferon research and brought about a renewed commitment to bring this exciting group of agents to clinical utilization.

When I was first asked to plan this volume, I realized that many promising approaches that may lead to the fulfillment of interferons' potential as effective chemotherapeutic agents had been neglected. I therefore decided to emphasize this phase of interferon research.

The authors, leaders in their fields, have prepared chapters on areas in which they hold positions of esteem. Each chapter is designed to be broad enough to be of value to the novice yet detailed enough to be useful as a reference source for the experienced interferon researcher.

Interferon and interferon inducers are presently undergoing clinical evaluation. This book is intended to serve as background for these studies, highlighting our progress and problems currently being encountered.

Dale A. Stringfellow

CONTENTS

CONTRIBUTORS

KURT BERG Department of Virology, Institute of Medical Microbiology, University of Aarhus, Aarhus, Denmark

ROBERT F. BETTS Infectious Disease Unit, Department of Medicine, University of Rochester School of Medicine, Rochester, New York

ALFONS BILLIAU Department of Human Biology, Division of Microbiology, Rega Institute, University of Leuven, Leuven, Belgium

MARY C. BREINIG* Department of Microbiology, Medical College of Virginia, Virginia Commonwealth University, Richmond, Virginia

RITA F. BUFFETT Department of Viral Oncology, Roswell Park Memorial Institute, Buffalo, New York

ROBERT B. COUCH Department of Microbiology and Immunology, Baylor College of Medicine, Houston, Texas

PIET DE SOMER Department of Microbiology, Division of Microbiology, Rega Institute, University of Leuven, Leuven, Belgium

R. GORDON DOUGLAS, JR. Infectious Disease Unit, Department of Medicine, University of Rochester School of Medicine, Rochester, New York

STEPHEN B. GREENBERG Departments of Medicine, and Microbiology and Immunology, Baylor College of Medicine, Houston, Texas

MAURICE W. HARMON Department of Microbiology and Immunology, Baylor College of Medicine, Houston, Texas

IVER HERON Institute of Medical Microbiology, Department of Immunology, University of Aarhus, Aarhus, Denmark

---

*Present affiliation: Department of Microbiology, Graduate School of Public Health, University of Pittsburgh, Pittsburgh, Pennsylvania.

MICHIO ITO Department of Viral Oncology, Roswell Park Memorial Institute, Buffalo, New York

HOWARD M. JOHNSON Department of Microbiology, University of Texas Medical Branch, Galveston, Texas

RUSSELL F. KRUEGER Merrell Research Center, Merrell-National Laboratories, Division of Richardson-Merrell Inc., Cincinnati, Ohio

HILTON B. LEVY Section of Molecular Virology, National Institute of Allergy and Infectious Diseases, National Institutes of of Health, Bethesda, Maryland

GERALD D. MAYER Merrell Research Center, Merrell-National Laboratories, Division of Richardson-Merrell Inc., Cincinnati, Ohio

PAGE S. MORAHAN Department of Microbiology, Medical College of Virginia, Virginia Commonwealth University, Richmond, Virginia

KURT OSTHER Biological Department, Alfred Benzon Ltd., Hvidovre, Denmark

DALE A. STRINGFELLOW Cancer and Virus Research, Experimental Biology Research, The Upjohn Company, Kalamazoo, Michigan

INTERFERON AND
INTERFERON INDUCERS

1

INTERFERONS: AN OVERVIEW

Dale A. Stringfellow
The Upjohn Company
Kalamazoo, Michigan

I. INTRODUCTION

Since its discovery in 1957 [1], interest in interferon as a mediator of antiviral resistance has steadily increased. During these years of exploration, the role of interferon as a natural regulator of various cellular functions has expanded beyond the initial area of mediation of antiviral resistance to include modulation of immune responsiveness and cellular growth and regulation. Thus its pharmaceutical potential now includes areas of cancer and viral chemotherapy and immune modulation. Yet the answers to questions as basic as what is the structure of this intriguing group of molecules and what is their natural physiological role are still not clear. This introductory chapter is a background for the chapters that follow and therefore will deal with interferon's "past" and how this fits into its future. Particular attention will be devoted to the antiviral action of interferon, its role in control of viral disease processes, the mechanism of antiviral action,

the properties of the interferon molecules, and how this information fits
into our present understanding of the interferon system.

II. DISCOVERY AND PROPERTIES

Host resistance to and recovery from virus infection is a complex phenomenon involving a wide range of known and currently unknown factors. One
such determinant is the nonspecific resistance initiated and mediated by
interferon. Interferon, or perhaps more accurately, interferons, are a
group of substances of cellular origin which render the cells of many verte-
brates incapable of supporting virus replication. The term interferon was
first applied to a soluble factor produced by the cells of chicken chorioallantoic membranes after exposure to inactivated influenza virus [1].
Exposure of the membranes to inactivated virus reduced their capacity to
support replication of infectious influenza virus and stimulated secretion
of the interferon.

Shortly after its discovery, Lindenmann et al. [2] determined that
interferon was a protein, or at least was susceptible to the action of proteolytic enzymes, and was nondialyzable yet could not be sedimented by
centrifugation at $100,000 \times g$ for 4 hr. Antiviral activity was retained when
solutions of interferon were subjected to pH extremes of 2 to 10, when heated
at 60°C for 1 hr, and when incubated with antiserum prepared against the
virus that had been used to stimulate its production. Inhibition of both RNA
and DNA viruses was also observed [3-5]. The fact that incubation of a
virus with interferon had no effect on viral infectivity led Lindenmann et al.
[2] to assert that interferon exerted its antiviral effects by rendering cells
incapable of supporting viral replication rather than interacting directly
with the intact virus particle. Shortly thereafter, Tyrrell [6] demonstrated
that interferon prepared in chickens had no detectable antiviral activity on
calf cells, thereby introducing the concept of species specificity.

Since the discovery of the original interferon, numerous reports have
described the induction of other viral-inhibitory substances which have
essentially the same characteristics. In culture, cells from humans, pigs,
chickens, cats, dogs, cows, rabbits, mice, rats, guinea pigs, sheep, hamsters, monkeys, tortoises, snakes, fish, and other animal species have
yielded interferon when exposed to an appropriate inducing agent. Interferon appears in the blood, lungs, brains, urine, spinal fluid, and other
tissues of animals following administration of various interferon inducers.
Although viruses or viral components were initially used to induce the
production of interferon, certain nonviral substances also stimulate its
production in vivo and in vitro. Among these nonviral interferon inducers
are endotoxins [7,8], polysaccharides [9], phytohemagglutinin [10],
bacteria [11], rickettsiae [12], protozoa [13], synthetic low-molecular-
weight compounds such as bis(diethylaminoethyl)fluoronone [14], synthetic

polynucleotides [15], as well as a number of polyanions [16,17] and basic dyes [18] (see Chapter 6).

Although it was originally anticipated that interferon or interferon-like substances could be characterized in terms of biological and/or physico-chemical properties such as pH and heat stability, molecular weight, and species specificity, it has become increasingly apparent that considerable variation exists between an interferon induced in one species or by a specific inducer and another induced under different conditions. Some interferons have varied in the degree to which they resist heat, inhibit virus production in cells from heterologous species, and resist degradation under either acid or alkaline conditions [19]. Therefore, some interferons are different from the original interferon isolated from the chorioallantoic membranes of embryonated chick eggs. Molecular weight determinations confirm these differences. Partial purification of interferons has revealed a remarkable heterogeneity in molecular weights and electric charges of different prepara-tions [20]. Interferons with different molecular sizes have been observed in the serum of animals or from mammalian cells in vitro when inoculated with either virus or nonviral inducers [21,22]. These reports indicated that there were usually two or more molecular species, one with a molecular weight greater than 100,000 and another smaller molecule ranging between 20,000 and 40,000. Ke and Ho [23] have reported that the molecular weights of interferon found in the serum of endotoxin inoculated rabbits were con-siderably greater than the 35,000 molecular weight molecule execreted in the urine. Carter [24] suggested that some interferons may be multimeric aggregates of a smaller common weight molecule, since shifting the salt concentration dissociated the high-molecular-weight species of mouse or human interferon into smaller common molecular weight components which were biologically active [25]. It is notable that Stewart et al. [26] recently reported that low-molecular-weight "subunits" of native interferons also display antiviral activity. Furthermore, although it was previously suggested that viral inducers stimulated the production of a relatively low-molecular-weight interferon (20,000-30,000 daltons) while nonviral inducers, particu-larly such agents as endotoxins, stimulate the release of a larger molecular species (90,000-120,000 daltons), it is possible that this may be a function of the conditions under which the interferon was induced. For example, in an animal given a single injection of an inducer, the molecular species of interferon in the serum differed markedly from those found in different organs [27], yet the different molecular species were apparently anti-genically similar as indicated by neutralization of biological activity with anti-interferon antibody.

More recent studies on the antigenicity of various interferon prepara-tions convincingly demonstrate that there are several types of interferon produced by a particular animal species. For example, there are at least three antigenically distinct types of human interferon: fibroblast, lympho-cyte, and immune or type II interferons [28-30; Chapter 2]. It is not clear, however, what function each distinct type of interferon plays in vivo. Havell [31] has suggested that human fibroblasts can produce both fibroblast and lymphocyte interferon, and conversely human lymphocytes make both types as well as type II (immune-induced) interferon. The function of each interferon is not clear. Possibly a particular (fibroblast) interferon is preferentially involved in cellular regulation while leukocyte or type II interferons are involved in immune regulation, although by definition each interferon species has antiviral activity.

Although interferons differ, most meet many of the physicochemical and biological properties which historically have been established to characterize interferons. These include species specificity, stability at a pH of 2.0, and nondializability yet nonsedimentability when centrifuged at 100,000 × g for 4 hr. There are also several properties which a substance must possess before it can be considered to be an interferon. Three of the most basic of these are (1) inactivation of antiviral activity by treatment with proteolytic enzymes but not by nucleases; (2) antiviral activity cannot be mediated through a direct interaction with the intact virus particle but must rather function by rendering otherwise susceptible cells incapable of supporting virus replication through a process requiring cellular protein and RNA synthesis; and (3) the interferon-like substance must be active against a wide range of viruses. Some of the discrepancies that have appeared in the literature regarding the properties and characteristics of interferons can be attributed, at least in part, to the crudeness of the interferon preparations used in most studies. A variety of techniques have more recently been applied to the concentration and purification of interferons. Characterization of the interferon in these preparations will hopefully resolve some of the conflicting reports, further clarify the molecular characteristics, and possibly lead to determination of the amino acid sequence of various interferons (see Chapter 2).

Lockart [32] and Hilleman [33] have postulated that interferons are a family of proteins of cellular origin which are capable of initiating a nonspecific intracellular inhibition of virus replication. Interferons may be differentiated according to their source, their spectrum of activity, and their physicochemical properties. They may be similar in many respects to enzymes and antibodies which are classified on the basis of their biological activities but include proteins which can vary considerably with respect to their molecular size, physicochemical properties, and biological properties.

III. THE INDUCTION PROCESS

Since its discovery, practically every major group of viruses has been found capable of inducing interferon production in suitable in vivo or in vitro systems. Thus the production of interferon is a general response of cells toward viral infections. On the other hand, in 1964 [7] interferon was detected in the serum of chickens that had been injected intravenously with Brucella abortus. Since then, other nonviral substances have been found capable of inducing the production of interferon, and viruses or viral components cannot be considered specific stimuli responsible for the induction phenomenon. The present discussion will initially consider the viral induction process, which will be expanded to consider other types of inducers.

Heller [34] and Wagner [35] furnished the first evidence concerning the mechanisms involved in the induction of interferon synthesis by demonstrating that the cellular interferon response to chikungunya virus could be inhibited by pretreating cells with actinomycin D. The principal activity of this antibiotic is the binding of guanine residues of double-stranded DNA, thereby preventing the formation of new messenger RNA (mRNA) and subsequently inhibiting protein synthesis. This evidence suggested that interferon was synthesized under host genetic control in response to a viral stimulus. Furthermore, if actinomycin D was introduced after mRNA was formed, it had no effect on interferon synthesis [36]. It was therefore assumed that interferon is produced by cells in response to virus infection by a mechanism involving derepression of a host cistron(s) to form an mRNA that codes for the production of interferon [37].

The precise event or stimulus which initiates cellular mRNA, and consequently interferon production, is presently unclear and the subject of considerable controversy. With RNA viruses it appears that the double-stranded replicative intermediate formed during the replication of a single-stranded RNA virus and the natural double-stranded RNA of other viruses are potent interferon inducers [38,39]. The induction of interferon by natural and synthetic polynucleotides has also been observed in a variety of mammalian cells in vitro or in whole animals [40]. Furthermore, Field et al. [15] reported that single-stranded polynucleotides were inactive at a concentration 10,000 times greater than that which induced viral interference with the helical double-stranded form. Likewise double-stranded DNA or DNA-RNA hybrids also have been reported to be ineffective as interferon inducers [40].

The importance of the double-stranded form has been challenged, however, by experiments which employed inactivated viruses as the inducer. Dianzani et al. [41] attempted to inhibit the replication of Newcastle disease virus (NDV) RNA with actinomycin D and therefore eliminate the double-stranded intermediate form. They concluded that, since no infectious virus was produced under the conditions employed, the viral RNA did not replicate and the interferon induced was due to single-stranded RNA. NDV was later found to carry its own transcriptase into the cell with its nucleic acid, which may have led to the formation of double-stranded intermediates even though no infectious virus was formed, and therefore the interferon induced may well have been due to a small amount of double-stranded RNA. This also could explain how ultraviolet-irradiated NDV can induce interferon since the replicase would not be affected by UV irradiation. More recently

Dianzani et al. [42] repeated their early studies using chikungunya virus as the inducer. This single-stranded RNA virus does not carry its own replicase with it, and therefore the interferon response induced using this virus was presumably induced by single-stranded RNA. Although the controversy has not been fully settled, double-stranded RNAs are effective interferon inducers and to a major degree are probably responsible for most RNA virus-induced interferon, although additional processes may be required [43,44].

How does our understanding of the ability of double-stranded viral RNA to induce interferon fit into the mechanism of induction by other substances? The specific answer to this question is not available. It is not clear whether inducers need to penetrate the cell or whether they are active at an external membrane site. Most evidence suggests that inducers such as polynucleotides need only interact with the cell surface to induce interferon production [45-48]. However, in these studies, polynucleotides were attached to insoluble matrices that could not enter the cell, but unfortunately polynucleotide was slowly released [46,47]. Therefore, even though the matrix-attached inducer could not enter the cell, the slow release of small amounts of inducer might be responsible for the interferon response. Recently, Borden and Leonhardt [49,50] have demonstrated that amphotericin B caused enhanced cellular production of interferon in response to a polynucleotide inducer. They postulated that amphotericin caused the cellular membrane to become "leaky" thereby permitting greater intracellular accumulation of inducer. These data, along with the ability of viral RNA to induce interferon, suggest that intracellular nucleotides can induce interferon.

How double-stranded RNAs, or for that matter other inducing agents (Chapter 6), stimulate cells to begin producing the mRNA(s) that code for the interferon protein is not understood. It appears that some inducers do combine with specific membrane or cytoplasmic receptor sites and that this attachment is inhibited by agents such as hormones [51]. Interpretation of these studies is complicated by the fact that most of the agents used stimulate membrane-associated adenylate cyclase causing an intracellular increase in cyclic AMP. Therefore the decreased responsiveness of such cells to interferon induction might simply be due to modulation of interferon production by cyclic AMP [52-55]. In addition, treatment of cells with interferon or interferon inducers stimulates production or cellular release of prostaglandin-like molecules [56]. Certain prostaglandins (i.e., series E prostaglandins) stimulate cyclic AMP levels in various types of cells, and the interrelationship between prostaglandins, cyclic nucleotides, and membrane receptor sites is still unclear. Also, prostaglandins do appear to be involved, independent of cyclic nucleotides, in modulation of interferon production by at least murine cells [57].

The mechanism by which various low-molecular-weight compounds, such as tilorone hydrochloride or various pyrimidines (see Chapter 6), stimulate cellular interferon production is even less well defined. Many inducers are active only in vivo or in complex multicellular in vitro cell culture systems [58], suggesting that several cell populations may be needed to initiate interferon production. For example, the pyrimidine inducer 2-amino-5-bromo-6-methyl-4-pyrimidinol (ABMP) stimulated high levels of interferon in vivo in the spleens and thymuses of mice or when added to murine spleen and thymus organ culture systems in vitro [58]. However, if macrophages (glass-adherent cells) were separated from lymphocytes (nonadherent cells), the ability of both cell populations to produce interferon in response to in vitro addition of ABMP was lost. These data suggest that cell-to-cell interaction or amplification may be necessary to achieve interferon induction with many inducing agents.

IV.   CONTROL OF INTERFERON
PRODUCTION

As with most biologically active molecules, natural control or regulatory mechanisms limit the amount of interferon cells normally make. High interferon levels appear to trigger the production of another cellular protein that inhibits further interferon synthesis, probably through suppression of further interferon mRNA production. The precise nature of the control protein is unknown. Speculation has included the antiviral protein(s) that interferon induces, interferon itself, or another as yet unidentified control protein [59-61]. Evidence for the existence of such a control system is based in large part on indirect evidence generated through the selective use of metabolic inhibitors. Cells can be manipulated to produce abnormally high levels of interferon (superinduction) by the addition of actinomycin D and cycloheximide shortly after (2-3 hr) stimulation by an inducer [62-66]. During the initial 2- to 3-hr period interferon mRNA is transcribed and translation is initiated. By adding actinomycin D at that time, production of the mRNA that codes for the control protein is inhibited, but cells can proceed with interferon mRNA translation, consequently producing much higher levels of interferon (up to 10 times more).

The control protein has not been satisfactorily isolated or identified, although Borden et al. [67,68] have reported that such a protein could be detected in vitro in murine L929 cell cultures induced to make interferon with NDV. During the early stages of interferon induction very little control protein was detected, while later on when cells were making less interferon, high levels of the control substance were detected. Interferon and the hyporeactivity factor were never completely separated physicochemically, but biologically a distinct separation was observed.

Expanding upon these observations, Stringfellow and Glasgow [69a] utilized an in vivo system to determine if such a control protein could be detected in the serum of mice infected with encephalomyocarditis (EMC) virus. They had earlier observed [69b] that EMC-infected mice developed

a severe state of hyporesponsiveness to interferon induction. A factor in
the serum was identified and characterized [70]. It had many of the properties of interferon (species specificity, pH stability, a molecular weight of
10,000-20,000, etc.) but had no demonstrable antiviral activity nor was
its ability to mediate hyporeactivity lost by incubation with anti-interferon
antibody. Since that time a similar factor has been identified in the sera
of mice infected with any of several viruses or carrying two types of lymphomas [71,72]. Tarr et al. [73] have identified a similar substance in
the serum of mice infected with cytomegalovirus, although in their studies
the hyporeactive factor was inactivated by incubation with anti-interferon
antibody. Whether the substances detected in vivo are the same as the control protein identified by Borden et al., and if these substances are proteins
that naturally control interferon production, is not yet known.

Recently, Stringfellow [57] reported that mice infected with EMC virus
developed a hyporeactive interferon response and that the response of these
mice could be restored to normal if inducers were administered with
prostaglandins. These data suggest that the hyporeactive state (at least
under these conditions) was reversible and that prostaglandins may be
involved in regulation of interferon responsiveness (cf. Chapter 6). The
administration of prostaglandins did not appear to influence the levels of
hyporeactive factors in the serum of infected mice but rather appeared to
reverse the effect of the substance. For example, mouse embryo fibroblast
cells incubated with hyporeactive factor from EMC-infected mice [57]
develop a 90% suppressed response; yet, when PGE2 (2 μg/ml) was added
to such cells, only a 10-20% suppression was observed. The interrelationship between prostaglandins, the control protein, and modulation of interferon production is currently under investigation.

V. MECHANISM OF ANTIVIRAL
   ACTIVITY

The antiviral activity of interferon is indirect since it can be prevented by
pretreating cells with actinomycin D or other inhibitors of protein synthesis
[74-76]. Interferon itself causes the host to produce mRNA for yet another
antiviral protein or polypeptide which functions as the actual antiviral agent.
Such a protein, however, has yet to be isolated in cells treated with interferon preparations [74-75], although Samuel and Joklik [76] found a
ribosomal-associated protein (molecular weight of 48,000) in interferon-
induced cells. While direct proof for the interferon-induced antiviral
protein is still lacking, circumstantial evidence supports this interpretation [77-80].

Soon after the discovery of interferon, it became apparent that it did
not interact with viruses directly nor did it prevent the absorption of viruses
to cells, viral uncoating, viral assembly, or release of virus particles
[81-84]. Instead, interferon appeared to act by preventing the synthesis

of progeny virus particles [85]. The precise mechanism by which the theorized antiviral protein induced by interferon prevents synthesis of new virus particles or viral proteins is not known. Marcus and Salb [86-88] reported that ribosomes derived from interferon-treated cells were capable of interacting with either viral or host mRNA. They observed, however, that there was a suppression of the translation of viral but not host mRNA. This led them to postulate that interferon-treated cells produced mRNA which then coded for a new protein which they called translation inhibitory protein (TIP). TIP supposedly was bound to cellular ribosomes; polysomes composed of host mRNA and TIP-attached ribosomes translated normally, while those composed of viral mRNA and TIP-attached ribosomes did not translate as efficiently, resulting in suppression of viral protein synthesis. Carter and Levy [89], working with a different cell virus system, found that ribosomes from interferon-treated cells failed to bind viral RNA at all, but normal ribosomes bound and translated viral RNA to form polysomes. Thus, although somewhat in contrast with Marcus and Salb, Carter and Levy argued that the primary site of interferon action was on the binding efficiency of viral RNA to cellular ribosomes, not on final viral RNA translation. Both groups did agree, however, that the action of interferon was directly on the ribosomes. Samuel and Joklik have reported the presence of a ribosomal-associated protein (48,000 mol. wt.) that was not present in ribosomal washes from untreated cells [76]. Whether this is the same TIP described by Marcus and Salb is not known at present. Additional work has confirmed and extended these observations [90-92], although no information is currently available on the mechanism by which ribosomes from interferon-treated cells selectively distinguish between viral and cellular mRNAs. In addition, recent studies suggest that interferon's action may involve modification or alteration of cellular tRNA or mRNA as well as ribosomes, making the mechanism of action even more complicated [93-95].

Taking another approach, Marcus et al. [96] have postulated that the antiviral action of interferon may be due to an inhibition of transcription rather than or in addition to translation. Using chick embryo fibroblast cell cultures which were infected with a strain of vesicular stomatitis virus (VSV), they, as did Manders et al. [97], demonstrated a decrease in VSV polymerase activity in interferon-treated cells and postulated that interferon might interfere with viral transcription rather than inhibition of translation of viral mRNA as previously speculated. Jungwirth et al. [98] and Hiller et al. [99], while investigating the anti-poxvirus state created by interferon, did not, however, observe a reduction in the amount of early viral RNA. Therefore, an explanation for the drastic inhibition of viral protein synthesis in interferon-treated cells could not be explained in their systems on the basis of a reduction in transcription of early RNA. Recent studies [100-106], however, confirmed the original observation of Marcus et al. [96] that interferon can alter transcription of viral RNA and that the reduction was not associated with more rapid degradation of viral mRNA. Increased degradation of viral mRNA may, however, in some cases explain the inhibition of viral protein synthesis in interferon-treated cells. Apparently, a nuclease is activated due to the presence of double-stranded RNA in interferon-treated cells [107-110]. Recently, Kerr et al. [111-112] identified a trinucleotide in interferon-treated cells exposed to double-stranded RNA that may be responsible for activation of a nuclease [113] which degrades mRNA and inhibits protein synthesis. Although the mechanism is not fully understood, evidence from a number of virus-cell systems indicates that the interferon-induced antiviral state is characterized by inhibition of both primary transcription and translation [106].

Recent studies also suggest that interferon may mediate, in specific instances, some of its antiviral activity through modification of membrane function. Billiau et al. [114] and Chang et al. [115] reported that in interferon-treated mouse cells the release of murine leukemia virus (MLV) was inhibited and that infectious virus particles accumulated at the cell surface. In these studies the ability of cells to release virus particles was inhibited, but viral protein synthesis was not affected. This suggests a third mechanism of interferon-mediated antiviral activity, namely alteration of cellular membrane function.

Interferon produced by animal cells apparently does not need to penetrate the cell to initiate establishment of antiviral resistance. Rather, interferon needs to be released or excreted by the cell and specifically binds to the cell membrane before antiviral resistance develops [116-118]. Evidence for this includes blocking the establishment of the antiviral state by cytochalosin B [119], cholera toxin, chorionic gonadotropin, and thyroid-stimulating hormone (TSH) [120,121]. Each of these substances was bound to or altered the cell membrane in such a fashion that attachment of interferon was inhibited. Also, incorporation of anti-interferon antibody into the culture media in which the cells were induced blocked establishment of the antiviral state, suggesting that interferon had to be externalized before the antiviral state could be initiated [122]. The existence and specificity of membrane receptor sites may be one explanation for the species specificity of interferon.

A working hypothesis concerning the induction and mechanism of interferon action can be postulated from the literature reviewed. This hypothesis does not attempt to explain the mode of action of all types of interferon inducers but uses an RNA virus as a convenient example. In the simplest concept a single-stranded RNA virus penetrates the cell, is uncoated, releases its RNA, and, using the original strand of RNA as a template, begins reproducing complementary strands of RNA that are essential for replication. Double-stranded RNA, formed in the process, is not normal to the cell, and this is presumed to provide the stimulus for cellular formation of interferon mRNA and interferon production. Newly synthesized interferon is released and either diffuses or is distributed to cells locally or at diverse sites by way of the blood stream, body fluids, or by direct cell contact. Apparently, interferon then attaches at specific membrane

receptor sites and initiates derepression of a host cistron that codes for a
new mRNA. This new mRNA in turn directs the synthesis of the antiviral
protein(s) that interferes with the production or release of progeny virus.
This interference can be either at the level of translation, transcription,
or viral particle release and theoretically does not affect the normal metabolic process of the cell, although some diverse effects on cellular metabolism and division due to interferon have been reported. These are possibly
due to the effect of interferon on cellular membrane and induction of endo-
nucleases.

VI. NONANTIVIRAL PROPERTIES
OF INTERFERONS

Besides their antiviral activities, interferons appear to have other effects
on cells. These include regulation of cellular functions such as phagocytosis,
antitumor activity of macrophages, production of antibodies and lymphokines
by lymphocytes, expression of cellular antigens, and cytotoxicity of cellular
immunity, in addition to effects on cellular macromolecular synthesis and
cell growth [123-130]. Conflicting reports have described both enhancement and suppression of cellular functions, probably reflecting the impurity
of the interferon preparations employed, different sources of interferon,
and variations in experimental methods and procedures. Nevertheless,
sufficient evidence now supports the notion that interferon plays a broader
role in cellular regulation than simply as a modulator of antiviral resistance,
and this has stirred interest in the natural physiological role of interferon.
Is its primary function antiviral, immune regulatory, or a critical part of
cellular homeostasis? Answers to these questions are elusive, but the
insight gained on the antiviral mechanisms of interferon may shed light on
some of its other cellular affects. The observation that interferons have
multiple effects on cells is not too surprising since the antiviral action
encompasses at least three mechanisms: inhibition of transcription and
translation of mRNA and inhibition of viral particle release from cellular
membranes. With such diverse effects interferon can hardly be considered
to be specific in its actions. For example, many of the nonantiviral properties of interferon may be associated with effects on cell membranes. Many
of the alterations listed are intrinsically associated with membrane function;
thus, an agent like interferon, which apparently does attach to and affect
the cellular membrane, could dramatically alter functions such as phagocytosis and antitumor activity of macrophages and lymphocytes. In fact,
it was recently reported that interferon activates the tumoricidal activity
of macrophages [131] and that prostaglandin E inhibited the activation
process [132]. These results again suggest that interferon acts on the
cellular membrane and that prostaglandins and/or cyclic nucleotides may
be involved in the activation process. Treatment of cells with interferon

or interferon inducers has been reported to induce prostaglandin production
by cells, suggesting that such molecules may be involved in regulation of
the interferon system. Many prostaglandins, particularly those of the E
series, stimulate membrane-associated adenylate cyclase activity resulting
in increased intracellular cyclic AMP levels [133-135]. These data suggest
that many of the nonantiviral and, for that matter, antiviral effects of interferon may be modulated by cyclic nucleotides and prostaglandins, and future
studies on the nonantiviral effects of interferon should consider this possibility.

VII. ROLE OF INTERFERON
IN HOST RESISTANCE

By its very nature interferon appears intimately involved in host defense
mechanisms. Little is presently known about the role of interferon in the
regulation of immune responsiveness (see Chapter 11) and the control of
neoplastic processes, but the role of interferon as a natural barrier to viral
infection is more clear.

For a virus to establish an infection successfully, it must replicate in
the initially infected cell. Then, the resulting progeny virus can spread to
infect other cells within the same tissue area, subsequently infecting tissues
at diverse sites or target organs. One of the first host responses to appear
in the initially infected tissues is interferon [136,137]. Interferon can be
detected in infected cells at about the same time that infectious, progeny
viruses are synthesized. Presumably, however, the interferon-sensitive
stage of virus replication has already been passed by the time interferon
is synthesized by the cell, and viral resistance mediated by interferon is
not established in the initially infected cell. As a result virus infection is
probably not affected in that cell, since inhibition of interferon production
by metabolic inhibitors does not significantly increase the virus yield from
cells during single-step growth curves [138].

Theoretically, following release of interferon from infected cells, it
diffuses to surrounding cells where it initiates activation of the antiviral
state. In this way, by reaching as yet uninfected cells, it is thought to
establish a barrier to further viral replication that limits viral dissemination. The degree of antiviral activity is probably dependent on the extracellular concentration of interferon as well as the sensitivity of the virus
to the action of interferon. Therefore, the cells in closest contact with the
infected interferon-producing cells are exposed to the highest concentration
of interferon and become more resistant to virus replication [139,140].
Protection of more distant cells and tissues does occur but apparently to
a lesser degree depending on the virus or strain of virus being used. The
interferon defense mechanism thus might be thought of as functioning in
one of two ways. First, interferon could act by limiting virus replication

at the site of initial entry thereby reducing the amount of virus produced
locally and subsequently reducing systemic spread. The second means of
antiviral action by interferon could be to diffuse or be transported to other
target cells and/or organs and establish an antiviral state in these as yet
uninfected cells thereby localizing tissue involvement. Obviously the defense
barriers established by interferon are in a delicate balance with other host
defense mechanisms such as the immune response (both cellular and humoral)
as well as other more nonspecific factors. Furthermore, the degree of
protection furnished is dependent upon the amount of interferon induced or
present as well as the relative susceptibility of the infecting virus to the
action of interferon.

In comparison, recovery, as measured by decreasing virus levels in
infected tissues, usually begins one or more days after interferon is first
detected [144,145]. The presence of interferon in target organs during
recovery has also been observed [146].

One common characteristic of tissues recovering from virus infection
is nonspecific resistance to viral superinfection, suggesting that nonspecific
defense mechanisms such as interferon may be correlated temporarily with
recovery from the established infection [141,142]. Supporting evidence
indicating that interferon is an important part of host defense to virus infection is available from many sources. In adequate quantities interferon can
inhibit the multiplication of many viruses in a variety of animal tissues in
vivo or in vitro and is generally present in infected tissues of animals prior
to and during the onset of recovery from virus infections [143]. These
studies have demonstrated that interferon can be produced as early as 1 hr
after virus infection and is generally demonstrable at high levels within
24-28 hr.

In comparison, recovery, as measured by decreasing virus levels in
infected tissues, usually begins one or more days after interferon is first
detected [144,145]. The presence of interferon in target organs during
recovery has also been observed [146].

Further evidence relating interferon to recovery is furnished by experiments that attempted to decrease the ability of animals to produce interferon
thereby anticipating that a corresponding increase in the severity of virus
infections would result. Baron and Isaacs [147] utilized such an experimental approach in an attempt to evaluate what role interferon plays in host
resistance to virus infection. They demonstrated that chick embryos younger
than 8 days had an "immature" interferon system and were very susceptible
to the lethal effects of influenza virus infection. As the age of the embryos
increased, there was a corresponding increase in both their ability to produce interferon and their resistance to the lethality of infection. A decreased
capacity to produce interferon, caused by altered temperature, reduced
oxygen tension, psychological stress, chemical inhibitors, different virus
strains, age, and treatment with steroid hormones and vasoactive amines,
has also, in some cases, led to impaired recovery of animals from virus
infections [148-150]. Furthermore, studies carried out in vitro have
indicated that impairment of the ability of cells to produce interferon enhanced the virulence of a variety of viruses. Two interesting studies were
reported by Fauconnier [151,152], who utilized rabbit anti-mouse interferon

antibody to reduce the protective efficacy of interferon in both in vivo and in vitro situations. Under in vitro conditions Fauconnier was able to reduce the amount of interference observed between several types of viruses (presumably mediated by interferon) by adding anti-interferon antibody to the system, thereby enlarging the plaque size of the infecting viruses. Similarly, in vivo an augmentation of viral virulence was observed when mice were treated with rabbit anti-mouse interferon antibody and were then infected with Semliki Forest virus. An increase in both cumulative mortality as well as virus levels in brain tissues was reported. A note of caution should be observed in the interpretation of many of these studies, however, since methods used to inhibit the interferon response were not entirely selective and may also have suppressed other host defenses such as the cellular immune response, which may, at least in part, have been responsible for the enhanced severity of infection.

Although most attention has been directed toward demonstrating a correlation between the amount of interferon produced, the sensitivity of the virus to interferon, and susceptibility to infection, another aspect of this relationship might well be the susceptibility of the cell itself to the action of interferon. For example, the effect of a specific decrease in the ability of mice to respond to the action of interferon was demonstrated in a series of studies involving a Group B arbovirus infection of two strains of mice. Both strains were capable of producing equivalent amounts of interferon, but one was more resistant to the establishment of the antiviral state by interferon and was therefore much more susceptible to the lethal outcome of infection with the arbovirus. This difference was not only observed in vivo, but cells obtained from each mouse strain demonstrated the same susceptibility and lack of interferon protection that had been seen in the intact animal [153]. Olivie and Boiron [154] have also demonstrated a similar pattern of altered sensitivity of mouse embryo cells infected in vitro with a murine sarcoma virus. Although both uninfected and murine sarcoma virus-infected cells produced equivalent levels of interferon in response to Newcastle disease virus (NDV), the infected cells were severely refractile to the antiviral activity of passively transferred interferon. When both uninfected and murine sarcoma virus-infected cells were treated with NDV-induced interferon and then challenged with vesicular stomatitis virus, no protection was observed in the murine sarcoma virus-infected cells while the uninfected cells were completely protected.

Added credence is given to the relationship of interferon to viral resistance when studies are considered which utilized passive transfer of exogenous interferon to protect or treat potentially susceptible animals or cells. In a variety of experimental settings exogenous interferon and interferon inducers, when administered either prophylactically or after establishment of infection with a variety of viruses (Chapters 4 and 5), have been effective in vivo and in vitro in both preventing and limiting virus infections (Chapters 6 through 10).

VIII. CONCLUSIONS

Although a great deal has been learned in the last 20 years, many questions about interferons are still far from being answered. Questions as basic as what the molecular nature or mechanism of antiviral action is remain unanswered. Interferon and its accompanying cellular antiviral resistance play a significant role in host defense against virus infection, may play a role in control of metastasis or malignancy, and may modulate immune responsiveness. However, rather than its being considered as the sole factor involved in host resistance, it is more realistic to visualize interferon as a member of a complex system of cellular and humoral barriers. The importance of interferon or any other member of the host's defense system in any particular disease probably depends upon the nature of the invasive organism as well as the condition of the host. A depression of any aspect of the cellular or humoral defense mechanisms, including interferon, could (again depending upon the nature of the causative agent) lead to a compromised state of resistance and concomitant increase in susceptibility to infection. The administration of exogenous interferon or potent nontoxic interferon inducers may be an ideal chemotherapeutic approach to the treatment of viral and possible neoplastic diseases. However, as discussed in the remaining chapters, the practical utilization of the interferon system faces many obstacles, although recent successes indicate that such an approach holds promise.

REFERENCES

1. A. Isaacs and J. Lindenmann, Proc. Roy. Soc., Ser. B 147:258-267 (1957).
2. J. Lindenmann, D. C. Burke, and A. Isaacs, Brit. J. Exp. Pathol. 38:551-562 (1957).
3. A. Isaacs, D. C. Burke, and L. Fadeeva, Brit. J. Exp. Pathol. 39: 447-451 (1958).
4. A. Isaacs, Virology 10:144-146 (1960).
5. A. Isaacs and G. Hitchcock, Lancet ii:69-71 (1960).
6. D. A. J. Tyrrell, Nature 184:452-453 (1959).
7. J. S. Youngner and W. R. Stinebring, Science 144:1022-1023 (1964).
8. M. Ho, Science 146:1472-1474 (1964).
9. W. J. Kleinschmidt, J. C. Cline, and E. B. Murphy, Federation Proc. 23:507 (1964).
10. E. F. Wheelock, Science 149:310-311 (1965).
11. W. R. Steinebring and J. S. Youngner, Nature 204:712 (1964).
12. H. E. Hopps, S. Kohno, M. Kohno, and J. E. Smadel, Bacteriol. Proc. pp. 115-116 (1964).
13. K. Y. Huang, W. W. Schultz, and F. B. Gordon, Science 162:123-124 (1968).

14. G. D. Mayer and R. F. Krueger, Science 169:1214-1215 (1970).
15. A. K. Field, A. A. Tytell, G. P. Lampson, and M. R. Hilleman, Proc. Nat. Acad. Sci. U.S. 58:1004-1010 (1967).
16. E. DeClercq and T. C. Merigan, Ann. Rev. Med. 21:17-47 (1970).
17. T. C. Merigan and M. J. Finkelstein, Virology 35:363-369 (1968).
18. J. Diederich, E. Lademann, and A. Wacker, Virusforschung 40:82 (1973).
19. R. A. Lockart, Jr., in Interferons (N. B. Finter, ed.), North Holland Publ., Amsterdam, 1966, pp. 1-20.
20. K. H. Fantes, in Interferons (N. B. Finter, ed.), North Holland Publ., Amsterdam, 1966, pp. 119-179.
21. T. J. Smith and R. R. Wagner, J. Exp. Med. 125:559-564 (1967).
22. T. C. Cesario, P. J. Schryer, and J. G. Tilles, Antimicrob. Agents Chemother. 11:291-298 (1977).
23. Y. H. Ke and M. Ho, J. Virol. 1:883-890 (1967).
24. W. A. Carter, Proc. Nat. Acad. Sci. U.S. 67:620-626 (1970).
25. W. A. Carter, Prep. Biochem. 1:55-61 (1971).
26. W. E. Stewart, T. Chudizio, L. S. Lin, and M. Wiranowska-Stewart, Proc. Nat. Acad. Sci. U.S. 75:4814-4818 (1978).
27. R. E. Levy-Koenig, R. R. Golgher, and K. Paucker, J. Immunol. 104:791-797 (1970).
28. E. A. Havell, C. A. Berman, K. Ogburn, K. Berg, K. Paucker, and J. Vilcek, Proc. Nat. Acad. Sci. U.S. 72:2185-2187 (1975).
29. E. A. Havell, Y. K. Yip, and J. Vilcek, J. Gen. Virol. 38:51-59 (1977).
30. J. S. Youngner and S. B. Salvin, J. Immunol. 111:1914-1922 (1973).
31. E. A. Havell, T. G. Hayes, and J. Vilcek, Abstr. Ann. Meeting Amer. Soc. Microbiol. p. 246 (1978).
32. R. A. Lockart, Jr., Progr. Med. Virol. 9:451-475 (1967).
33. M. R. Hilleman, J. Cell Physiol. 71:43-60 (1968).
34. E. Heller, Virology 21:652-656 (1963).
35. R. R. Wagner, Trans. Assoc. Amer. Physicians 76:92-101 (1963).
36. R. R. Wagner, Amer. J. Med. 38:726-737 (1965).
37. A. Buchan and D. C. Burke, Biochem. J. 98:530-536 (1966).
38. A. K. Field, G. P. Lampson, A. A. Tytell, M. M. Nemes, and M. R. Hilleman, Proc. Nat. Acad. Sci. U.S. 58:2102-2108 (1967).
39. W. F. Long and D. C. Burke, J. Gen. Virol. 6:1-12 (1970).
40. C. Colby, Progr. Nucleic Acid Res. Mol. Biol. 11:1-21 (1971).
41. F. Dianzani, S. Gagoni, C. E. Buckler, and S. Baron, Proc. Soc. Exptl. Biol. Med. 133:324-330 (1970).
42. F. Dianzani, A. Pugliese, and S. Baron, Proc. Soc. Exp. Biol. Med. 145:428-433 (1974).
43. C. J. Gauntt, Infec. Immun. 17:711-718 (1973).
44. R. Z. Lockart, Jr., N. L. Bayliss, S. T. Toy, and F. H. Yin, J. Virol. 2:962-970 (1968).

45. J. Taylor-Papadimitriou and J. Kallos, Nature [New Biol.] 245: 143-145 (1973).
46. P. M. Pitha and J. Pitha, J. Gen. Virol. 21:31-39 (1973).
47. E. DeClercq and P. De Somer, J. Gen. Virol. 22:271-280 (1974).
48. L. Bachner, E. DeClercq, and M. N. Thang, Biochem. Biophys. Res. Commun. 63:476-481 (1975).
49. E. C. Borden and P. H. Leonhardt, Antimicrob. Agents Chemother. 9:551-570 (1976).
50. E. C. Borden, Abstr. Ann. Meeting Amer. Soc. Microbiol. p. 264 (1978).
51. F. Besancon, H. Ankel, and S. Basu, Nature 259:576-578 (1976).
52. F. N. Reizin, V. M. Roikhel, and M. P. Chumakov, Arch. Virol. 49: 307-315 (1975).
53. M. Jensen, Proc. Soc. Exp. Biol. Med. 130:1-8 (1969).
54. H. M. Johnson, Nature 265:154-156 (1977).
55. F. Dianzani, P. Neri, and M. Zucca, Proc. Soc. Exp. Biol. Med. 140:1375-1380 (1972).
56. M. Yaron, I. Yaron, D. Gurari-Rotman, M. Revel, H. R. Lindner, and U. Zor, Nature 267:457-459 (1977).
57. D. A. Stringfellow, Science 201:376-378 (1978).
58. D. A. Stringfellow, Antimicrob. Agents Chemother. 11:984-992 (1977).
59. S. Rousset, J. Gen. Virol. 22:9-20 (1974).
60. M. C. Breinig, J. A. Armstrong, and M. Ho, J. Gen. Virol. 26: 149-158 (1975).
61. P. B. Sehgal and I. Tamm, Proc. Nat. Acad. Sci. U.S. 73:1621-1625 (1976).
62. J. Vilcek, T. G. Rossman, and F. Varacelli, Nature 222:682-683 (1969).
63. J. Vilcek, Ann. N.Y. Acad. Sci. 173:390-403 (1970).
64. Y. H. Tan, J. A. Armstrong, Y. H. Ke, and M. Ito, Proc. Nat. Acad. Sci. U.S. 67:464-470 (1970).
65. P. B. Sehgal, I. Tamm, and J. Vilcek, Virology 70:256-259 (1976).
66. P. B. Sehgal, I. Tamm, and J. Vilcek, Science 190:282-284 (1975).
67. E. C. Borden and F. A. Murphy, J. Immunol. 106:134-142 (1971).
68. E. C. Borden, E. V. Prochownik, and W. A. Carter, J. Immunol. 114:752-756 (1975).
69a. D. A. Stringfellow and L. A. Glasgow, Infec. Immun. 10:1337-1342 (1974).
69b. D. A. Stringfellow and L. A. Glasgow, Infec. Immun. 6:743-747 (1972).
70. D. A. Stringfellow, Infec. Immun. 11:294-302 (1975).
71. D. A. Stringfellow, Infec. Immun. 13:392-398 (1976).
72. D. A. Stringfellow, E. R. Kern, D. K. Kelsey, and L. A. Glasgow, J. Infec. Dis. 135:540-552 (1977).
73. G. C. Tarr, J. A. Armstrong, and M. Ho, Infec. Immun. 19:903-907 (1978).

74. R. M. Friedman and J. A. Sonnabend, Nature 203:366-367 (1964).
75. S. Levine, Virology 24:586-588 (1964).
76. C. E. Samuel and W. K. Joklik, Virology 58:476-491 (1974).
77. F. Dianzani, C. E. Buckler, and S. Baron, Virology 39:491-496 (1968).
78. W. E. Stewart and R. Z. Lockart, J. Virol. 6:795-799 (1970).
79. J. Vilček and F. Varacelli, J. Gen. Virol. 13:185-188 (1971).
80. W. K. Joklik, Texas Repts. Biol. Med. 35:364-269 (1977).
81. M. Ho and J. F. Enders, Proc. Nat. Acad. Sci. U.S. 45:385-389 (1959).
82. J. Vilček, Nature 187:73-74 (1960).
83. R. R. Wagner, Virology 13:323-337 (1961).
84. D. H. Metz, Cell 6:429-439 (1975).
85. J. Taylor, Biochem. Biophys. Res. Commun. 14:447-451 (1964).
86. P. I. Marcus and J. M. Salb, Virology 30:502-516 (1966).
87. P. I. Marcus and J. M. Salb, Cold Spring Harbor Symp. Quant. Biol. 31:335-344 (1966).
88. P. I. Marcus and J. M. Salb, in The Interferons (G. Rita, ed.), Academic Press, New York, 1968, pp. 111-127.
89. W. A. Carter and H. B. Levy, Science 155:1254-1256 (1967).
90. W. A. Carter and H. B. Levy, Biochem. Biophys. Acta. 155:437-443 (1968).
91. R. M. Friedman, D. H. Metz, R. M. Esteban, D. A. Torell, L. A. Ball, and I. M. Kerr, J. Virol. 10:1180-1198 (1972).
92. S. L. Gupta, M. L. Sopori, and P. Lengyel, Biochem. Biophys. Res. Commun. 54:777-783 (1973).
93. A. Zilberstein, B. Dudock, H. Berissi, and M. Revel, J. Mol. Biol. 108:43-54 (1976).
94. M. Revel, Texas Repts. Biol. Med. 35:212-220 (1977).
95. G. C. Sen, R. Desrosiers, L. Ratner, S. Shaila, G. E. Brown, B. Lebleu, E. Slattery, M. Kawakita, B. Cabrer, H. Taira, and P. Lengyel, Texas Repts. Biol. Med. 35:221-229 (1977).
96. P. I. Marcus, D. L. Engelhardt, J. M. Hunt, and M. J. Sekellick, Science 174:593-598 (1971).
97. E. K. Manders, J. G. Tilles, and A. S. Huang, Virology 49:573-580 (1972).
98. C. Jungwirth, I. Horak, G. Bodo, J. Lindner, and B. Schultz, Virology 48:59-70 (1972).
99. G. Hiller, C. Jungwirth, G. Bodo, and B. Schultz, Virology 52:22-29 (1973).
100. P. I. Marcus and M. J. Sekellick, Virology 69:378-393 (1976).
101. W. J. Bean and R. W. Simpson, J. Virol. 9:286-289 (1972).
102. C. J. Gauntt, Biochem. Biophys. Res. Commun. 47:1228-1236 (1972).
103. S. L. Gupta, W. D. Graziadei, H. Weideli, M. L. Sopori, and P. Lengyel, Virology 57:49-63 (1974).

104. D. H. Metz, M. J. Levin, and M. N. Oxman, J. Gen. Virol. 32: 227-240 (1976).

105. M. N. Oxman and M. J. Levin, Proc. Nat. Acad. Sci. U.S. 63: 299-302 (1971).

106. M. N. Oxman, Texas Repts. Biol. Med. 35:230-238 (1977).

107. G. E. Brown, B. Lebleu, H. Kowakita, S. Shaila, G. C. Sen, and P. Lengyel, Biochem. Biophys. Res. Commun. 69:114-122 (1976).

108. B. Lebleu, G. C. Sen, S. Shaila, B. Carver, and P. Lengyel, Proc. Nat. Acad. Sci. U.S. 73:3107-3111 (1976).

109. G. C. Sen, B. Lebleu, G. E. Brown, M. Kawarita, E. Slattery, and P. Lengyel, Nature 264:370-373 (1976).

110. R. M. Friedman, Bacteriol. Rev. 41:543-567 (1977).

111. I. M. Kerr, R. E. Brown, and L. A. Ball, Nature 250:57-59 (1974).

112. I. M. Kerr and R. E. Brown, Proc. Nat. Acad. Sci. U.S. 75:256-260 (1978).

113. C. Baglioni, M. A. Minks, and P. A. Maroney, Nature 273:684-687 (1978).

114. A. Billiau, V. G. Edy, H. Sobis, and P. DeSomer, Int. J. Cancer 14:335-340 (1974).

115. E. H. Chang, S. J. Mims, T. J. Triche, and R. M. Friedman, J. Gen. Virol. 34:363-367 (1977).

116. B. Berman and J. Vilcek, Virology 57:378-386 (1974).

117. C. Chang, A. Gregoire, J. Lamaitre-Moncuit, P. Brown, F. Besancon, H. Surarez, and R. Cassingena, Proc. Nat. Acad. Sci. U.S. 70: 557-561 (1973).

118. C. Chang, Biomedicine 24:148-157 (1976).

119. K. L. Radke, C. Colby, J. R. Kates, H. M. Krider, and D. M. Prescott, J. Virol. 13:623-630 (1974).

120. F. Besancon and H. Ankel, C. R. Acad. Sci. Paris [B] 283:1807-1810 (1976).

121. L. D. Kohn, R. M. Friedman, J. M. Holmes, and G. Lee, Proc. Nat. Acad. Sci. U.S. 73:3695-3699 (1976).

122. V. E. Vengris, B. D. Stollar, and P. M. Pitha, Virology 65:410-417 (1975).

123. W. A. Fleming, T. A. McNeill, and M. Killen, Immunol. 23:429-437 (1972).

124. W. Braun and H. B. Levy, Proc. Soc. Exp. Biol. Med. 141:769-773 (1972).

125. R. M. Donahoe and K. Huang, Scand. J. Infec. Dis. 4:101-104 (1972).

126. I. Gresser, C. Bourali, I. Chouroulinkov, D. Fontaine-Brouty-Boye, and M. Thomas, Ann. N.Y. Acad. Sci. 173:694-707 (1970).

127. J. C. Cerrottini, K. T. Brunner, P. Lindahl, and I. Gresser, Nature [New Biol.] 242:152-153 (1973).

128. E. DeMaeyer, J. Infec. Dis. 133:A63–A65 (1976).
129. P. Lindahl, I. Gresser, P. Leary, and M. Tovey, Proc. Nat. Acad. Sci. U.S. 73:1284–1287 (1976).
130. H. Dahl and M. Degre, Nature 257:799–801 (1975).
131. R. M. Schultz, J. D. Papamatheakis, and M. A. Chirigos, Science 197:674–676 (1977).
132. R. M. Schultz, N. A. Paulidis, W. A. Stylos, and M. A. Chirigos, Science 202:320–321 (1978).
133. R. W. Butcher, Advan. Biochem. Psychopharmacol. 3:57 (1970).
134. R. R. Gorman, J. Cyclic Nucleotide Res. 1:1–9 (1975).
135. S. Bergstrom, H. Danielson, and B. Samuelsson, Biochem. Biophys. Acta 90:207–211 (1964).
136. S. Baron, Advan. Virus Res. 10:39–64 (1963).
137. A. Isaacs, Advan. Virus Res. 10:1–38 (1963).
138. R. M. Friedman, Nature 201:848–849 (1964).
139. F. Dianzani and S. Baron. Nature 257:682–684 (1975).
140. F. Dianzani, I. Viano, M. Santiano, M. Zucca, and S. Baron, Proc. Soc. Exp. Biol. Med. 155:445–452 (1977).
141. S. Baron, J. Gen. Physiol. 56:184–211 (1970).
142. S. Baron, Arch. Intern. Med. 216:84–93 (1970).
143. S. Baron, H. B. duBuy, C. E. Buckler, and M. L. Johnson, Proc. Soc. Exp. Biol. Med. 117:338–341 (1964).
144. S. Baron, C. E. Buckler, R. V. McCloskey, and R. L. Kirschstein, J. Immunol. 96:12–16 (1966).
145. B. R. Murphy and L. A. Glasgow, J. Exp. Med. 127:1035–1052 (1968).
146. M. Boxaca, L. B. DeGuerrero, and V. L. Savy, Arch. Ges. Virusforsch. 40:10–16 (1973).
147. S. Baron and A. Isaacs, Nature 191:97–98 (1961).
148. S. Baron and G. E. Buckler, Science 141:1061–1063 (1963).
149. J. Ruiz-Gomez and J. Sosa-Martinez, Arch. Ges. Virusforsch. 17:295–299 (1965).
150. J. Mendelson and L. A. Glasgow, J. Immunol. 96:345–352 (1966).
151. B. Fauconnier, C. R. Acad. Sci. Paris [B] 271:1464–1466 (1970).
152. B. Fauconnier, Arch. Ges. Virusforsch. 31:266–272 (1970).
153. B. H. Hanson, H. Koprowski, S. Baron, and C. E. Buckler, Microbios 1B:51–68 (1969).
154. M. Olivie and M. Boiron, C. R. Acad. Sci. Paris [B] 274:1106–1108 (1972).

2

PRODUCTION, PURIFICATION, AND PROPERTIES OF HUMAN INTERFERONS

Kurt Berg and Iver Heron

University of Aarhus
Aarhus, Denmark

Kurt Osther

Alfred Benzon Ltd.
Hvidovre, Denmark

I. INTRODUCTION

During the last decade the production of human interferons for clinical
purposes has given rise to a great deal of effort from several groups.
The most successful work until now has unequivocally been done by Profes-
sor Cantell's group (Helsinki), who, as early as 1967 [1], started the
systematic exploitation of the "art of producing human leukocyte interferon"
using human buffy coats. Since Cantell proved that it was indeed possible
to produce large quantities of human leukocyte interferon [$> 10^{11}$
interferon units (U)/year], many new groups will undoubtedly begin to

emerge. For example, human leukocyte interferon is now being produced in Denmark, using a modification of the "Cantell procedure" (for details, see Section II.A).

Since one limitation to production of leukocyte interferon is the number of buffy coats available, the use of transformed lymphocytes for the production of human interferon has been explored. Several groups are working along these lines, for example, Bridgen's group [2] and N. B. Finter and K. H. Fantes, Wellcome Research Laboratories, United Kingdom (personal communication). The Wellcome group has now developed techniques that enable them to produce large quantities of high-titered (20,000-40,000 U/ml) lymphoblastoid interferon in >1000-liter tanks. Finally, the production of human fibroblast interferon will be mentioned. Considerable progress has been made by C. M. Tan and co-workers (personal communication), who very recently found a high-producing fibroblast cell line that is trisomeric with respect to chromosome No. 5 (associated with interferon production). Thus, crude, unconcentrated fibroblast interferon can now be obtained with titers in the range of 200,000-800,000 U/ml. It should also be pointed out that interferon may possibly be produced by bacteria that have had the proper chromosome(s) incorporated into their genomes by a genetic recombination technique. For example, preliminary reports indicate that insulin produced by such a technique may be available for commercial sale in 1980.

II. PRODUCTION AND PURIFICATION OF HUMAN INTERFERONS FOR CLINICAL PURPOSES; FURTHER PURIFICATION FOR LABORATORY EXPERIMENTS

The aim of this section is to provide a brief view of the present state of "the art of producing interferons in clinical amounts." This will be described in some detail for human leukocyte interferon (HuLeIF), human lymphoblastoid interferon (HuLyIF), and human fibroblast interferon (HuFiIF). Since HuLeIF is the only species of interferon which has been used clinically to any great extent, a more detailed description of this interferon will be presented. After the production has been described, purification of interferons in clinical amounts will be briefly mentioned. Further experimental purification on a small scale (up to 10^7 U) will also be considered in some detail. This scheme will be used for the three types of interferons described.

A. Human Leukocyte Interferon

Production on a large scale for clinical purposes is essentially done (in our laboratory) as described by Cantell and co-workers [4-6,40,41,71], with minor modifications. For further information, see the excellent reviews by Strander [39] and Mogensen and Cantell [73].

In brief, blood (in plastic bags) taken from voluntary donors is immediately chilled in crushed ice until centrifugation can be performed. (It may
also be shipped in boxes with crushed ice to a central production laboratory
for further processing.) After centrifugation (2-4° C), about 15 ml of "buffy
coat" is expressed from the plastic bag. Considerable variations in the
volume of the buffy coat can occur (10-30 ml). The buffy coats are collected
during the daytime and kept at 2-4° C overnight (pooled) to be used the next
morning. Two-day-old buffy coats cannot be used.

Contaminating erythrocytes must be completely removed since they
will otherwise react with Sendai virus (hemagglutinate), would lyse (proteolytic enzymes would be released into the medium), and toxic products will
interfere with the interferon yield (<500 U/ml). Removal of erythrocytes
is performed by lysis using ammonium chloride (9 volumes 0.83% NH_4Cl
to one volume buffy coat for 15 min at 2° C, centrifuge at 2-4° C, resuspend
in PBS, and repeat the procedure). The cells are resuspended in the incubation medium and counted.

The leukocytes are finally suspended in round-bottom 2-liter flasks
with 10^7 cells/ml. A total volume of 900 ml is important, and each flask
should be loosely covered with alufoil with magnetic stirring at 37.5° C
(water bath). The suspension is primed with 100 U/ml for 1-2 hr (37.5° C).
This step is important. After the priming period, Sendai virus is added
to a final concentration of 100-150 hemagglutination units (HAU)/ml of
leukocyte suspension. After 15-20 hr, the suspension is centrifuged
(160 × g for 10 min). The pellet is discarded. The supernatant is kept
at -40° C until further processing. The titers of crude interferon are usually
around 25,000-50,000 U/ml. At present, the normal weekly production in
our laboratory amounts to 15 bottles, and the total weekly production comes
to 400-700 × 10^6 U. Based on these figures, it can be calculated that one
buffy coat gives about 1-3 × 10^6 U.

Interferon is thawed and pooled, and potassium thyocyanate (as a 5 M
solution) is added with stirring until the final concentration reaches 0.5 M
(4° C). The pH is slowly lowered by dropwise addition (with stirring) of
1 N HCl and 0.1 N HCl to pH 4.5, whereby a precipitate is formed (more
than 98% of the interferon is found in the precipitate together with 45% of
the proteins). After centrifugation, the interferon may be treated in two
ways: (1) The precipitate is dissolved in about one-tenth of the original
crude volume in PBS; the pH is adjusted to 7.5 by means of an additional
0.1 N NaOH (important, otherwise the precipitate will not be dissolved)
and dialyzed extensively against PBS. This type of preparation, which is
called crude leukocyte interferon (CIF), is normally too crude to be used
in humans. Specific activity is about 10^4 U/mg protein. (2) The precipitate
is dissolved in ethanol and, by increasing the pH stepwise to 5.8, the major
part of the impurities precipitate. By further increasing the pH, most of
the interferon precipitates out at pH 8. The last precipitate is dissolved
in PBS (about 20-40 ml) and dialyzed extensively against PBS. This partially
purified interferon (PIF) has a specific activity of about 0.5-1 × 10^6 U/mg

protein. The recovery is 50-60% (based on the crude interferon solution). It is ampulled (in 3×10^6 IFU portions) and kept at -20°C until use. This type of material is stable for more than 10 months at -20°C.

The PIF material has been very well tolerated by more than 15 patients (administered intramuscularly). The only side effect we have noticed [3], along with Torben Fog (personal communication), is the well-known fever reaction, which is in accordance with the findings of others, for example, H. Strander's group (personal communication). The fever often reaches 38-39°C and lasts for 1-3 hr. After 2-8 injections, the fever reaction gradually disappears.

The PIF preparations from two different laboratories (Cantell's and our own) have been compared in sodium dodecyl sulfate-polyacrylamide gel electrophoresis (SDS-PAGE) (slab gradient) to determine similarities or differences in the protein composition (Figure 1). The protein patterns are quite similar (the input for both types of PIF preparations had a specific activity close to 1×10^6 U/mg protein). The CIF preparations also show identity (Figure 1). No antigenic differences were found between the interferon batches (determined by interferon neutralization tests).

In principle, troubleshooting looks relatively simple, and that is probably the reason why many people have started to follow up the success of Cantell. In practice, however, relatively few laboratories have succeeded in getting a real and steady production going (between 300-1000 million U/week). The reason is clearly harbored in the many small and delicate technicalities which are "hidden" in this type of procedure. For example, great care must be taken to almost completely remove the erythrocytes. Ca^{2+} (and similar divalent ions) must be avoided, otherwise clumping will occur. One also has to consider the quality of the water, etc. Even the form of the flask is of great importance: the flask must be round-bottomed, 2 liters in size, and have a broad neck (5 cm in diameter). The stirring has to be kept at a very constant level: not too quickly, which is harmful to the leukocytes, and not too slowly, as clumping will then occur. The virus is probably the most important variant in the whole "game." Great care should be taken to obtain a good Sendai virus pool [1,4,5,6] without bacterial contamination. Pools should be made from 10-12 eggs; keep the virus at 4°C and wait for a bacteriological screening (which should be negative). Inclusion of egg substrate should not be forgotten; alternatively, the virus batches can be checked by means of special screening plates made only with egg substrates. The virus may also be kept at -70°C after addition of agamma serum (as a stabilizer). The diluted virus suspensions should be handled carefully (virus is unstable when diluted).

Although the HA technique does vary among laboratories, it has been found in three independent laboratories that only when a virus with an HA titer >4000 per milliliter is used will a good production of interferon be possible (15,000-100,000 IFU/ml crude interferon). Too high concentrations of egg proteins will probably interfere with the yield. During the

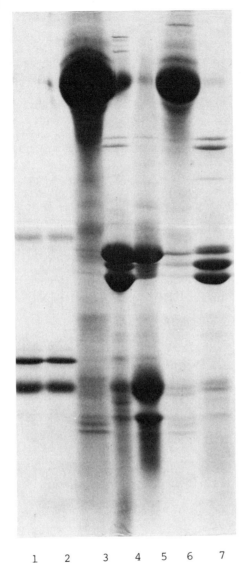

25,000

17,800

12,400

1 2 3 4 5 6 7

FIGURE 1. SDS-PAGE, thin slab of HuLeIF (24 cm-long gels). Slots
No. 1 and 2: Molecular markers (mol. wt. 12,400, 17,800, and 25,000).
Slot No. 3: CIF 83A (Cantell). Slot No. 4: PIF (Cantell). Slot No. 5:
PIF-1 (Table 3), not a typical PIF preparation due to variation in the
ethanolic precipitation procedure (the titer was about 1×10^6 U/ml). Slot
No. 6: CIF (KO, KB). Slot No. 7: PIF (KO, KB). The titers of CIF in slots
No. 3 and No. 6 were about the same (400,000 U/ml). The corresponding
PIF had titers of 1-4 $\times 10^6$ U/ml. Based on the protein bands (slots No. 4
and 7) it can be seen that the two PIF preparations are very similar with
respect to the impurities.

whole production period great care must be taken to minimize bacterial
contamination. If too high a level is reached, proteolytic enzymes will be
released, and loss of biological activity will inevitably occur. Crude interferon preparations are routinely frozen in batches of 10 liters (-40°C) before
being processed to PIF, but other laboratories (for example, that of Cantell)
just keep the CIF at 4°C. During the last eight months, we have had a
routine production of crude human leukocyte interferon of 25,000-35,000
U/ml (a total of about 500 × 10^6 U/week).

It should, undoubtedly, be possible to improve the above-mentioned
system considerably by further manipulation of the priming procedure,
virus, media, etc. For example, one may consider the possibility of pretreating the leukocytes with polycations before the virus is added [7]. The
pH of the leukocyte suspension is crucial. It should be in the vicinity of
7.2 (7.1-7.3); after the induction of interferon the pH may drop to 6.8. A
too high pH level may indicate a poor choice of buffer and give rise to cell
death. There are no reports on the successful use of the superinduction
technique in the production of human leukocyte interferon (see Vilček on
the human fibroblast system, Section II.C).

Further purification of human leukocyte interferon is often desirable.
When exploring different aspects of interferon, including the binding of
interferon to membranes, the action of interferon, etc., it is most desirable
to have as pure an interferon preparation as possible. Many laboratories
will very often be asked the now classical question by the referee: "Is the
phenomenon you have observed a result of interferon itself, or is it due to
some unknown impurities present in unknown quantities?" Extensive efforts
have therefore been devoted to purifying interferon. At present, no one
has reported a complete purification of human leukocyte interferon. The
best specific activity obtained is 10^8-10^9 U/mg protein. In the following
section several methods will be outlined that will, hopefully, serve as a
guide for those who wish to purify interferon to a level that the referee may
accept.

Gel filtration of concentrated crude leukocyte interferon (CIF) has
routinely been done in our laboratory with very good results, using Ultrogel
AcA 5/4 (Pharmacia, column K 2.6/100 at 4°C, employing 1 M urea (including 0.1% ethanolamine) in PBS, pH = 7.2 (recovery of about 100% in each
run). A typical profile is shown in Figure 2. About 90-95% of the impurities
are located in the protein peak, which is followed by the interferon activity.
The specific activity is close to 10^6 U/mg protein, and in many respects
this type of material resembles the PIF material. When dealing with small
amounts of crude leukocyte interferon (1-20 × 10^6 U/ml), the gel filtration
technique should be the first choice. Incidentally, this type of material
was tolerated very well in one patient, as was PIF (2 × 10^6 U/dose).

Törmä and Paucker [43] reported a similar purification procedure
for leukocyte interferon using PIF plus sodium dodecyl sulfate (SDS) in a
gel filtration, ending up with a specific activity of 5-10 × 10^6 U/mg protein

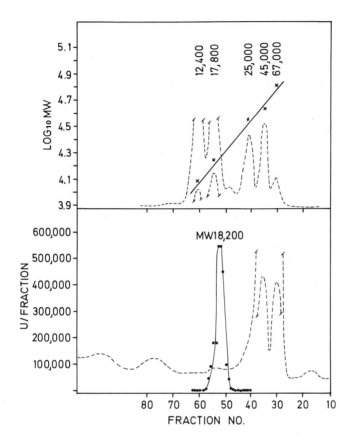

FIGURE 2. Gel filtration of crude human leukocyte interferon (CIF). Ten ml of CIF, 4×10^6 U in total (in PBS). was loaded directly on an Ultrogel AcA 5/4 column (100 $\times$ 2.5 cm; K 2.6/100, Pharmacia) at 4°C (buffer: 1 M urea including 0.1% ethanolamine, in PBS, pH 7.2). Fractions size 8 ml; flow rate 35–40 ml/hr. Recovery 95–100%; specific activity about 10^6 U/mg protein. The column was equilibrated by means of standard markers. Key: solid curve, U/fraction (in 69/19 B units); dashed curve, OD_{280}.

(100–140% recovery). One major drawback with this method is the presence of SDS, which has to be removed before additional affinity chromatography can be performed [8]. How close a PIF preparation is related to a gel-filtered CIF preparation remains to be seen (experiments in progress).

    Hydrophobic chromatography has been extensively exploited by Sulkowsky and co-workers [9–13]. Mostly, they have been working with relatively small amounts of interferon (10,000–100,000 U) without obtaining great

improvements in specific activity. The main purpose of their work has
been more in the direction of divulging the hydrophobic properties of human
leukocyte interferon. They have not yet been able to find a matrix which
will clearly be useful in purification when crude HuLeIF is the starting
material. For example, phenyl-Sepharose is able to bind interferon (several
hundred thousand units), but unfortunately most other proteins are also
bound and eluted with the interferon—thus the purification factor is only
twofold (K. Berg, unpublished data). Of course, this situation could change
drastically if a new matrix which was far more selective would appear.
The whole picture might also change drastically if a more purified interferon
preparation were used as a starting material (for example, a gel-filtered
CIF). Thus, it is still too early to rule out this type of technique for large-
scale purification of clinical amounts of material.

Since most interferons are bound to <u>Con A</u>, it has been widely claimed
that interferons are glycoproteins [56]. Jankowski et al. [10] demonstrated
that leukocyte interferon was not bound to a Con A column (the same has
been found in our laboratory). One might speculate whether this behavior
of leukocyte interferon in contrast to other interferons could be due to the
rather crude material (specific activity $= 10^4$ U/mg protein) which has been
used in these experiments. In a crude HuLeIF preparation the glycoprotein
content could be very high, causing competition between interferon and
extraneous glycoproteins for binding sites on Con A.

By using three types of different purity human leukocyte interferon
(specific activity 10^4, 10^6, 6×10^7 U/mg protein), we found that all the
interferon was passed through the Con A column as long as the specific
activity was below 10^6 U/mg protein. At a specific activity of 6×10^7 U/mg
protein, we could indeed bind most of the activity to the Con A column, but
on subsequent elutions only 5% was recovered. Therefore it is difficult to
make any conclusions since the protein content was rather low (about 3-5
µg/ml). Thus nonspecific binding or inactivation may very well have
occurred.

Until now, the most promising technique for the purification of human
leukocyte interferon has been <u>antibody affinity chromatography</u>, which was
introduced by Anfinsen et al. [14] and Berg et al. [15]. The principle of
antibody affinity chromatography is that antibodies to interferon are bound
to a matrix (for example, Sepharose 4B) and packed into a column. At
neutral pH, the immobilized antibodies will react with the crude interferon
preparation that is loaded on the column at 4°C. By lowering the pH to 2.4,
the antigen–antibody (immobilized) complex is dissociated, and the purified
antigen (interferon) is released. By equilibrating the column with "loading
buffer," the column can be used repeatedly. Antibody columns will last
for 1-2 years (and can be used more than 100 times). When not in use, the
columns are stored in PBS (4°C) with penicillin, streptomycin, gentamycin,
and chloromaphenicol (1% of each). The column should be cleaned (loading
buffer plus eluting buffer plus loading buffer) before it is actually loaded

with crude interferon. By this technique, fairly large volumes of interferon can be handled (up to 500×10^6/U, depending on the size of the column and the antibodies). For further details, the reader is referred to Anfinsen et al. [14] and Berg et al. [15].

The crucial point in antibody affinity chromatography is the antibodies. In theory, the antibodies should be monospecific, i.e., the antibodies should react only with the interferon proteins. In practice, antibodies are raised in sheep or rabbits by a prolonged injection schedule using only partially purified interferon. In order to remove antibodies that bind non-interferon proteins, the antiserum is cleaned by absorption. The absorption can, in principle, be performed by two methods: (1) by employing those contaminants thought to be most important by binding them to a Sepharose matrix and then passing the crude antiserum (or immunoglobulins) through such a column several times [16]; or (2) by binding the contaminants to Bentonite [17] using batchwise absorption. A combination of (1) and (2) may be used, starting with the batchwise procedure. The contaminants should include human serum proteins, egg–allantoic fluid, buffy coat extracts, whole buffy coats, etc., as previously described [14, 15,17].

By the use of indirect hemagglutination procedures, it is possible to follow the removal of the different known contaminants [17], although one should not put too much emphasis on this technique [16]. By the use of the best absorbed antiserum, a column was constructed [15], and crude human leukocyte interferon was purified in one step up to about 10×10^6 U/mg protein.

In theory, the very best antigen mixture to use for absorption of anti-interferon would be a crude interferon preparation that harbors all the impurities. Such an absorption, however, might also remove anti-interferon antibodies during repeated absorption. Most fortunately, this does not happen. Berg et al. [18] showed that the major part of the antibodies remained in solution, even after the immunoglobulins were passed through a "CIF column" (CIF bound covalently to Sepharose) for more than 10 times. The absorbed antiserum was in turn coupled to Sepharose 4B, and the column was loaded with crude leukocyte interferon. Specific activity in the eluate was about $30\text{–}40 \times 10^6$ U/mg protein (Table 1, experiment Nos. 299, 303, 313).

When gel filtration was combined with affinity chromatography, interferon of two to three times higher specific activity was obtained, as seen from Table 1, experiment No. 420 (specific activity about 10×10^8 U).

It was disclosed that probably 5–10% of the interferon is "masked" as far as the antigenic properties are concerned. When performing antibody affinity chromatography of CIF, about 10% of the input was always found in the wash [8]. If the CIF was first prepurified by gel filtration (in 1 M urea with 0.1% ethanolamine), dialyzed and loaded on the affinity column (input 100% of the original starting crude material), less than 0.1% was

TABLE 1. Purification of Human Interferons by Antibody-Affinity Chromatography

Exp. No.	Type of interferon	Interferon input (U × 10^{-6})	Volume (ml)	Specific activity of input (U/mg protein)	Wash total (U)	Eluate total (IFU × 10^{-6})	Specific activity of eluate (U/mg protein) × 10^{-6}	Recovery (%)	Purification factor
299	CIF	3	25	10^4	8 × 10^5	4.2	43	140	6000[a]
303	CIF	1.5	2.5	10^4	6 × 10^5	1.8	33	120	4000[a]
313	CIF	2	5	10^4	6 × 10^5	2.4	31	120	3100[b]
420	Gel-filtered CIF	4.5	50	5 × 10^5	2 × 10^3	3.0	90	66	180[b]
285	Crude Namalva	1.6	150	6 × 10^3	1.7 × 10^4	2.6	23	90	3800[b]
296	Crude Namalva	1.05	150	4 × 10^3	8 × 10^4	0.95	8.6	90	4000[a]
301	Human fibroblast	4	50	8 × 10^5	8 × 10^5	3.6	103	90	250[a]

[a]Based on specific activity of peak fraction.
[b]Based on the pool eluate.

found in the wash. This indicated that (1) the antigenic sites were masked by some proteins which were removed with 1 M urea plus gel filtration, and (2) since the biological site was not disturbed (the interferon was measurable), the location of the antigenic sites might be different from the biological site(s) (see discussion in Section IV). Alternatively, "unmasking" takes place during the biological assay.

Sequential antibody affinity chromatography of leukocyte interferon has recently been described [8]. Initially, normal antibody affinity chromatography was performed. The eluate was dialyzed against the loading buffer, then passed through a "control column" which was directed mainly against the impurities, and the last wash (which in principle contained most of the interferon) was loaded again directly on the anti-interferon column. As far as removal of the impurities was concerned, the principle worked; but, unfortunately, most of the interferon activity was lost during the procedure.

One of the ultimate means to check the purity of a given protein preparation is Sodium dodecyl sulfate—polyacrylamide gel electrophoresis (SDS-PAGE). Several papers by Stewart and co-workers have dealt with electrophoresis of human interferon [19-21,72]. We are at present using a thin slab version of SDS-PAGE (20-24 cm long gels, 8-20% acrylamide gradient) loaded with 80-µl samples. The results of a gel-filtered antibody affinity-purified leukocyte interferon preparation are shown in Figure 3. It can clearly be seen that proteins are not located only at the interferon peaks. When using shorter gels, the interferon activity and the proteins coincided (not shown). When re-examining the preparation in longer gels (24 cm), the visible protein bands and the interferon peaks could be separated. This emphasizes that great care should be exercised in the interpretation of these types of experiments. Interferon recoveries from such experiments are usually about 50%, based on the total input on the gel. This is somewhat lower than reported by others [2]. In order to see stained interferon protein bands, we would estimate that more than $2-5 \times 10^6$ U have to be applied on one gel. This amount of interferon happens to be the same as was very recently described by De Maeyer-Guignard et al. [22] in the mouse system, when they obtained visible, stained interferon protein bands.

The anticellular effect of leukocyte interferon as described by Stewart and co-workers [20] was also measured at the same time. As illustrated in Figure 3, the two curves, interferon and thymidine uptake, were opposite as expected, except at fraction No. 34 (mol. wt. 35,000). There was no interferon activity in peak 34, and on several occasions the anticellular effect could be detected. We have, however, not been able to isolate the anticellular activity (at fraction No. 34). One might speculate whether a high local concentration of SDS would give rise to the observed phenomenon, or whether we are dealing with a protein which is very unstable (present in very small concentrations).

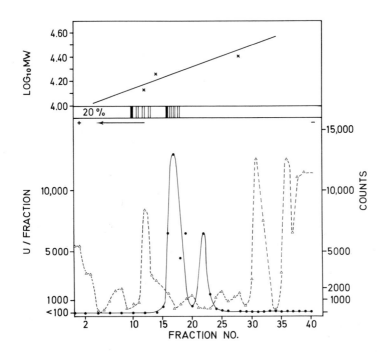

FIGURE 3. SDS-PAGE of purified human leukocyte interferon (PIF). About
2×10^6 U was purified by means of gel filtration, dialysis, and antibody
affinity chromatography. After concentration (visking tube + aquacide II)
and dialysis versus electrophoresis buffer (diluted threefold), there were
115 µg in 175 µl together with 2.5×10^6 U in total (specific activity about
20×10^6 U/mg protein); 80 µl were mixed with 10 µl glycerol, including
bromphenol blue as a tracking dye. After the electrophoresis was performed,
the gel was cut into 2 mm pieces, eluted in 0.01% SDS at 4°C for 2 days,
and titrated for interferon activity. Low interferon titers (5-40 U/fraction)
were found in fractions 4-15. The anticellular activity was measured by
means of a human lymphoblastoid B-cell line (Daudi), which was cultured
in microtiter plates. The interferon samples were added to the cells at
the beginning of cell propagation, and the cell proliferation was measured
by thymidine uptake. Key: solid curve, interferon units/fraction; dashed
curve, [^{14}C]thymidine uptake.

B. Human Lymphoblastoid (Namalva) Interferon

Since one limitation to the amount of PIF that can be produced is the number of buffy coats available, it would be important if a substitute cell source could be found. Strander et al. [42] investigated if it was possible to make use of transformed lymphocytes in the production of human lymphoblastoid interferon. They screened about 21 human lymphoblastoid cell lines and found one which was a remarkably good interferon producer, namely, the Namalva cell line. Titers of about 10,000 U/ml could be obtained. W. B. Finter and K. H. Fantes (personal communication) have taken up the production of Namalva interferon in large tanks (>1000 liters), and they now produce crude interferon with titers of about 20,000-40,000 U/ml. Bridgen et al. [2] have also reported production of Namalva interferon in 800-liter tanks using techniques similar to those of Finter and Fantes, although their yield per ml seems much lower (2000 U/ml).

In theory, the procedure is very simple. The Namalva cells are grown as a suspension culture (from 100 ml up to 1000 liters) until a density of 5×10^6 cells/ml is reached. The cells are resuspended in medium, and the interferon induction is done essentially as described in the previous section, except that a twofold higher amount of Sendai virus (300 HAU/ml in the final cell suspension) is recommended. We have also checked the production on a "semi-micro" scale (50-100 ml) and found it very easy to obtain titers of about 12,000-15,000 U/ml. It is advisable before starting to grow the cells for interferon production, to clone the original suspension in order to ensure a good and healthy starting cell population (J. Zeuthen, personal communication).

The crude Namalva interferon is precipitated by means of trichloroacetic acid (TCA) as follows (K. H. Fantes, personal communication): 1/20 volume of 50% TCA (adjusted to pH 2.5) is added to the crude interferon and, after 4°C overnight, is centrifuged. The precipitate can either be dissolved in PBS (1/10 volume) and dialyzed extensively versus PBS to give crude concentrated Namalva interferon, or it can be dissolved (homogenized) in 94% ethanol using one-fifth of the original interferon volume. By raising the pH to 5.1, many contaminating proteins are precipitated together with a small amount of interferon. By further raising the pH to 7.5, the interferon is precipitated out of the ethanolic solution. It is redissolved in a small volume of PBS and dialyzed extensively. The recovery is normally about 40-50% when working with crude interferon of a reasonable titer $\geq 10,000$ U/ml). If lower titers of crude interferon are obtained, the recoveries will drop to below 15%.

Such purified Namalva interferon could be suitable for clinical purposes. If the Namalva cells are grown in the presence of calf serum, special precautions must presumably be taken against any residual amounts of calf serum proteins that may provoke a serious allergic reaction even when present in extremely small amounts (ng). If media without calf serum proteins that would not give rise to any allergic reactions can be developed, a bright future appears for the usage of Namalva interferon. Most likely the danger of using materials from transformed cells will be cleared up shortly, especially if considering the use of PIF-like materials for human trials. As an initial step, "Namalva PIF" should be used in cancer patients, and based upon these trials further analyses and decisions could be made.

Further Purification of Namalva Interferon

K. H. Fantes has reported (personal communication) that, in ion exchange chromatography, crude Namalva interferon can be 30-fold purified by loading (100-300 ml) on a sulfopropyl (SP-Sephadex C25 column [size 10 ml]) at pH 4.0. Recovery is about 50-80%. Similar reports have been published by Bridgen et al. [2] and G. Bodo (personal communication).

Gel filtration of Namalva interferon has also been reported by Fantes, using Ultrogel AcA 5/4 (which proved to be the very best gel) with quantitative recovery (at pH 3.5). Purification 50-150-fold (specific activity about 10^6 U/mg protein).

Antibody-affinity chromatography has been reported by Bridgen et al. [2], K. H. Fantes (personal communication), and Berg et al. [23]. They found that Namalva interferon can be purified up to 20×10^6 U/mg protein with about 80% recovery (Table 1, experiment Nos. 285 and 296). If gel filtration and antibody-affinity chromatography are combined, a 3-6-fold higher specific activity is obtained (K. Berg, unpublished data).

By combining antibody-affinity chromatography with SP-Sephadex chromatography, together with isoelectric focusing followed by SDS-PAGE, a specific activity up to 10^8-10^9 U/mg protein will most likely be obtained. By employing a suitable ligand, it might be possible to make some short cuts in the purification procedure, ending up with pure interferon proteins. Undoubtedly, we shall very soon see the final purification of Namalva interferon.

C. Human Fibroblast Interferon

The production of human fibroblast interferon has during the last decade attracted much attention. Originally, Vilček and Havell [24] introduced "superinduction," which rendered possible the production of large amounts of fibroblast interferon with titers above 10,000 U/ml. Billau et al. [25] have also begun the production of fibroblastoid interferon. They screened 18 continuous human cell lines for the ability to produce interferon, using Newcastle disease virus (NDV) or superinduction with poly I:poly C, and found one line (MG-63) of osteosarcoma origin which was able to produce more than 50,000 U/ml. It was possible to produce 10^9 IFU in 5 weeks, using 364 bottles of cells. If the MG-63 cell line could be adapted to grow as a suspension culture, giving the same high titers, one can envisage that fibroblastoid interferon could be produced in huge quantities (on a similar scale as Namalva interferon). Of course, the same reservations can be raised with regard to the use of interferon produced from transformed cells as mentioned in Section II.B.

Mozes et al. [26] reported that increased interferon production in human fibroblasts could be obtained by employing UV-irradiated cells instead of superinduction (irradiation plus superinduction gave smaller yield than irradiation alone). Knight [27] recently published a paper on the purification and production of human fibroblast interferon using the "Vilček technique" for the production of interferon.

Very recently, the work of Berthold et al. [28] gave rise to renewed speculation on the production of human fibroblast interferon for clinical application. By employing cells that are trisomeric in chromosome No. 5, they succeeded in making crude unconcentrated interferon with titers up to 500,000 U/ml. Briefly, monolayer cultures of C-10 cells were induced with poly I: poly C plus cylohexamide for 4 hr. Three hours later actinomycin D was added, and interferon was harvested. The crude interferon preparation was found to be very labile. It was stabilized by precipitation with 50% ammonium sulfate and kept as such for months at 4°C. Prior to use, it was redissolved in PBS and dialyzed. Again it would be very desirable if one could accommodate the C-10 cells to a suspension culture.

Purification of human fibroblast interferon has been described by several groups. Several techniques have been applied with remarkable success. Generally speaking, a principal difference seems to exist between fibroblast and leukocyte interferons. Fibroblast interferon, as opposed to leukocyte interferon, will often bind to a wide variety of affinity matrices. For example, fibroblast interferon binds to Con A (strongly), to octyl-sepharose, to poly-U Sepharose, to blue Sepharose, to serum albumin Sepharose [although this last type of binding is not so reproducible (E. Sulkowsky, personal communication)], to glass beads, etc. Crude leukocyte interferon will, however, only bind to one of these matrices (blue Sepharose). Whether this is the result of fundamental molecular differences between fibroblast interferon and human leukocyte interferon remains to be seen. For the time being, one cannot completely rule out that differences in the impurities present in the two preparations might somehow interfere with the apparently different behavior of the interferons (see, for example, under Section II.A, the Con A column) owing to competition between impurities and interferon proteins with regard to the binding sites on a given matrix.

Knight [27], for the first time, completely purified human fibroblast interferon by using a combination of "classical" physicochemical procedures. First, the interferon was fractionated and concentrated by means of ammonium sulfate. It was then fractionated on a BioGel P-150 column and purified on a carboxymethyl-Sepharose column followed by a preparative SDS-PAGE. After elution and concentration, it was analyzed on SDS-PAGE (thin slab gradient); only one band appeared after staining (molecular weight 20,000). Specific activity was 2×10^8 U/mg protein, and total recovery was about 8%.

Berthold et al. [28] have also purified human fibroblast interferon (produced from C-10 cells), using the Con A affinity approach combined with SDS-PAGE. First they loaded a Con A column with crude, concentrated interferon and eluted, resulting in 30% recovery; specific activity was 2×10^7 U/mg protein. The elution of interferon also gave rise to Con A protein, which could be abolished by a subsequent phenyl-Sepharose affinity chromatography. This purified preparation was lyophilized (without losing interferon activity), and a preparative SDS-PAGE was performed (recovery about 16% based on the input on SDS-PAGE; total recovery based on original input was 4%); a final specific activity of $2-10^8$ U/mg protein was obtained. Only one band was found in an analytical SDS-PAGE (slab). This material was also labelled, and it was shown that the radioactivity was at the same location as the interferon proteins. Thus it appears that pure labelled human fibroblast interferon can now be produced in 20 μg quantities.

Albumin-Sepharose columns were introduced by Huang et al. [29] with promising results. They obtained a high specific activity (over 1×10^7 U/mg protein) and quantitative recovery. Presumably, the method involves hydrophilic binding between the matrix and interferon (the interferon is loaded at pH 7.2 at low ionic strength and eluted with 20% ethylene glycol). The method was later found to be erratic and, for the time being, has been abandoned (E. Sulkowski, personal communication).

Hydrophobic chromatography, which was originally introduced by Sulkowsky and co-workers [9,10,30,31,36], is a very useful method for purifying small amounts of interferon (5000-100,000 U). The specific activities obtained are usually about 10^5 U/mg protein, depending on the amount and source of the interferon. Recovery is about 100%. Octyl-Sepharose, phenyl-Sepharose, ω-carboxypentyl-Sepharose, etc. can be used as matrices.

The Ciba-cron blue F3Ga-Sepharose column, introduced by Janowsky et al. [32], is also a very useful approach for purifying 50,000-500,000 U/mg to a specific activity of about 10^6 U/mg protein (recovery about 100%). In brief, the column is loaded with crude interferon in 0.02 M sodium phosphate at pH 7.4, including 0.15 M NaCl, washed with the same buffer, including 1 M NaCl, and finally eluted with 50% ethylene glycol (including 1 M NaCl). It is very important that the dialysis is done thoroughly; otherwise the interferon does not bind to the column. The columns should also be washed extensively with 10-15 bed volumes of buffer before loading the interferon.

The Con A-Sepharose column was introduced by Besançon and Bourgeade [33] and Davey et al. [34,35]. The principle makes use of the fact that glycoproteins will very often bind to Con A due to the right sugar composition on the interferon molecule (hydrophobic interaction might also be involved

[35]. In practice, the interferon is loaded in 0.02 M sodium phosphate (pH 7.4) containing 0.15 M NaCl (loading buffer). By adding 0.1 M α-D-mannopyranoside (αDMP) to the loading buffer, some impurities are eluted from the column. By further adding 20% ethylene glycol, all the interferon is eluted (quantitative recovery) with a specific activity of 5×10^7 U/mg protein. Such a purified preparation was not homogeneous on SDS-PAGE (E. Sulkowski, personal communication).

The Con A column leaks off Con A proteins during use. To minimize the leakage, the column should first be washed with the loading buffer followed by the elution buffer (if necessary, this "cycle" can be repeated). The column will still leak Con A protein (at a lower level compared to the "unwashed" Con A column). To get rid of the contaminating Con A proteins (in a purified interferon preparation), the eluate should be dialyzed back to 0.02 M PBS, 0.15 M NaCl, and then rechromatographed on phenyl-Sepharose (E. Sulkowski, personal communication). This method can process up to about 500×10^6 U on a small column (20-ml size).

Controlled pore glass beads have recently been described by Edy et al. [37]. In principle, the crude interferon is loaded on a 10-ml column filled with controlled pore glass (CPG-10-350, Electro-Nucleonics, Inc., Fairfield, N.J.). Most of the impurities escape the column during washing, and by lowering the pH to about 2, 60% of the interferon can be recovered (specific activity 1-5 $\times 10^6$ U/mg protein). Since no leakage of the column matrix occurs, it may become possible by this method to purify fibroblast interferon for clinical trials.

Zinc chelate affinity chromatography has very recently been introduced by Edy et al. [38] with even greater success. Approximately 60% of the interferon could be recovered (final specific activity close to 10^8 U/mg protein). The interferon is loaded on a small column (6 ml) at pH 7.2 (in 0.02 M sodium, potassium phosphate buffer plus 0.15 M NaCl) and eluted with a pH gradient (pH 6-4). It will be interesting to see the number of protein bands that develop on an SDS-PAGE of such purified material.

Antibody affinity chromatography of fibroblast interferon has also been employed in our laboratory, using an antiserum which was directed against human leukocyte interferon (cf. Berg et al. [18] and Section IV). The crude fibroblast interferon was purified up to 10^8 U/mg protein in one step (recovery 70%). The eluate was subsequently checked on an SDS-PAGE (slab methods) and several protein bands were revealed, of which one located in the range where biological activity was determined. Thus we observed a specific activity of purified fibroblast interferon in the same range as Knight [27] found with pure fibroblast interferon, but contrary to his, our preparation was not homogeneous (four bands in all). Since the recovery in Knight's procedure is rather low (5%) as compared with ours, we would expect his homogeneous preparation to be "contaminated" with pure, but inactive interferon proteins. Therefore the specific activity of the homogeneous preparation could, at least theoretically, be on the same level as our heterogeneous one.

Anfinsen et al. [14] suggested that the impurities present in a human leukocyte interferon preparation might be antigenically different from the corresponding impurities in a fibroblast interferon preparation. If so, it should be possible to purify fibroblast interferon on an antileukocyte column (the so-called denominator principle). Berg et al. [15] could not confirm this interesting idea, since they obtained almost the same specific activity when loading an antileukocyte column with fibroblast interferon or leukocyte interferon. We later found, however, that, when using a highly absorbed antiserum (absorbed by means of crude interferon immobilized on Sepharose [8]) the "denominator principle" was working as far as the impurities were concerned. Mock-fibroblast interferon proteins were indeed passing through an antileukocyte column, provided that the absorption was pursued to the extreme [8]. In contrast a mock-leukocyte interferon preparation was bound to the antileukocyte column.

D. Immune Interferon

The induction of interferon(s) was originally described as a cell response to viral infection [74]. Such interferon is named "classical" interferon, antiviral-induced leukocyte interferon or type I interferon. Human "immune" interferon (also called type II interferon) is an interferon-like substance [75-77] produced from immunocompetent cells (in vivo and in vitro). There are several reports on the production of human immune interferon in vitro [75-79]. In brief, lymphocytes are exposed to, for example, antilymphocyte serum [75], phytohemagglutanin (PHA) [76], Con A (K. Berg, unpublished data), or other mitogens [78, 79] with a varying degree of success. Normally the titers are in the low range (20-500 U/ml).

The criteria used when evaluating whether a given interferon preparation is of immune interferon origin are the same as those used for type I interferon, except that (a) type II has to be destroyed at low pH (2.5) and (b) the antigenic properties of type II are different from type I. Very often the first prerequisite is only partially fulfilled, probably due to a partial contamination of the immune interferon preparation with type I.

A partial (low) neutralization is sometimes obtained when immune interferon is tried with antitype I interferon. Very often the investigator wants to observe a special effect of immune interferon in a given system; therefore it would be important to be sure that the immune interferon preparation is not contaminated with type I. We would expect that by passing a mixture of type I and II through an anti-interferon column, all the type I should be bound (provided that type I, or part thereof, is not "masked"; see Section II. A). Thus, after such a passage the wash, which in theory should contain only type II interferon, can be checked versus low pH and in a neutralization test. Such a procedure is for the time being explored in our laboratory with promising results (experiments in progress).

There have been some reports that type II interferon binds to a blue Sepharose C16B column (Mizrahi's group, personal communication) using 0.02 M sodium phosphate pH 7.4. It could be eluted (and 20-fold purified) using a higher salt concentration (1 M NaCl) and 50% ethylene glycerol.

No reports on further purification of type II interferon are available. Falcoff et al. [75] reported a molecular weight of 50,000 obtained by a gel filtration.

E. Concluding Remarks

The research on interferon has expanded during the past 20 years from the field of basic virology to the fields of biochemistry, cell biology, immunology, and clinical medicine. The clinical interest in interferon is based on a wide spectrum of actions (antitumor and antiviral activity) together with few side effects of this "natural" compound.

The mass production of human leukocyte interferon has been thoroughly described earlier in this section. It was mentioned that large amounts of material, suitable for patients, can now be produced. The material is very well tolerated by the patients, and the stability of leukocyte interferon appears to be satisfactory. Thus HuLeIF may soon (1-3 years) become a practical clinical tool in medicine.

The major limitation for mass production on an industrial scale is the amount of buffy coats available. One way out of this dilemma is most likely to be the Namalva cells, which for the first time make it possible to produce interferon in "industrial amounts." The main problems remaining to be solved are (1) the "danger" of using proteins from a transformed cell-line and (2) the possible allergic reactions which minute amounts of calf serum proteins could provoke, although this problem might not be so great (K. H. Fantes, personal communication). For example, it is highly likely that there are also minute amounts of egg proteins in current PIF material which, nevertheless, are tolerated very well. There have been reports that fibroblast interferon is not as stable as leukocyte interferon when given to man, since it was difficult to detect any interferon in serum after injection of 5×10^6 U. Whether this is due to an actual breakdown of fibroblast interferon, or if the fibroblast interferon is more readily bound to cell surfaces compared to HuLeIF, remains to be seen.

Human immune interferon might reveal anticellular and immunoregulatory properties which could be very useful for the future treatment of patients. This new aspect of interferon is currently under intense investigation, and we shall undoubtedly fairly soon see some new principles and use of this interferon.

Finally, it should be mentioned that the ways and means by which interferons are administered to patients for the time being appear too unsophisticated. A large amount of interferon is given to a patient, and it is "hoped" that a certain part of the interferon reaches the specific target that is involved in the illness. It would be much better, at least on paper, to envisage techniques developed that would permit us to direct our interferon to the specific targets. For example, one could think of using a certain type of lyposomes (carrying the interferon), which preferentially would be absorbed by the liver, for treating hepatitis patients, etc. [80].

III. STABILITY OF HUMAN INTERFERONS
(INCLUDING DENATURING CONDITIONS)

One of the major impediments to production, purification, and clinical evaluation of interferon as an antiviral and antitumor agent has been its notorious instability, particularly in a relatively pure form (specific activity above 10^7 U/mg protein, depending on the total amount of interferon present). The instability was not "limited" to the purified interferon preparations. We have occasionally experienced that crude human leukocyte interferon batches have suddenly (over 3-7 days at 4°C) lost most of the activity (from 25,000 U/ml to below 2000 U/ml). The reason for this loss has not been fully explained, although there appear to be some hints that proteolytic activity might be an important cause. For example, a number of HuLyIF (Namalva) interferon preparations were checked for proteolytic activity using Azocoll (Calbiochem) as a substrate. The manufacturer claims that practically all known proteolytic enzymes will react with the substrate, which is made from numerous peptides with a dye bound to the peptides. A proteolytic activity will split the peptides and release the dye. By measuring the optical density (OD) at 520 nm in the supernatant, an "expression" of the proteolytic activity is obtained. It was hoped that a high proteolytic activity (high OD) would correspond to a low interferon titer. As can be seen from Table 2, these expectations were clearly not met, although proteolytic enzymes, undoubtedly, might sometimes play an important role in the stability of interferon.

Several other interferon batches were also checked; among these were PIF and CIF (from Cantell) and PIF-1 (from another laboratory; see Table 3). PIF-1 was never used for any clinical purposes, since it lost its activity going from 1×10^6 U/ml down to 20,000 U/ml during a period of three weeks (at 4°C). It appeared that proteolytic activity might have been the determinating factor for the instability observed. A retrospective examination of the protocol also revealed that there had been a minor bacterial contamination during the production (of PIF-1). It is noteworthy (Table 3) that the level of proteolytic activity in PIF (Cantell) is lower compared to CIF 83A. Thus during the purification procedure (including the ethanolic precipitation), proteolytic activity is removed along with other impurities. Crude interferon preparations appear to have almost the same level of proteolytic activity as CIF, despite the fact that interferon activity is increased 10- to 20-fold in the latter.

TABLE 2. Correlation between Stability (or High Yield)
of Interferon and Proteolytic Activity

Namalva interferon		Proteolytic "activity"	
Batch no.	U/ml 69/19B units	(OD 520)[a]	Mean value
402	5,000	2.279 2.045	2.162
416	5,000	0.460 0.390	0.425
418	1,600	0.494 0.459	0.476
435	11,300	0.370 0.383	0.376
439	20,000	0.729 0.754	0.742
443	15,000	0.542 0.545	0.543

[a]Measured by using a calculating absorptiometer (LKB 7400).

On a number of occasions, proteolytic inhibitors, such as soybean trypsin inhibitor (STI), Trasylol, etc., were added without the slightest effect on the stability of leukocyte interferon. This is in contrast to the findings of Berthold et al. [28], who reported that they were able to stabilize fibroblast interferon by means of Trasylol.

A proteolytic attack of human leukocyte interferon has also recently been advocated by Chadha et al. [62]. Using molecular sieving of crude HuLeIF, they revealed an apparent molecular weight of 26,000. However, after denaturation (guanine + mercaptoethanol; Mogensen and Cantell [44]), a molecular weight of 21,000 was observed. The reactivated interferon (mol. wt. 21,000) gave only a single peak in SDS-PAGE, confirming that a single molecular species was generated during the denaturation and reactivation procedures. Based on these findings, the authors suggested that the interferon molecule underwent a proteolytic cleavage, probably by a protease present in the extracellular fluid. Thus a peptide fragment dissociates from the parent molecule when HuLeIF is denatured in the presence of a reducing agent, resulting in a drop of 5000 in molecular weight (without any loss of antiviral activity in the parental molecule). No interferon activity was found in the small fragment (mol. wt. 5000). It might also be argued that the loss in molecular weight (5000) is due to a break in an S—S bond.

TABLE 3. Proteolytic Activity Determined in HuLeIF Preparations

Samples	OD reading[a]	Activity $\times 10^{-3}$	Interferon titer
Control	0.100	—	0
PIF-1 (uncentrifuged)	1.370	0.035	20.000
PFI-1 (centrifuged)	1.090	0.028	20.000
CIF 83A (Cantell)	0.800	0.015	400.000
PIF (Cantell)	0.210	< 0.005	2×10^6
Crude HuLeIF 95B (HKN)	1.370	0.030	9.000
Crude HuLeIF 95C	1.160	0.025	5.400
Crude HuLeIF 95D	1.388	0.034	5.400
Crude HuLeIF 95E	0.410	< 0.005	16.000
Crude HuLeIF 96C	0.709	0.005	48.000
Crude HuLeIF 96D	0.706	0.005	5.400
Crude HuFiIF (12099/138)	0.318	< 0.005	20-40.000

[a]The OD reading is expressed as milligrams of trypsin per milliliter, comparing the OD value with a trypsin standard curve obtained by using different but known amounts of trypsin.

During the reactivation, the small part is unable to come into the right molecular configuration, which thus results in the loss in molecular weight of 5000.

It has been reported that an increase of the serum concentration, together with a decrease of proteolytic activity, might stabilize crude interferon, but the pattern was not clear (K. H. Fantes, personal communication). We found that CIF and PIF were more stable at -20°C; Cantell et al. [71] normally keep their interferon preparations at +4°C. For the last 10 months we have not encountered the instability problem, probably because of more rigorous rules in the laboratory concerning bacterial contamination, including a more streamlined procedure. Thus we can essentially confirm the findings of Cantell et al. that leukocyte interferon, when handled properly, appears to be stable for months (> 10 months).

Several reports have been published in connection with the stability of human interferon under denaturating conditions. Some of the data are summarized in Table 4. Generally speaking, the interferon activity is

TABLE 4. Stability of Interferon

	Type of interferon		
	Human leukocyte	Namalva	Human fibroblast
Heat (100° C) 1 min	99.5% destroyed	>98% destroyed	>98% destroyed
Heat (100° C) in guanidine HCl	70% destroyed	ND[a]	100% destroyed
Addition of SDS	100-150% recovery	100% recovery	20-60% recovery
SDS + heat (100° C) 1 min	150-250% recovery	ND	25-100% recovery
Heat followed by C_2H_5SH + SDS ("heat resurrection")	0% recovery	ND	25-125% recovery
Proteolytic activity in crude interferon	++	++	+
Inhibition of proteolytic activity by Trasylal or STI[b]	No inhibition	No inhibition	Inhibition
Mol wt in SDS-PAGE	17,800 and 21,000	18,000 and 21,000	20,000
Mol wt by gel filtration	26,000 (21,000) (17,800)	23,000	20,000- 25,000

[a]ND = not done.
[b]Soybean trypsin inhibitor.

lost when interferon is heated to 100° C (1 min). Partially purified leukocyte interferon (PIF) showed a remarkable stability at 56° C [44]. After three days at 56° C no loss was seen (CIF dropped one log in activity in 12 hr at 37° C). These results [44] are in concord with the data shown in Table 3 concerning the proteolytic activity of different interferon preparations. Although it is tempting to speculate whether the higher instability

in CIF observed by Mogensen and Cantell [44] was due to a higher proteolytic activity compared to PIF, it is still too early to make such a conclusion.
For example, it might be expected that a partial inactivation of proteolytic
enzymes would occur at 56° C.

It is clearly documented [44] that interferon contains S—S bonds which
are important for the expression of the biological activity. By breaking up
these bonds (by means of mercaptoethanol alone) the biological activity disappears [44]. By breaking the S—S bonds in the presence of 8 M urea (or
5 M guanidine chloride), the biological activity can be recovered after
dialysis against PBS. The urea (or guanidine) functions as a protein-folding
agent which permits the reduced interferon molecule to return to the proper
configuration before reoxidation (done by dialysis against PBS) has occurred.
Based on anti-interferon neutralization tests, the antigenic composition of
leukocyte interferon seems to remain unchanged after such treatment
(K. Berg, unpublished data).

In 1974 Stewart et al. [45] introduced an interesting principle concerning the "resurrection" of interferon. Interferon was boiled (and inactivated);
mercaptoethanol, urea, and SDS were added, and the mixture was boiled
again. After subsequent dialysis the investigators [45] found that most of
the activity was recovered in a stable form. Resurrection worked only for
fibroblast interferon (human and mouse), but not for HuLeIF (Table 4).
Although recovery does vary (also in our hands), it is an interesting observation that it is possible to resurrect "dead" (boiled) interferon. On a number
of occasions, we have tried to see if such resurrected interferon preparations are more stable in subsequent purification steps (affinity chromatography, etc.). We have not, however, found any marked improvements, and
since our recoveries from the resurrection procedure generally were low
(25-30%) we stopped pursuing this technique. The antigenic properties of
interferon assessed by antibody affinity chromatography remain unchanged
after such treatment.

The fact that the biological activity of human interferons can be either
completely or, at least, partially recovered after SDS treatment (see Table
4) has aided considerably in the molecular weight determination of all types
of interferon by means of SDS-PAGE. Treatment of protein mixtures with
SDS, followed by boiling (or modest heating, for example, to 56° C), breaks
noncovalent bonds whereby proteins, complexing with or masking interferon,
are dissociated from the interferon molecule. It seems likely that such
random binding of foreign proteins to interferon was responsible for the
variation in the reported molecular weights obtained by means of gel filtration [46-48].

Stewart et al. [49,50] were the first to report calculation of interferon
molecular weight by means of SDS-PAGE. They found biological activity
in two peaks of human leukocyte interferon, corresponding to molecular
weights of 21,000 and 15,000, respectively. In addition to these findings
they also disclosed that the two peaks differed, as far as stability was con-

cerned, in SDS under reducing conditions and in their degree of hetero-
specificity on rabbit cells.

We have also examined PIF on an SDS-PAGE (slab gel, 24 cm long,
gradient of polyacrylamide 9-20%) and found slightly higher values (mol.
wt. 17,800 and 23,000). Thus we can also, essentially, confirm the findings
of Stewart. Knight [27] recently reported that the molecular weight of
pure interferon in SDS-PAGE is about 20,000 (only a single peak). This
is in agreement with others, including Reynolds and Pitha [51] and Vilček
et al. [52].

Edy et al. [53] recently reported that a minor fraction of human fibroblast interferon resembled human leukocyte interferon in being renaturable
after treatment with guanidine hydrochloride. However, antigenically, and
by its low activity on heterologous cells, it resembled human fibroblast
interferon.

Cartwright et al. [54] reported that fibroblast interferon could be
stabilized against many inactivating forces (mechanical disturbances,
filtering processes, etc.) by means of simple sulfhydryl reagents such as
N-acetylcysteine. The use of such easily removable and relatively nontoxic stabilizers may help in the preparation and purification of fibroblast
interferon for clinical use.

No reports are available on the stability of purified Namalva interferon
(Namalva PIF); but most likely stability properties similar to those of
normal leukocyte interferon (PIF) would be expected, although there have
been problems in adjusting the alcoholic precipitation procedure to Namalva
interferon (K. H. Fantes, personal communication).

Interferon proteins are considered to be glycoproteins. Originally,
Schonne et al. [55] observed a decreased charge heterogeneity of rabbit
interferon upon isoelectric focusing following treatment with neuraminidase.
They proposed that interferon most likely was a glycoprotein (possessing
varying amounts of sialic acids). This observation was further substantiated
by Dorner et al. [56], who, after incubation of rabbit interferon with neuraminidase, found only one (broad) peak at pH 6.3. This type of interferon
regained its original heterogeneous character after re-incorporation of
sialic acid residues in the presence of sialyl transferase. The studies of
Schonne et al. [55] and Dorner et al. [56] showed that terminal sialic
residues may be removed without loss of antiviral activity. Dorner et al.
[56] also showed that the next carbohydrate residue in the polysaccharide
chain, galactose, could be successively oxidized with galactose oxidase
and reduced with sodium borohydride without loss of activity. Human fibroblast interferon has also been suggested to be a glycoprotein [27,30,33,34,
55-59]. Thus mouse, rabbit, and human fibroblast interferon all bind to
lectins with a known sugar specificity. It is therefore tempting to speculate
whether human leukocyte interferon should also be a glycoprotein. The
evidence for this is less compelling. Neither crude human leukocyte interferon [59,73] nor PIF would bind to Con A [73].

Isoelectric profiles of human leukocyte interferon before and after treatment with neuraminidase show differences much less pronounced than those obtained after a similar treatment of rabbit interferon [56, 60, 61, 73]. Bose et al. [58] were able to remove a fragment (mol. wt. 4000) from the interferon molecule by treating HuLeIF with glycosidases, thus indicating the presence of a sugar moiety on the interferon molecule. On the other hand, it cannot be completely ruled out that a possible proteolytic activity present in the crude interferon preparation could be responsible for the loss in molecular weight. This would, in a way, be in harmony with the recent results of Chadha et al. [62].

Recently, Stewart et al. [63] demonstrated that it was possible to convert the heterogenous leukocyte interferon to one peak (in isoelectric focusing) by means of chemical oxidation (using periodate). They could also show that the 21,000-molecular-weight species was converted to the 15,000 species. The latter was suggested to be the most stable species of HuLeIF. The same loss (in molecular weight) was reported by Bose et al. [58] and by Chadha et al. [62], using different approaches. At present, it appears that the two species of leukocyte interferon (mol. wt. 15,000 and 20,000) can be converted to one species (mol. wt. 15,000) by as varied treatments as (1) chemical cleavage or "oxidation" (using periodate), (2) protein denaturation or "reduction" (using guanidine and mercaptoethanol), and (3) enzymatic cleavage (using glycosidases and neuraminidase). It would be interesting to combine treatments 1-3 to see whether all the phenomena described are unrelated or whether we are dealing with different aspects of the same molecule.

IV. ANTIGENIC PROPERTIES

For many years, it has been widely accepted that interferons were species-specific as far as the antiviral activity was concerned. That is to say, mouse interferon will only protect mouse cells, not human cells, etc. This theorem has gradually been modified, especially after Gresser et al. [64] showed that HuLeIF had a higher antiviral activity on bovine cells compared to human cells. With regard to antigenicity of interferons, the "species specificity theorem" appears still to be valid, since no antiserum against interferon from another species has been shown to neutralize, for example, HuLeIF (or vice versa). In 1964, Paucker [65] showed that anti-mouse interferon failed to neutralize chick interferon.

Ogburn et al. [17] reported that mouse interferon (from L cells) produced by means of two different inducers (poly I: poly C or NDV) was bound equally well to an anti-mouse interferon column, suggesting that there were no antigenic differences among interferons produced in response to different inducers acting on the same cell. The same was also found by Havell et al. [66] in the human system.

Later it was found that antigenic differences exist among interferons produced in different cell types of the same species. This was first demonstrated by Youngner and Salvin [67], who found an interferon-like substance present in serum from sensitized mice after injection with the sensitizing antigen. This substance, which presumably is produced from circulating lymphocytes, could not be neutralized with antibodies raised against virus-induced mouse L-cell fibroblast interferon (which is not surprising, as we shall see shortly). The authors called the interferon-like substance made by this immunostimulation type II interferon ("immune interferon") as opposed to the conventional type I interferon ("classical or viral interferon").

Berg et al. [15] showed that human leukocyte and fibroblast interferons were dissimilar with respect to antigenicity. This was probably most clearly demonstrated by subjecting leukocyte and fibroblast interferons to antibody affinity chromatography, using two different columns made by means of antileukocyte interferon and antifibroblast interferon. When loading leukocyte interferon on an antifibroblast column, practically no interferon (< 1-2%) was bound. When loading fibroblast interferon on an antileukocyte column, more than 95% of the interferon was bound to the column. Based on these findings, it was suggested that the antigenic composition of fibroblast interferon (F form) was different from leukocyte interferon (L form). This was also confirmed by interferon neutralization studies [15,66]. That the antileukocyte serum can neutralize both types of interferon can probably be ascribed the "buffy coat preparation," which is composed of a wide variety of cells, whereas the fibroblast cell belongs to a much more homogeneous cell population. Thus during the interferon induction, both forms of interferon (L and F forms) are produced in the buffy coat system, and only one form (the F form) is produced in the fibroblast system. Of the total amount of interferon activity in leukocyte interferon, the L form amounts to about 99% and the F form to 1%. Apparently, this small amount of the F form is sometimes sufficient to evoke an antibody response in rabbits. This was documented, for example, by Havell et al. [66] and Berg et al. [15] by means of the interferon neutralization test: The anti-interferon serum (for example, as twofold dilutions) is mixed with 10 U of the interferon. If the antiserum neutralizes the interferon, the mixture (interferon + antiserum) will not protect cells against a challenge virus (or vice versa).

It might seem peculiar that antifibroblast interferon cannot neutralize leukocyte interferon, since the very same antifibroblast serum is used to bind the F form present in leukocyte interferon [15]. These results are, nevertheless, in good agreement. When using the antifibroblast interferon as an immunosorbent in an antibody affinity chromatography, the total amount of the F form put on will be bound by the column. Thus upon dilution this interferon will still behave as fibroblast interferon with respect to antigenicity. When crude leukocyte interferon is diluted to a concentration of 10 U/ml, the F form is not recognized by the antifibroblast interferon,

since it is only present in small amounts (0.1 U/ml) as compared with the
L form (about 9.9 U/ml).

Havell et al. [66] were also able to isolate the antifibroblast interferon
activity that was present in a selected antileukocyte interferon by "reverse"
affinity chromatography. First, they immobilized fibroblast interferon to
Sepharose (they could demonstrate that the beads had a titer of about 400
U/0.1 ml reacted beads). After loading the antileukocyte serum (which had
a titer of about 100–200 against both forms of interferon), they were able
to elute antifibroblast interferon (which could not neutralize leukocyte interferon).

In conclusion, it has thus been proven that human leukocyte interferon
is made up of two species: the L form (~99%) and the F form (~1%). The
latter is most likely identical with, or very closely related to, the fibroblast
interferon produced by fibroblast cells, as summarized in Table 5.

Recently, Paucker et al. [68] showed that the F and L forms can also
be distinguished by using rabbit cells instead of human cells in the neutralization of leukocyte interferon (when employing sheep anti-interferon).
They proposed a model in which a single interferon molecule contains
multiple binding sites, each of which is capable of interacting with cells
of different species.

Namalva interferon, which is produced by a transformed B-cell line
(Namalva), is very similar to leukocyte interferon with respect to molecular
weights and isoelectric points, as shown in Table 5. As far as antigenic
properties are concerned, however, there is a distinct difference between
leukocyte and Namalva interferons. About 15% of the total interferon activity
in Namalva interferon is represented by the F form, whereas, in leukocyte
interferon, only about 1% of the activity is represented by the F form.
This was elegantly shown by Havell et al. [69], employing antibody affinity
chromatography with "monospecific" antisera. When passing crude Namalva
interferon on an antifibroblast column, about 13% of the interferon could be
bound and subsequently eluted by lowering the pH. This corresponds very
well with the neutralization results. Only when using a mixture of anti-
interferon sera (antifibroblast plus antileukocyte sera) was it possible to
neutralize Namalva interferon (using "monospecific" sera; J. Vilček, personal communication).

It might be asked if the F form (in Namalva interferon) is identical
with fibroblast interferon as regards molecular weight and isoelectric
points. This identity could easily be demonstrated by first passing crude
Namalva interferon through an antifibroblast column. This purified F form
could then be further analyzed to see if full (or partial) identity exists.

Very few reports have been published on the possible correlation between the antiviral activity and the antigenicity of interferon. An important
question might be asked: Will the antigenic determinant(s) on the interferon molecule be located on the same site as the biological (antiviral)
activity? Mogensen and Cantell [70] reported that carboxymethylation

TABLE 5. Antigenic Properties of Interferons

Type of interferon	Neutralized with			SDS-PAGE (mol wt)	Isoelectric point(s), pI	F form (%)	L form (%)
	Anti-fibroblast IF (%)	Anti-leukocyte IF (%)	Anti-fibroblast + anti-leukocyte				
Fibroblast	100	0–100	100	20,000	6.8–7.3	100	0[a]
Leukocyte	0	100	100	21,000 (23,000) 15,000 (17,000)	5.4–6.4 (7) Three components	1	99
Namalva	Partial	Partial	100	21,000 (23,000) 15,000 (17,500)	5.4–6.3 (7) Three components	15	85
Immune	ND[b]	0	ND	ND	ND	—	—

[a]In a preliminary report, Havell et al. (Amer. Soc. Microbiol. Abstr., 1978) find that fibroblast interferon contains a small portion of the L form.
[b]ND = not done.

of mercaptoethanol-reduced HuLeIF destroyed its antiviral activity and antigenicity, suggesting the same location for the two properties. In this laboratory, we have on several occasions observed that inactive interferon could not compete in neutralization tests with active interferon of similar purity (K. Berg, unpublished data). In order to explore a possible relationship between antigenicity and antiviral activity, the following experiment was performed. Crude HuLeIF was bound to two different matrices: activated Sepharose 4B (AS) and epoxy-Sepharose 4B (ES), both purchased from Pharmacia. About 50% of the proteins were bound in both instances. CIF-ES had absolutely no antiviral activity when the beads were tried on human cells. CIF-AS had a distinct activity (in a dilution higher than 1:100). Antigen columns were made using the two gels. Anti-interferon (titer about 100,000 interferon-neutralizing units/ml) was loaded on each column, and, after a thorough wash, the columns were eluted (no neutralizing activity could be found in the very last fractions of the wash). From both antigen columns anti-interferon could be eluted specifically. Thus one of the gels (CIF-ES) had no biological activity but was still able to neutralize (bind) anti-interferon specifically. (No anti-interferon activity was found in an eluate after loading the antigen columns with normal rabbit serum.) One explanation could be that the antigenic and biological site(s) might have different locations on the interferon molecule. If this proves to be so, it makes the interpretation of radioimmunoassay very difficult—if not impossible—even with pure interferon.

ACKNOWLEDGMENT

This work was supported by a grant from The Danish Cancer Society.

REFERENCES

1. K. Cantell, H. Strander, G. Hadhazy, and H. R. Nevanlinna, How much interferon can be prepared in human leukocyte suspensions. In The Interferons: Proceedings of the International Symposium held at Siena, 1967 (G. Rita, ed.), Academic Press, New York, 1968, pp. 223-232.

2. P. J. Bridgen, C. B. Anfinsen, L. Corby, S. Bose, K. Zoom, V. T. Rüegg, and C. E. Buckler, Human Lymphoblastoid Interferon. Large scale production and partial purification. J. Biol. Chem. 252: 6585-87 (1977).

3. I. S. Christophersen, R. Jordal, K. Osther, A. Hammer, J. Lindenberg, P. H. Petersen, and K. Berg, Interferon treatment of neoplastic diseases: A preliminary report. Acta Med. Scand. 204:471-476 (1978).

4. K. Cantell, Preparation of human leukocyte interferon. In Standardization of Interferon and Interferon Inducers: Proceedings of the International Symposium held in London, 1969 (F. T. Perkins and R. H.
Regamey, eds.), Karger, Basel, 1970.

5. H. Strander and K. Cantell, Further studies on the production of interferon by human leukocytes in vitro. Ann. Med. Exp. Biol. Fenn. 45:
20-29 (1967).

6. H. Strander and K. Cantell, Production of interferon by human leukocytes in vitro. Ann. Med. Exp. Biol. Fenn. 44:265-273 (1966).

7. B. Larsen, personal communication (1978).

8. K. Berg, Sequential antibody affinity chromatography of human leukocyte interferon. Scand. J. Immunol. 6:77-86 (1977).

9. J. K. Chen, W. J. Jankowski, J. A. O'Malley, E. Sulkowski, and
W. A. Carter, Nature of the molecular heterogeneity of human leukocyte interferon. J. Virol. 19:425-434 (1976).

10. W. J. Jankowski, M. W. Davey, J. A. O'Malley, E. Sulkowski, and
W. A. Carter, Molecular structure of human fibroblast and leukocyte
interferons: Probe by lectin and hydrophobic chromatography. J. Virol.
16:1124-30 (1975).

11. J. W. Huang, C. I. Hejna, E. Sulkowski, W. A. Carter, G. H. Silver,
H. Munayyer, and P. Cane, Human interferon-albumin interaction:
The influence of albumine conformation. Virology 65:268-271 (1975).

12. J. K. Chen, W. J. Jankowski, J. A. O'Malley, E. Sulkowski, and
W. A. Carter, Nature of the molecular heterogeneity of human leukocyte interferon. J. Virol. 19:425-434 (1976).

13. M. W. Davey, J. W. Huang, E. Sulkowski, and W. A. Carter, Hydrophobic binding sites on human interferon. J. Biol. Chem. 250:348-349
(1975).

14. C. B. Anfinsen, S. Bose, L. Corley, and D. Gurari-Rotman, Partial
purification of human interferon by affinity chromatography. Proc.
Nat. Acad. Sci. U.S. 71:3139-42 (1974).

15. K. Berg, C. A. Ogburn, K. Paucker, K. E. Mogensen, and K. Cantell,
Affinity chromatography of human leukocyte and diploid cell interferons
on sepharose-bound antibodies. J. Immunol. 114:640-644 (1975).

16. K. Paucker, K. Berg, and C. A. Ogburn, Purification of mouse inter-
feron by antibody affinity chromatography. In Effects of Interferon on
Cells, Viruses and the Immune System (A. Geraldes, ed.), Academic
Press, New York, 1975, pp. 639-657.

17. A. Ogburn, K. Berg, and K. Paucker, Purification of mouse interferon
by affinity chromatography on anti-interferon globulin-sepharose.
J. Immunol. 111:1206-1218 (1973).

18. K. Berg, R. Hamilton, and I. Heron, Purification of human interferon
by antibody affinity chromatography, using highly absorbed anti-
interferon. Scand. J. Immunol. 8:429-436 (1978).

19. W. E. Stewart, II, and J. Desmyter, Molecular heterogeneity of
    human leukocyte interferon: Two populations differing in molecular
    weights, requirements for renaturation and cross-species antiviral
    activity. Virology 67: 68-73 (1975).
20. W. E. Stewart, II, I. Gresser, M. G. Tovey, M.-T. Bandu, and
    S. LeGoff, Identification of the cell multiplication inhibitory factors
    in interferon preparations as interferons. Nature 262: 300-302 (1976).
21. W. E. Stewart, II, L. S. Liu, M. Wiranowska-Stewart, and K. Cantell,
    Elimination of size and charge heterogeneities of human leukocyte
    interferons by chemical cleavage. Proc. Nat. Acad. Sci. U.S. 74:
    4200-4204 (1978).
22. J. DeMaeyer-Guignard, M. G. Tovey, I. Gresser, and E. DeMayer,
    Purification of mouse interferon by sequential affinity chromatography
    on poly(U) and antibody-agarose columns. Nature 271: 622-625 (1978).
23. K. Berg, R. Alacam, R. D. Hamilton, and I. Heron, Texas Repts.
    Biol. Med. pp. 187-193 (1977).
24. J. Vilček and E. A. Havell, Stabilization of interferon messenger
    RNA activity by treatment of cells with metabolic inhibitors and lower-
    ing of the incubation temperature. Proc. Nat. Acad. Sci. U.S. 70:
    3909-3913 (1973).
25. A. Billiau, V. G. Edy, H. Heremans, J. van Damme, J. Desmyter,
    J. A. Georgiades, and P. De Somer, Human interferon: Mass produc-
    tion in a newly established cell line, MG-63. Antimicrob. Agents
    Chemother. 12: 11-15 (1977).
26. L. W. Mozes, E. A. Havell, M. L. Gradoville, and J. Vilcek,
    Increased interferon production in human cells inadiated with ultra-
    violet light. Infec. Immun. 10: 1189-91 (1974).
27. E. Knight, Interferon: Purification and initial characterization from
    human diploid cells. Proc. Nat. Acad. Sci. U.S. 73: 520-523 (1976).
28. W. Berthold, C. Tan, and Y. H. Tan, Purification and in vitro labelling
    of human fibroblastoid interferon. J. Biol. Chem. in press (1978).
29. J. W. Huang, M. W. Davey, C. J. Hejura, W. van Muenchhausen,
    E. Sulkowsky, and W. Carter, Selective binding of human interferon
    to albumin immobilized on agarose. J. Biol. Chem. 249: 4665-4667
    (1974).
30. M. W. Davey, W. A. Sulkowski, and W. A. Carter, Binding of human
    fibroblast interferon to concanavalin A-agarose: Involvement of carbo-
    hydrate recognition and hydrophobic interaction. Biochemistry 15:
    704-713 (1976).
31. E. Sulkowski, M. W. Davey, and W. A. Carter, Interaction of human
    interferons with immobilized hydrophobic amino acids and dipeptides.
    J. Biol. Chem. 251: 5381-5385 (1976).
32. W. J. Janowsky, W. von Muenchhausen, E. Sulkowski, and W. A.
    Carter, Binding of human interferons to immobilized Cibacron Blue
    F36A. Biochemistry 15: 5182 (1976).

33. F. Besançon and M-F. Bourgeade, Affinity of murine and human inter-feron for Concanavalin A. J. Immunol. 113:1061-1063 (1974).
34. M. W. Davey, E. Sulkowski, and W. A. Carter, Hydrophobic inter-action of human interferon with concanavalin A-agarose. J. Biol. Chem. 249:6354-6355 (1974).
35. M. W. Davey, E. Sulkowski, and W. A. Carter, Binding of human fibroblast interferon to concanavalin A-agarose: Involvement of carbo-hydrate recognition and hydrophobic interaction. (Manuscript in preparation, 1976.)
36. M. W. Davey, E. Sulkowski, and W. A. Carter, Hydrophobic inter-action of human, mouse and rabbit interferons with immobilized hydrocarbons. J. Biol. Chem. 251:7620-7625 (1976).
37. V. G. Edy, I. A. Brande, E. De Clercq, and P. De Somer, Purifica-tion of interferon by adsorption chromatography on controlled pore glass. J. Gen. Virol. 33:517-521 (1976).
38. V. G. Edy, A. Billiau, and P. De Somer, Purification of human fibro-blast interferon by zinc chelate affinity chromatography. J. Biol. Chem. 252:5934-5935 (1977).
39. H. Strander, Production of interferon by suspended human leukocytes. Thesis, Balder AB, Stockholm, 1971.
40. H. Strander and K. Cantell, Studies on antiviral and antitumor effects of human leukocyte interferon in vitro and in vivo. In The Production and Use of Interferon for the Treatment and Prevention of Human Virus Infections: Proceedings of a Tissue Culture Association Workshop held at Lake Placid, 1973 (C. Weymouth, ed.), Tissue Culture Assoc., Rockville, Md., 1974, pp. 49-56.
41. K. Cantell and S. Hirvonen, Large-scale production of human leukocyte interferon containing 10^8 units per ml. J. Gen. Virol. 39:541-543 (1978).
42. H. Strander, K. E. Mogensen, and K. Cantell, Production of human lymphoblastoid interferon. J. Clin. Microbiol. 1:116-117 (1975).
43. E. Törmä and K. Paucker, Purification and characterization of human leukocyte interferon components. J. Biol. Chem. 251:4810-4816 (1976).
44. K. E. Mogensen and K. Cantell, Human leukocyte interferon: A role for disulphide bonds. J. Gen. Virol. 22:95-103 (1974).
45. W. E. Stewart, II, E. De Clercq, and P. De Somer, Stabilisation of interferons by defensive reversible denaturation. Nature 249:460-461 (1974).
46. J. S. Youngner and W. R. Stinebring, Comparison of interferon pro-duction in mice by bacterial endotoxin and statolon. Virology 1:310 (1966).
47. T. C. Merigan and W. J. Kleinschmidt, Different molecular species of mouse interferon induced by statolon. Nature 208:667 (1965).

48. T. C. Merigan and W. J. Kleinschmidt, A second molecular species of mouse interferon in mice injected with statolon. Nature 212: 1383 (1966).

49. W. E. Stewart, II, Distinct molecular species of interferons. Virology 61: 80 (1974).

50. W. E. Stewart, II, P. De Somer, V. G. Edy, K. Paucker, K. Berg, and C. A. Ogburn, Distinct molecular species of human interferons: Requirements for stabilization and reactivation of human leukocyte and fibroblast interferons. J. Gen. Virol. 26: 327-331 (1975).

51. F. H. Reynolds and P. M. Pitha, Molecular weight study of human fibroblast interferon. Biochem. Biophys. Res. Commun. 65: 107 (1975).

52. J. Vilček, E. A. Havell, and S. Yamazaki, Antigenic, physicochemical, and biological characterization of human interferons. Ann. N.Y. Acad. Sci. 284: 703-710 (1976).

53. V. G. Edy, J. Desmyter, A. Billiau, and P. De Somer, Stable and unstable forms of human fibroblast interferon. Infec. Immun. 16: 445-448 (1977).

54. T. Cartwright, O. Senussi, and M. D. Grady, Reagents which inhibit disulphide band formation stabilize human fibroblast interferon. J. Gen. Virol. 36: 323-327 (1977).

55. E. Schonne, A. Billiau, and P. De Somer, The properties of interferon IV. Isoelectric focusing of rabbit interferon (NDV-RK13). In Standardization of Interferon and Interferon Inducers: Proceedings of the International Symposium held in London, 1969 (F. T. Perkins and R. H. Regamey, eds.), Karger, Basel, 1970, pp. 61-68.

56. F. Dorner, M. Scriba, and R. Weil, Interferon: Evidence for its glycoprotein nature. Proc. Nat. Acad. Sci. U.S. 70: 1981-1985 (1973).

57. E. Knight, Heterogeneity of purified mouse interferons. J. Biol. Chem. 250: 4139-4143 (1975).

58. S. Bose, D. Gurari-Rotman, U. T. Ruegg, L. Corley, and C. B. Anfinsen, Apparent dispensability of the carbohydrate moiety of human interferon for antiviral activity. J. Biol. Chem. 251: 1659-1662 (1976).

59. W. J. Janowski, M. W. Davey, J. A. O'Malley, E. Sulkowski, and W. A. Carter, Molecular structure of human fibroblast and leukocyte interferons: Probe by lectin and hydrophobic chromatography. J. Virol. 16: 1124-1130 (1975).

60. K. E. Mogensen, L. Pyhälä, E. Törmä, and K. Cantell, No evidence for a carbohydrate moiety affecting the clearance of circulating human leukocyte interferon in rabbits. Acta Pathol. Microbiol. Scand. 82B: 305-310 (1974).

61. J. Morser, J. P. Kabayo, and D. W. Hutchinson, Differences in sialic content of human interferons. J. Gen. Virol. in press (1978).

62. K. C. Chadha, M. Sclair, E. Sulkowski, and W. A. Carter, Molecular size heterogeneity of human leukocyte interferon. Biochemistry 17: 196-200 (1978).

63. W. E. Stewart, II, L. S. Liu, M. Wiranowska-Stewart, and K. Cantell, Elimination of size and charge heterogeneities of human leukocyte interferons by chemical cleavage. Proc. Nat. Acad. Sci. U.S. 74: 4200-4204 (1977).

64. I. Gresser, M.-T. Bandu, D. Brouty-Boye, and M. Tovey, Pronounced antiviral activity of human interferon on bovine and procine cells. Nature 251:543-545 (1974).

65. K. Paucker, The serological specificity of interferon. J. Immunol. 94:371-378 (1964).

66. E. A. Havell, B. Berman, C. A. Ogburn, K. Berg, K. Paucker, and J. Vilček, Two antigenically distinct species of human interferon. Proc. Nat. Acad. Sci. U.S. 72:2185-2187 (1975).

67. J. S. Youngner and S. B. Salvin, Production and properties of migration inhibitory factor and interferon in the circulation of mice with delayed hypersensitivity. J. Immunol. 111:1914-1922 (1973).

68. K. Paucker, B. J. Dalton, C. A. Ogburn, and E. Törmä, Multiple active sites on human interferons. Proc. Nat. Acad. Sci. U.S. 72: 4587-4591 (1975).

69. E. A. Havell, Y. K. Yip, and J. Vilček, Characteristics of human lymphoblastoid (Namalva) interferon. J. Gen. Virol. 38:51-59 (1977).

70. K. E. Mogensen and K. Cantell, Loss of specific antigenicity of carboxymethylation of mercaptoethanol-reduced interferon on human leukocyte origin. Intervirology 2:52-55 (1974).

71. K. Cantell, S. Hirvonen, K. E. Mogensen, and L. Pyhala, Human leukocyte interferon: Production, purification, stability and animal experiments. In The Production and Use of Interferon for the Treatment and Prevention of Human Virus Infections: Proceedings of a Tissue Culture Association Workshop held at Lake Placid, 1973 (C. Weymouth, ed.), Tissue Culture Assoc., Rockville, Md., 1974, pp. 35-38.

72. W. E. Stewart, II, and J. Desmyter, Molecular modification of interferon: Attainment of human interferon in a conformation active on cat cells, but inactive on human cells. Virology 70:451-458 (1976).

73. K. E. Mogensen and K. Cantell, Production and preparation of human leukocyte interferon. Pharmacol. Therap. 1:369-381 (1977).

74. A. Isaac and J. Lindenmann, Virus interference. I. The interferon. Proc. Roy. Soc. Biol. 147:258 (1957).

75. E. Falcoff, R. Falcoff, L. Catinot, A. De Vomecourt, and J. Sancean, Synthesis of interferon in human lymphocytes stimulated in vitro by antilymphocytic serum. Eur. J. Clin. Biol. Res. 1:20-26 (1972).

76. M. J. Valle, G. W. Jurdan, S. Haahr, and T. C. Merigan, Characteristics of immune interferon produced by human lymphocyte cultures compared to other human interferon. J. Immunol. 115:230-233 (1975).

77. E. F. Wheelock, Interferon-like virus inhibitor induced in human leukocytes by phytohemagglutinin. Science 169:310 (1965).

78. L. B. Epstein, The effect of interferons on the immune response in vitro and in vivo. In Interferons and Their Actions (W. E. Stewart, II, ed.), CRC Press, Ohio, 1977, pp. 92-126.

79. H. M. Hirth, M. Schwenteck, H. Becker, and H. Kirchner, Interferon production and lymphocyte cultures stimulated by Corynebacterium parvum. Clin. Exp. Immunol. in press (1978).

80. C. La Bounardière, Donneés préliminaires sur l'effet protecteur de l'interféron couplé: Des liposomes dans le modèle souris-virus de l'hépatite murine. Ann. Microbiol. (Inst. Pasteur) 129A:397-402 (1978).

3

EXOGENOUS INTERFERON:
STABILITY AND PHARMACOKINETICS

Stephen B. Greenberg, Maurice W. Harmon, and Robert B. Couch

Baylor College of Medicine
Houston, Texas

I. INTRODUCTION

The prospect for use of exogenous interferon in human disease necessitates an evaluation of the relative stability of different types of preparations and of the pharmacokinetics of this antiviral agent. Not only is this information needed for clinical trials of preparations, but any eventual preparation, distribution, and use of commercial material will require knowledge of stability of the preparation. In addition, design of schedules for optimal clinical utilization must be based on an understanding of the absorption, distribution, metabolism, and excretion of this biological substance within the host animal.

Although originally described as stable in an acidic solution, studies have demonstrated the susceptibility of interferon to inactivation by thermal and mechanical stress. The instability of some interferon preparations in various body fluids has also been demonstrated. Thus, although incomplete, information on the stability of different human interferon preparations to a variety of different conditions is available.

Recent reviews have emphasized our lack of understanding of the pharmacokinetics of interferon and indicated a need for additional research in this area [1-3]. Those factors affecting the absorption, distribution, and metabolism of interferon, as well as pharmacological and clinical conditions which define its utility, need to be determined. These two subjects, the stability of human interferon and its pharmacokinetics in animals and man, are the subjects of this review.

II. STABILITY

It has been known for some time that distinct structural differences exist among interferons of different animal species. Antibody directed against interferon from one animal species generally fails to neutralize interferon produced by other animal species [4]. Moreover, Youngner and Salvin [5] recognized that more than one structurally distinct interferon could be made by the same animal species when they demonstrated that interferon induced in sensitized mice with tuberculin was not neutralized by antiserum against virus-induced mouse L-cell interferon.

More recently, it was found that human interferon produced by leukocytes differed in several respects from human interferon produced by fibroblast cells. Antiserum against fibroblast interferon neutralized homologous interferon but not leukocyte interferon [6, 7]. Antiserum to leukocyte interferon showed the greatest neutralizing activity against homologous interferon, but some neutralizing activity toward fibroblast interferon was also evident [6, 8]. This was shown to be due to a minor component in the leukocyte interferon which had the antigenic specificity of fibroblast interferon and thus acted as a separate immunogen [8-10].

In addition to antigenically distinct human interferons (leukocyte and fibroblast), differences in molecular weight and/or charge occur within each type. Leukocyte interferon is heterogeneous with respect to both molecular weight [10-13] and charge [14-16]. Fibroblast interferon thus far has appeared to be homogenous in molecular weight [17] but heterogeneous in charge [18, 19].

Because of this known heterogeneity of interferon preparations, any consideration of the stability of interferons should keep in mind that each of the molecular species that comprise an interferon preparation may exhibit a unique stability. Thus, what would appear to be partial stability to a certain treatment may in fact be complete stability of one component(s) and total lack of stability of another component(s) of that preparation.

A. Thermal Stability

Early reports concerning the heat stability of human leukocyte and fibroblast interferons indicated that both were somewhat labile [20]. More recent data, however, indicate that interferon produced by leukocytes is generally more stable than interferon produced by fibroblast cells (Table 1 [17,20-26]). Crude interferon preparations heated at 56°C resulted in a 50% loss of leukocyte interferon activity after 10 min, while fibroblast interferon lost 50% of its activity after only 2-3 min [21]. De Somer et al. [23] found that crude fibroblast interferon exposed to 56°C lost 90% of its activity after 30 min, although it was stable at -20°C or 4°C. Havell and Vilček [24] found a 50% loss of crude fibroblast interferon activity after 30 min at 56°C. In contrast, Mogensen and Cantell [25] found crude leukocyte interferon required exposure to 56°C for 12 hr before a 90% reduction in activity was noted.

   Mogensen and Cantell also presented evidence that partially purified leukocyte interferon was more stable to heating than the crude preparation [25]. For the purpose of this review, interferon preparations with a specific activity equal to or greater than 10^6 U/mg protein are considered partially purified. In a partially purified state, leukocyte interferon was completely stable to heating at 70°C for 100 min, whereas crude leukocyte interferon lost more than 99% of its activity under the same conditions. Evidence suggested that aggregation of interferon with other proteins was responsible for the apparent loss of activity, since centrifugation of heated, crude interferon at 80,000 × g for 1 hr resulted in a pellet (interferon does not normally sediment upon high-speed centrifugation) which, when treated with 4 M guanidine hydrochloride, resulted in full recovery of interferon activity. This aggregation phenomenon of crude leukocyte interferon may be responsible for the limited heat stability of the leukocyte interferon preparations reported in other studies [21].

   It was recently shown that the concentration of interferon preparations may also influence their stability toward heat. Knight [17] indicated that crude fibroblast interferon was stable for 1 to 2 months at 4°C while partially purified interferon in dilute solutions (< 10 μg/ml) lost 50-75% of its activity in 24 hr at 4°C. This observation was confirmed and extended by Sedmak and Grossberg [26]. Partially purified fibroblast interferon, in concentrations of 500, 50, and 5 μg protein/ml, was incubated at 37°C for 24 hr and the amount of activity lost was 57%, 90%, and >97%, respectively. The effect of concentration on heat stability was also shown to apply to partially purified leukocyte interferon [26]. After heating at 68°C for 30 min, interferon in concentrations of 500, 50, and 5 μg protein/ml lost 24%, 42%, and 83% of their activity, respectively.

TABLE 1. Thermal Stability of Human Interferons

Interferon concentration[a]	Conditions and results		Ref.
	Leukocyte interferon	Fibroblast interferon	
$1–9 \times 10^5$ U/mg protein	37°C, 200 min: 50% loss 56°C, 5–7 min: 50% loss		20
$2–8 \times 10^2$ U/mg protein		37°C, 200 min: 50% loss 56°C, 5–7 min: 50% loss	
$1–2 \times 10^3$ U/ml (crude)	56°C, 10 min: 50% loss		21
$1–2 \times 10^3$ U/ml (crude)		56°C, 2–3 min: 50% loss	
Not stated (crude)		56°C, 30 min: 50% loss	24
Not stated (crude)		-20°C, months: no loss 4°C, months: no loss[b] 4°C, 8 days: 30% loss 20°C, 8 days: 30% loss 37°C, 1–1.5 days: 50% loss 56°C, 30 min: 90% loss	23
1.8×10^4 U/mg protein	37°C, 6 weeks: 90% loss 45°C, 3 weeks: 90% loss 56°C, 12 hr: 90% loss 56°C, 3 days: no loss		25
1×10^6 U/mg protein			

Concentration[a]	Thermal stability	Reference
Not stated (partially purified)	45°C, 1 hr: no loss 56°C, 1 hr: no loss	22
Not stated (crude)	45°C, 1 hr: no loss 56°C, 1 hr: 70% loss	17
4–20×10^3 U/ml (crude) 1×10^7 U/mg protein	4°C, 1–2 months: no loss 4°C, 24 hr: 50–75% loss (<10 μg/ml)	
2×10^6 U/mg protein	68°C, 30 min: 24% loss (500 μg/ml) 68°C, 30 min: 42% loss (50 μg/ml) 68°C, 30 min: 83% loss (5 μg/ml)	26
Not stated (partially purified)	37°C, 24 hr: 57% loss (500 μg/ml) 37°C, 24 hr: 90% loss (50 μg/ml) 37°C, 24 hr: >97% loss (5 μg/ml)	

[a]The concentrations of interferon preparations were expressed as units (U)/mg protein (specific activity) or U/ml. Interferon preparations were considered partially purified if the specific activity was equal to or greater than 10^6 U/mg protein.

[b]This preparation was tested for thermal stability in the freeze–dried state. All other preparations were tested in the liquid state.

B. Mechanical Stability

Human interferon has also been shown to be subject to inactivation by
mechanical stress, a particular problem during processing and purification
of fibroblast interferon. Havell and Vilček [24] found that vigorous mechanical stirring of crude fibroblast interferon resulted in an 80% loss of activity
after 5 min. DeSomer et al. [23] found the activity of crude fibroblast
interferon was reduced 99% after rotation in tubes at 25 revolutions per
minute (rpm) for 24 hr at 4°C. Edy et al. [27] compared the susceptibility
of fibroblast and leukocyte interferon to mechanical stress. Interferon
preparations were rotated end-over-end at 50 rpm in glass-stoppered glass
tubes at a temperature of 4°C. A greater than 90% loss of activity was noted
with fibroblast interferon, while leukocyte interferon was completely stable
to the same treatment.

Cartwright et al. [28] observed mechanical inactivation of partially
purified fibroblast interferon in a rotational viscometer. Depending upon
the time exposed and the shearing rate, fibroblast interferon lost from
70 to >99% of the original activity. Loss of activity was not due to absorption
to surfaces, since inactivation occurred when siliconized glass and various
plastic or stainless steel tubes were used. Denaturation at a gas/liquid
interface and oxidation were also eliminated as probable causes for inactivation, since activity was lost in completely filled and sealed vessels as well
as when inert gases were used in the container. Inactivation appeared to
be solely caused by shearing forces. Changes in either of the two variables
governing the amount of shear force in the viscometer (rotational speed
and the width of the annular gap) had the predicted effect on inactivation of
fibroblast interferon. Crude human leukocyte interferon was completely
stable under the same conditions.

C. Stabilization to Thermal and Mechanical Stress

The demonstration of the susceptibility of human interferons to heat and
mechanical stress stimulated the search for agents or conditions which
would protect interferon from inactivation. Marshall et al. [20] were the
first to demonstrate that heating of interferon at low pH (3.5) tended to
preserve biological activity when compared to heating at neutral pH. Based
on their studies of the stabilizing effect of low pH on mouse interferon [29,
30], Sedmak et al. [31] evaluated the stabilizing effect of low pH (2.0) on
partially purified human fibroblast interferon. This interferon preparation
contained added cytochrome c to prevent absorption to surfaces [18]. At
−20°C, no difference was noted between the preparations maintained at pH
2.0 and pH 7.0. However, at 4°C, the pH 2.0 preparation lost only 5% of
its activity after 46 weeks of storage, whereas the pH 7.0 sample lost 93%
of its potency. At 20°C, the pH 2.0 sample was again the most stable.

After 2 weeks, 50% of the antiviral activity was lost at pH 2.0 as opposed
to 90% loss of activity after only 1 week by the sample held at pH 7.0. This
stabilizing effect of low pH was evident at pH values of 2 and 3 but was lost
as the pH was increased to 4 [31]. As noted earlier, fibroblast interferon
in dilute solution was less stable to heat than interferon in more concentrated
solutions; this was also shown to be the case at pH 2.0 [26,31].

The detergent sodium dodecyl sulfate (SDS) has also been shown to
stabilize human leukocyte interferon against heat inactivation [32]. Stewart
et al. [33] reported that crude human leukocyte and fibroblast interferons
differ in their stability to heat (100°C for 2.5 min) in the presence of SDS
under reducing or nonreducing conditions. Leukocyte interferon was stabilized by SDS alone, whereas fibroblast interferon was only partially protected from inactivation. Leukocyte interferon was protected less efficiently
in SDS under reducing conditions, while fibroblast interferon was more stable
in SDS with mercaptoethanol and urea added. These results were confirmed
by Vilček et al. [10].

Two molecular weight subspecies of leukocyte interferon have been
described. Stewart and Desmyter [11] reported that these two subspecies
were also distinguishable on the basis of their stability to heat in SDS alone
or SDS under reducing conditions. Leukocyte interferon boiled in SDS and
electrophoresed in SDS-polyacrylamide gels revealed 2 peaks of activity:
a major peak at 15,000 daltons, and a minor peak at 21,000 daltons. When
leukocyte interferon was boiled in SDS under reducing conditions and subjected to electrophoresis, only the minor peak (21,000 daltons) of activity
was obtained.

As noted, fibroblast interferon was not stabilized against boiling by
SDS alone. However, at 25°C, SDS alone did stabilize partially purified
human fibroblast interferon [17].

Experience with mouse interferon suggested that chaotropic salts, i.e.,
salts whose anions increase the solubility of the nonpolar regions of proteins,
would protect interferon against thermal inactivation [30]. This was found
to be the case with partially purified human fibroblast interferon in a high
temperature (68°C) test [31]. However, at the temperatures most likely
to be used for storage of interferon for clinical use (4°C, 20°C), chaotropic
salts did not stabilize fibroblast interferon.

Freeze-dried preparations of crude fibroblast interferon retained 50%
of their original activity after 24 hr of heating at 90°C [31]. Thus they
are much more stable to heating than liquid preparations. No difference
was noted between pH 2.0 and pH 7.0 freeze-dried preparations.

The thermal stability of crude freeze-dried fibroblast interferon was
not enhanced by addition of extraneous proteins. However, in the case of
immunoaffinity purified interferon (which contained 25 μg/ml cytochrome c)
thermal stability was increased by added protein. In a linear nonisothermal
test [34] in which the temperature was increased from 50 to 90°C, freeze-
dried purified interferon (with 25 μg/ml cytochrome c) was nearly completely

inactivated by the time the temperature reached 80°C. Addition of more protein in the form of bovine albumin, cytochrome c, gelatin, or ovalbumin to freeze-dried purified interferon conferred essentially complete stability to 90°C [31].

Another protein denaturant that distinguishes between human leukocyte and fibroblast interferon is guanidine hydrochloride in concentrations of 4-8 M. Human leukocyte interferon is stable to this reagent, while the majority of fibroblast interferon is inactivated [27]. The same minor portion of fibroblast interferon that was stable to guanidine hydrochloride was also stable to mechanical stress [27]. Edy et al. [35] recently provided evidence for stable and unstable forms of fibroblast interferon. The stable fraction of fibroblast interferon differs from the bulk of fibroblast interferon in the extent or nature of glycosylation.

Protection of fibroblast interferon from mechanical-stress-induced inactivation was accomplished using reagents that inhibit disulfide bond formation. Cartwright et al. [36] demonstrated that DL-thioctic acid, in concentrations of 0.1-1.0 mM, completely stabilized crude and partially purified fibroblast interferon to mechanical inactivation. Thioctic acid, however, had divergent effects on thermal stability. At 56 and 37°C, it accelerated inactivation, but at 4°C it stabilized biological activity [36]. It was shown that thioctic acid could be easily removed from the preparation by dialysis, whereas other stabilizers, such as SDS, cannot be removed.

The nonionic detergent Tween 80, in concentrations of 0.1-1.0%, also protected fibroblast interferon from mechanical inactivation [23]. Sedmak et al. [31] confirmed that observation with Tween 80 concentrations as low as 0.001%. They also demonstrated stabilization with 10 mM thioctic acid and 0.01-0.1% SDS. However, they were unable to demonstrate the protective action of low pH on mechanical inactivation [31].

It is apparent that rapid inactivation of human fibroblast interferon results from thermal and mechanical stresses. Leukocyte interferon is much more stable to these forces. Reagents that protect interferon from thermal inactivation do not necessarily provide protection against mechanical shear forces, which suggests unique mechanisms are responsible for the two types of inactivation. Thermal inactivation may be due to changes in the covalent structure of the proteins [37]. Instead of stabilizing interferon in its native configuration, thermal stabilizing conditions may generate unfolded molecules which, upon cooling and neutralization or removal of the reagent, may refold into the biologically active form [30]. For example, Stewart et al. [33] demonstrated that leukocyte interferon whose biological activity had been destroyed by heat could be completely reactivated by brief reheating in the presence of SDS. Inactivated fibroblast interferon required reheating in the presence of SDS under reducing conditions [33].

Inactivation by mechanical stress appears to be due to shearing forces that promote formation of molecular aggregates through the generation of intermolecular disulphide bonds [28,36]. Thioctic acid effectively prevented formation of such bonds. This hypothesis is compatible with the protective effects of Tween 80 and acid pH. Tween 80, by its detergent action, and acid pH, by protonation, may prevent formation of intermolecular disulphide bonds [23,27].

D. Stability in Body Fluids

The inhibition of interferon action by a nontoxic biological fluid was first demonstrated by Vilček and Lowy [38], who found that 40% fetal calf serum significantly inhibited the activity of chick embryo cell interferon. The inhibition was greatest if the fetal calf serum was added to cells along with interferon rather than immediately before or after interferon treatment. Rossman and Vilček [39] found that chick embryo cell interferon was also inhibited by normal sera from a variety of other animal species, including human serum. The amount of suppression of interferon action increased with increasing concentrations of serum and decreased with increasing concentrations of interferon. Preliminary characterization of the inhibition suggested it may be associated with a lipoprotein.

Cesario and Tilles [40] found that human fibroblast interferon incubated with human urine expressed less antiviral activity than interferon exposed to control medium. The loss of interferon activity began immediately upon exposure to urine and was completed within 30 min. Dialyzed urine did not inactivate interferon, and, of the dialyzable components of urine tested, only phenol reduced interferon titers. Cesario et al. [41] subsequently demonstrated that fibroblast interferon was inactivated by several human body fluids, including serum, cerebrospinal fluid, bile, stool extract, and saliva. Pleural fluid did not appear to inactivate fibroblast interferon.

Work in our laboratory indicated that nasal secretions contained an inhibitor of human fibroblast interferon [42]. Increasing quantities of nasal secretions resulted in increased inhibition of fibroblast interferon but showed no inhibitory activity toward leukocyte interferon (Figure 1). The inhibitory activity toward fibroblast interferon could be overcome with increasing concentrations of fibroblast interferon. Three of the major proteins intrinsic to nasal secretions (i.e., albumin, lysozyme, and IgA) did not appear to be responsible for the inhibition. Preliminary characterization of the inhibitor suggested it could be a lipoprotein.

Cesario [43] has recently tested several human body fluids against both fibroblast and leukocyte interferons. Leukocyte interferon was quite resistant to cerebrospinal fluid and serum (10-17% inactivation), while fibroblast interferon lost 74% and 97% of its activity, respectively. In response to bile and urine, leukocyte interferon lost 56% and 57% of its activity, while fibroblast interferon lost nearly 97% and 93% of its activity, respectively. Saliva reduced the leukocyte interferon titer by 45%, while fibroblast interferon lost 67% of its initial titer.

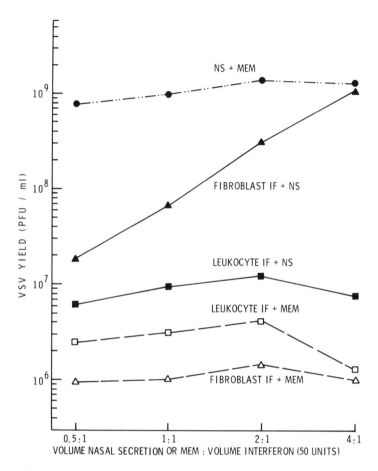

FIGURE 1. Effect of increasing volumes of nasal secretions (NS) or minimum essential medium (MEM) on the antiviral activity of human fibroblast
and leukocyte interferon (IF). (Reprinted from Ref. 42, by courtesy of the
Society for Experimental Biology and Medicine.)

E. Conclusions

From the data reviewed, it is apparent that the two major conditions responsible for loss of interferon activity are thermal and mechanical stress. It
is also evident that a number of factors influence the stability of interferon
to these stresses; these include the type of interferon (leukocyte or fibroblast), the concentration, and the relative purity of the preparation. Fibroblast interferon is quite susceptible to inactivation by heat and mechanical

stress, while leukocyte interferon is stable to these stresses, even when partially purified.

Conditions have been described that stabilize interferon to thermal and mechanical stress. Maintenance of a low pH and incorporation of thioctic acid should be particularly useful in the purification and concentration of fibroblast interferon. Storage of interferon in dilute solution, even for short periods of time, should be avoided.

The human interferon preparations tested for stability were not purified to homogeneity. It is evident that when completely purified interferon preparations become available, studies of stability to thermal and mechanical stress, as well as responses to stabilizing conditions, will have to be repeated.

Loss of interferon activity during storage may be largely avoided by using freeze-dried preparations. Purified interferon preparations may require the addition of a stabilizing protein. Accelerated storage tests have established that freeze-dried preparations have suitably long shelf lives for the long-term storage of interferon for clinical use [31].

With respect to stability in body fluids, there appear to be no major drawbacks to the use of leukocyte interferon. However, clinical use of fibroblast interferon may be limited if activity must be maintained in cerebrospinal fluid, serum, bile, urine, or nasal passages.

III. PHARMACOKINETICS

Data on the pharmacokinetics of interferon induced in animals by both viral and nonviral inducers have been reported previously [44]. These early observations were made by assaying for interferon in various body fluid compartments. Over the past 10-15 years, exogenous interferon preparations have been given to animals, and antiviral activity has been measured under a variety of conditions. This review will summarize those studies in animals and humans that employed only exogenous interferon and provided information on the pharmacokinetics of this antiviral agent (see Tables 2 and 3, respectively).

A. In Animals

Initial experiments on the pharmacokinetics of interferon in animals employed interferon prepared in mouse brain tissue (Table 2). The rapid loss of intravenously administered interferon in the mouse was demonstrated in four different reports [45-48]. These studies suggested that interferon was distributed to some but not all tissues of the body and that repeated injections did not lead to accumulation of interferon. However, Nuwer et al. [49], using mouse L-cell interferon injected intravenously every hour

TABLE 2. Pharmacokinetics of Exogenous Interferon (IF) Preparations in Animals

Interferon preparation	Animal model	Dose and route of administration	Serum level (half-life)	Comments	Ref.
Mouse brain	Mouse	NS[a] i.v.[b]	<30 U/3 ml at 1 hr[c]	30-fold loss per hour; clearance equivalent to 96.6% per hour	45
Mouse brain	Mouse	18,000 U i.m.[b] 11,400 U i.v.	0 U at 15 min 78 U at 1 hr >100 U at 1 hr 0 U at 2 hr	Repeat i.v. dose 2 hr later showed similar pattern of loss	46
Mouse brain	Mouse	13,000 U i.v. i.p.[b]	3,840 U at 1 min 80 U at 1 hr <10 U at 3 hr <13 U at 1 min 20 U at 3 hr	After i.v. injection, IF measured in peritoneal fluid; after intraperitoneal injection, serum level of IF detected, as well as in extracts of spleen, kidney, and lung	47
Mouse brain	Mouse	340 U i.v. 150 U i.v.	28 U at 5 min 20 U at 5 min	Approximately 40% recovered in kidney, liver, lung; no IF recovered in brain, spleen, or muscle	48
Mouse L cell	Mouse	750–4,500 U i.v. (q. 1 hr × 5)	(1 min)	Clearances slower after second to seventh injections	49

Interferon	Species	Dose	Route	Level measured	Comments	Ref.
Mouse cell	Mouse	3,850 U (q. 1 hr × 7)	p.o.[b]	4 U	Similar results with both 5- and 8-day-old mice, but not with adult mice; rabbit IF, given orally, also gave low serum levels	50
		1,400 U	p.o.	2 U		
Chick embryo	Chicken	5,000 U (q. 1 hr × 5)	i.v.	217 U/4 ml at 40 sec	No evidence of accumulation with repeated doses	87
				70 U/4 ml at 10 min		
				0 U at 1 hr		
Rabbit (NDV induced)[b]	Rabbit	100,000 U	i.v.	(11 min)	7–13% recoverable at 1 min after inoculation	51
Rabbit (NDV induced)	Rabbit	119,500 U	i.v.	356 U at 1 min	6.9–12.5% in plasma, 87–93% in tissues, distribution throughout entire extracellular space	52
		163,840 U	i.v.	256 U at 1 min		
		119,500 U	i.v.	256 U at 1 min		
Rabbit	Rabbit	1.5×10^6 U	i.v.	7,945 U at 1 min		56
		1.5×10^5 U	i.v.	1,000 U at 1 min		
		1.5×10^4 U	i.v.	82 U at 1 min		
Rabbit	Rabbit	4.3×10^3 U	i.c.[b]	ND[d]	150–250 U at 30 min after injection in CSF[e], half-life in CSF is approximately 1 hr; tailing effect with respect to concentration and time	61
		1.8×10^3 U	IVent[b]	ND		
		NS[a]	i.v.	(11 min)		
Human leukocyte	Mouse	17,500 U	i.m.	600 U at 1 hr	Mean level of IFU/ml of serum 348	57

Table 2 (continued)

Interferon preparation	Animal model	Dose and route of administration	Serum level (half-life)	Comments	Ref.
Human leukocyte	Guinea pig	175,000 U i.m.	200 U at 1 hr	Mean level of IFU/ml of serum 221	57
Human leukocyte	Sheep	30×10^6 U i.m.	600 U at 1 hr	Mean level of IFU/ml of serum 168	57
Human leukocyte	Rabbit	1.75×10^6 U i.m.	150 U at 1 hr	Mean level of IFU/ml of serum 148	57
Human leukocyte (crude) Human leukocyte (purified)	Rabbit	30×10^6 U i.m. 3×10^6 U i.m. 30×10^6 U i.m. 3×10^6 U i.m.	800 U at 1 hr 200 U at 1 hr 2,000 U at 1 hr 600 U at 1 hr	"Purified" IF preparation; faster clearance than "crude" IF	54
Human leukocyte	Rabbit	2×10^6 U i.v. 2×10^5 U i.v. 2×10^4 U i.v.	8,900 U at 1 min 1,100 U at 1 min 86 U at 1 min	Early clearance not affected by dose; no difference in results using "crude" or "purified" human IF; tailing effect more pronounced with increasing dose; after repeated (1 q. 24×5) injections of 3×10^6 U, no change in peak or trough	56

Human leukocyte	Rabbit	3×10^6 U $0.3\text{-}30 \times 10^6$ U 3×10^6 U 2.5 and 6×10^6 U	i.v. i.m. s.c.[b] p.o.	(13 min) 200 U at 1 hr 200 U at 3 hr Not detectable	IF levels not directly proportional to dose given; i.m. IF measured in serum longer than i.v. IF; repeat injections demonstrated same clearance rate	55
Human leukocyte	Rat	5×10^5 U 5×10^5 U	i.v. i.m.	150 U at 6 hr 600 U at 1 & 6 hr	Significant levels of IF in lymph after i.v. or i.m. injection	56
Human fibroblast Human leukocyte	Rabbit	10^6 U 10^6 U	i.v. i.m. i.v. i.m.	200 U at 1 hr 64 U at 1 hr 1,000 U at 1 hr 64 U at 1 yr	30 min after i.v. dose, <30 U/g of IF detected in liver when serum was 800 U/ml	58
Human leukocyte	Monkey	30×10^6 U 30×10^6 U 10×10^6 U	i.v. i.m. i.c.	60 U at 24 hr (7.1 hr)[f] 600 U at 24 hr 600 U at 2-12 hr	30-fold difference between IF concentration in serum and CSF; 20 U/ml in CSF at 24 hr after i.v. or i.m. dose; 20,000 U/ml in CSF at 24 hr after i.c. dose	59
Human leukocyte	Gibbon	3×10^6 U 3×10^6 U 3×10^6 U	i.v. i.m. s.c.	4 U at 24 hr (17 min) 40 U at 24 hr 20 U at 48 hr	Almost complete recovery of drug at 3 min; tailing effect noted after 3 hr; i.m. response similar to s.c.	60

Table 2 (continued)

Interferon preparation	Animal model	Dose and route of administration	Serum level (half-life)	Comments	Ref.
Human leukocyte	Rhesus monkey	5×10^5 U i.m.	200 U at 2 hr		88
Human leukocyte	Chimpan-zee	4,000 U i.n.[b]	ND	4 and 40 U recovered after 5 min; 5- to 50-fold reduction in recovered IF over 1 hr	63

[a]NS = not stated.
[b]i.v. = intravenous; i.m. = intramuscular; s.c. = subcutaneous; p.o. = orally; i.p. = intraperitoneal; i.c. = intracisternally; IVent = intraventricularly; i.n. = intranasally; NDV = Newcastle disease virus.
[c]U = units of IF in reference standard units for the species of interferon used, unless otherwise stated.
[d]ND = not done.
[e]CSF = cerebrospinal fluid.
[f]Method of interferon assay and use of 69/19 reference standard are not stated.

for five injections, found the pattern of clearance to be slower after repeated injections.

The first studies with orally administered interferon suggested that this route of administration would not be feasible. Adult mice were given mouse L cell, mouse serum interferon, or rabbit interferon orally [50]. None of the recipient animals had detectable serum interferon at 1 hr after the last feeding. However, when 5- or 8-day-old mice were inoculated orally with interferon every hour for seven doses, low levels of both mouse and rabbit interferon were detected in serum. This finding is consistent with the apparent ability of young animals to absorb proteins from the intestinal tract.

The distribution of rabbit interferon injected into rabbits extended the initial observations made with mice. In the earliest reports, the half-life of intravenously administered rabbit interferon was calculated to be 11 min. These single injection studies showed that there was a rapid disappearance of detectable interferon and that the interferon was distributed in plasma and tissues, as well as throughout the entire extracellular space [51,52].

Human leukocyte interferon prepared from the buffy coats of blood donors has been injected intramuscularly into various animals and the serum levels assayed with time [53-58]. Cantell and Pyhälä [55] demonstrated a similar distribution pattern of human leukocyte interferon in mice, guinea pigs, rabbits, and sheep. Peak serum levels in all animals were found some 1-3 hours after injection of the interferon preparations, and low levels were found between 12 and 24 hours later.

It was also shown that the rapid clearance of the human leukocyte interferon was not affected by the dose injected and followed a pattern similar to that of rabbit interferon [56]. A serum half-life of 13 min was found, and repeated injections (1 every 24 hr × 5) did not alter the peak or trough levels of interferon. When the interferon preparations were administered intravenously, Cantell and Pyhälä [56] observed a delayed final disappearance of interferon, or a tailing effect, which was more pronounced with increasing interferon doses.

In a dose response experiment, Cantell and Pyhälä [55] injected 0.3 to 30.0 × 10^6 units of human leukocyte interferon intramuscularly into rabbits and tested their serum for interferon at various times after inoculation. Although the serum levels were not directly proportional to the dose employed, increasing peak levels of interferon were found with the higher administered dose. In the same series of studies, a comparison was made between the intramuscular and subcutaneous routes of administration. Both intramuscularly and subcutaneously injected interferon gave similar curves, although the peak level of interferon came later with the subcutaneous route. In addition, interferon could be detected in serum for a longer time when given either intramuscularly or subcutaneously than when given intravenously.

Edy et al. [58] gave human fibroblast and leukocyte interferon to rabbits both intravenously and intramuscularly. A similar pattern of clearance was found for each interferon preparation. In addition, they could detect no interferon in the liver, which was removed when the serum level was 800 U/ml.

Studies using primates given human leukocyte interferon have reported conflicting results. Habif et al. [59] found a half-life of 7.1 hr in monkeys, while Skreko et al. [60] demonstrated a half-life of 17 min in gibbons. The reason for these conflicting results is not completely clear, although 10 times more interferon was injected into the monkeys than into the gibbons. Nevertheless, after intramuscular administration of human leukocyte interferon, the peak levels and pattern of loss were similar in both monkeys and gibbons.

Two animal studies have attempted to look at the transport of interferon across the blood-brain barrier. In the first study by Ho et al. [61], interferon was given intracisternally or intraventricularly into the central nervous system of rabbits. In both cases low levels of interferon were found in the cerebrospinal fluid for several hours after injection. The half-life in the cerebrospinal fluid appeared to be approximately 1 hr, but there was a similar delayed disappearance as described earlier for serum levels with respect to both concentration and time. In a similar study in monkeys, intracisternally administered interferon was found in the serum from 2 to 12 hr after injection, although a 30-fold difference was found between the interferon concentration in the serum and the cerebrospinal fluid [59]. From these results, Habif et al. [59] suggest that a blood-brain barrier exists for interferon.

There have been several studies in which interferon has been applied topically to mucous membranes [62,63]. In these studies, determinations of the rate of clearance or the detection of interferon in serum have been limited. Johnson et al. [63] measured the recovery of human leukocyte interferon after topical application to the nasal mucosa of chimpanzees. In 10 chimpanzees, there appeared to be a 5- to 50-fold reduction in the recovered interferon over 1 hr. These results suggested that interferon applied locally to the nasal mucosa is rapidly removed and that the clearance of locally applied interferon might alter the dose requirement of interferon necessary for antiviral activity in the nasal cavity.

B. In Humans

Most of the human studies with exogenously administered interferon have measured serum levels after a single dose and have employed patients with some underlying disease, such as Hodgkin's disease, lymphoma, or leukemia (Table 3). In most studies, information obtained in animals was used as a guide in choosing dosage ranges and routes of administration.

Varying serum levels of human leukocyte interferon have been found after parenteral administration. Strander et al. [64] found a peak serum level of 200 U only 1 min after intravenous administration of 4.5×10^5 U, suggesting a short half-life. Emodi et al. [65] also found evidence of a short half-life after intravenous administration. These investigators also demonstrated a peak level of 800 U about 8 hr after 30×10^6 U were given intravenously over an 8-hr period. When patients with herpes zoster and Hodgkin's disease were given human leukocyte interferon intravenously over a 12-hr period, an initial half-life of 2.8 hr was observed [66]. Jordan et al. [66] suggested that their longer half-life was the result of tissue binding and release of interferon and would not have been apparent in the single-dose experiments.

Intramuscular administration of interferon in humans resulted in a pattern of distribution and clearance similar to that found in the animal studies. A peak level 5-8 hr after injection with detectable levels present at 24 hr has been demonstrated. Cantell et al. [57] predicted from their studies that some 150,000-200,000 U/kg would be needed to maintain serum levels at 100 U/ml. These predictions have been confirmed by recent studies in herpes zoster patients given varying doses of human leukocyte interferon intramuscularly [67]. A mean peak serum interferon level of 238 U/ml was found in patients who had received 1.7×10^5 U/kg intramuscularly. No accumulation of interferon was found with repeated doses except when the highest dosage schedule (5.1×10^5 U/kg/day) was used. With this dosage, the serum interferon level fell by only 5% during the third to sixth day of treatment when a 50% lower dose of interferon was being administered.

Three patients with advanced breast cancer who received daily injections of human leukocyte interferon ($4.0-6.0 \times 10^4$ U/kg per day) intramuscularly were studied for serum interferon levels (M. W. Harmon, S. B. Greenberg, and J. Gutterman, unpublished observations). Serum interferon levels were measured before and 3, 6, 12, and 24 hr after injection (Figure 2). After the first injection, a mean peak level of 55 U/ml was found 3 hr after inoculation. The mean peak level increased to 330 U/ml after the seventh injection, and there was no evidence of serum accumulation over the next 21 daily intramuscular injections. These data are consistent with those obtained by other investigators and indicate that no significant accumulation of interferon occurs in patients with intact hepatic and renal function.

Other preparations of interferon have only recently been studied in human subjects, and available results suggest that there are differences in the pharmacokinetics of human leukocyte and human fibroblast interferon. In a recent study by Edy et al. [68], no interferon was found in the serum of individuals who were given 3×10^6 U of human fibroblast interferon intramuscularly. In addition, only one of five patients who were given 1.8×10^7 U of human fibroblast interferon had low but detectable levels of interferon in the serum 1 and 3 hours after injection. The reasons for the apparent

TABLE 3. Pharmacokinetics of Exogenous Interferon Preparations in Humans

Interferon preparation	Underlying disease	Dose and route of administration	Serum level (half-life)	Comments	Ref.
Human leukocyte	Malignancy	4.5×10^5 U i.v.[a]	200 U[b] at 1 min 65 U at 15 min	Results from one patient	64
Human leukocyte	Virus infections and tumor	30×10^6 U i.v. (over 5 min) 30×10^6 U i.v. (over 5 hr) 1×10^6 U i.m.[a] 1×10^6 U s.c.[a]	(15 min) 800 U at 8 hr 100 U at 2 hr 100 U at 4 hr	Tailing effect between 1 and 4 hr; i.v. dose disappeared by 36 hr; s.c. and i.m. gave similar curves; no IF detected in CSF[d] when serum level 150 U/ml	65
Human leukocyte	Hodgkin's disease; osteogenic sarcoma	5×10^6 U i.m. 5×10^6 U i.m. 2.5×10^6 U i.m.	50 U at 5 hr 42 U at 5 hr 60 U at 5 hr	Calculated that between 150,000–200,000 U/kg would be needed to maintain serum level at 100 U/ml	55
Human leukocyte	Malignancy with herpes zoster	80×10^6 U i.v. (over 12 hr) 80×10^6 U i.m. 6.4×10^6 U i.m. 6.4×10^6 U i.m.	300 U at 12 hr 200 U at 8–12 hr 32 U at 10 hr 17 U at 14 hr	Initial half-time was 2.8 hr after i.v. and 4.8 hr after i.m.; urine level of 24–50 U/ml in 1 pt; no CSF level in the patient with 278 U/ml in serum	66
Human leukocyte	Malignancy with herpes zoster	4.2×10^4 U/kg/day i.m. 1.7×10^5 U/kg/day i.m. 5.1×10^5 U/kg/day i.m.	52 ± 61 U at 4 hr 238 ± 21 U at 4 hr 455 ± 48 U at 4 hr	No accumulation except at highest dosage schedules	67

Human leukocyte	Congenital cytomegalovirus	$1.7-3.5 \times 10^5$ U/kg/day i.m.	145 U and 460 U	40 and 60 U in urine of two patients	80
Human fibroblast	NS[f]	3×10^6 U i.m. 1.8×10^7 U i.m.	10 U at 1, 3, or 6 hr 8 U at 1 hr 20 U at 3 hr	Only one of five patients given highest dosage of fibroblast IF had detectable serum levels	68
Human leukocyte	Normal volunteers	35,000 U/dose i.n.[a]	ND[c]	300 U in nasal wash 2 to 15 hr after IF administration	62
Human fibroblast	Normal volunteers	6×10^5 to i.n. 48×10^6 U	ND	No nasal secretion IF detected 2-14 hr after intranasal application	69
Human leukocyte	Normal volunteers	4000 U i.n.	ND	200 U at 30 and 60 min after inoculation	63
Human leukocyte	Disseminated neonatal herpes	6×10^5 U i.t.[a] (q. 12 hr × 6 day)	100 U at 1 hr after 7th dose	Patient also received IUDR[e] treatment at autopsy, herpes virus recovered from brain, although CSF titers varied from 800-8,000 U/ml; 1000 U/ml at 12 hr in CSF after first dose; 10,000 U/ml at 12 hr in CSF after second dose	71

[a] i.v. = intravenous; i.m. = intramuscular; s.c. = subcutaneous; i.t. = intrathecally; i.n. = intranasally.
[b] U = units of IF in reference standard units for the species of interferon used, unless otherwise stated.
[c] ND = not done.
[d] CSF = cerebrospinal fluid.
[e] IUDR = idoxuridine.
[f] NS = not stated.

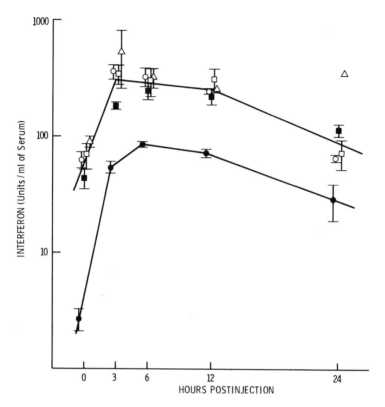

FIGURE 2. Serum interferon levels (U/ml) 0, 3, 6, 12, and 24 hr after
intramuscular injection of 3×10^6 U daily. Levels were measured before
and after the first dose (●—●), the seventh dose (○—○), and the fourteenth
dose (■—■), the twenty-first dose (□—□), and the twenty-eighth dose
(△—△). (M. W. Harmon, S. B. Greenberg, and J. Gutterman, unpublished
observations.)

differences in preparations are not fully known, but an inhibitor of human
fibroblast interferon has been demonstrated to be active in serum [41,43].
    Little information is presently available on the pharmacokinetics of
topically applied human interferon in humans. Merigan et al. [62] gave
human leukocyte interferon to normal volunteers by nasal spray prior to
a rhinovirus challenge. In those studies, 300 U of interferon were recovered
in nasal washes from 2 to 15 hr after a dose of interferon. A recent study
with human fibroblast interferon given by nasal drops to human volunteers
indicated that no interferon could be detected from 2 to 14 hr after intranasal application [69]. This is in contrast to the findings with human leuko-

cyte interferon and suggests, again, that the human fibroblast interferon preparation differs in fundamental ways from human leukocyte interferon.

In a recent study in normal volunteers in which human leukocyte interferon was applied locally to the nasal mucosa by nasal drops, we found a 5- to 50-fold reduction in recovered interferon from 5 to 60 min after application [63]. These results are similar to those found in the chimpanzee study and suggest that mucociliary clearance factors are important in the rate of disappearance of locally applied preparations. Although no serum interferon was detected from 10 to 60 min after local application of 80,000 U of human leukocyte interferon in three volunteers [70], additional studies are needed to see if locally applied interferon can be detected in the blood.

Although there are a few instances in which cerebrospinal fluid levels of interferon were measured after parenteral administration, only one published report has appeared in which human leukocyte interferon has been administered intrathecally [71]. In the one reported patient, human leukocyte interferon was administered intrathecally in a dose of 6×10^5 U every 12 hr for 2 days and then daily for 4 days. Because the patient was suffering from disseminated herpes simplex infection, he was also receiving idoxuridine treatment. Repeated measurements of the serum revealed approximately 100 U of interferon after injection. At the same time, the cerebrospinal fluid levels of interferon varied from 800 to 8000 U/ml. The investigators believe these results indicate that a blood-brain barrier does exist for interferon but that the barrier may be overcome by increasing the dose.

C. Mechanism of Serum Clearance

Studies in both animals and man have demonstrated that interferon is rapidly cleared from the blood stream after intravenous injection. This rapid clearance has been thought to be due to the glycoprotein nature of interferon [72-74]. As a glycoprotein, interferon contains sialic acid on the terminal end of the carbohydrate chain [75, 76]. It was recently shown that asialo-interferon disappears from the blood more rapidly than native interferon [72]. In contrast, another study reported no effect on the clearance of human leukocyte interferon in rabbits after neuraminidase treatment of the interferon preparation [16]. Because of conflicting results, Bose and Hickman [77] determined whether removal of the major portion of the carbohydrate moiety would alter the survival of interferon in the circulation. The rate of disappearance of three different interferon preparations, native lymphoblastoid interferon, neuraminidase-treated, and glycosidase-treated interferon, from the serum of rats was measured (Figure 3). A half-life of 9 min was found for both the native as well as the deglycosidated interferon. The half-life of the asialo-interferon was approximately 3 min, and it appeared to disappear more rapidly than the native interferon. Treat-

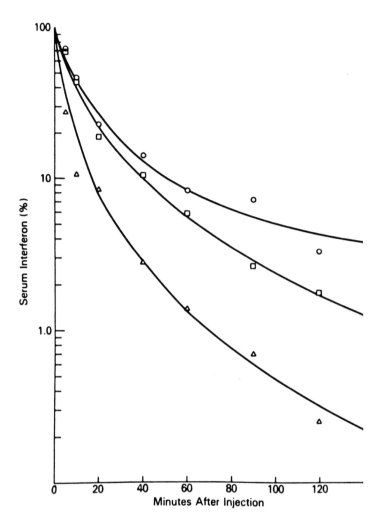

FIGURE 3. Clearance rates of native (□–□), neuraminidase-treated
(△–△), and glycosidase-treated (○–○) human lymphoblastoid interferon
preparations after their intravenous administration at 5×10^5 U doses in
rats. Each point is the average value obtained from six animals. (Reprinted
from Ref. 77, by courtesy of the American Society of Biological Chemists.)

ment with neuraminidase removes sialic acid from the native interferon and exposes the galactose residue of the carbohydrate moiety. These terminal galactose residues appear to be specific determinants for the hepatic recognition of interferon and other normally circulating serum glycoproteins [75]. Thus, these investigators agree with the work of Bocci indicating the probable importance of the liver as the organ for clearance of interferon from the circulation [74]. In addition, their results indicate that the carbohydrate moiety of the presently used interferon preparations can be removed without impairing the ability of interferon to survive in the circulation.

D. Side Effects

Various side effects in patients receiving human leukocyte interferon have been reported. The most commonly reported clinical side effect has been a febrile response occurring 2-4 hr after the initial parenteral dose of interferon [54,64-66]. This febrile reaction appears to be somewhat dose-related and decreases with repeated injections [3]. Fever has been observed in most patients who have received 4.2×10^4 U/kg per day or greater and with high doses of interferon (1.7×10^5 U/kg per day). The first injection may also be associated with nausea, vomiting, myalgias, and chills. One patient who received a rapid intravenous injection of human leukocyte interferon experienced a hypotensive episode [64], but this has not been observed after slow intravenous infusions in other patients. Transient hypotension was also seen in two patients after they received their first dose of 3×10^6 U intramuscularly; however, subsequent doses had no effect on their blood pressure (J. Gutterman, personal communication). In patients who have received repeated injections over weeks to months, a feeling of lassitude and malaise has been reported to occur, and the magnitude of these symptoms appeared to be lessened when more purified preparations of interferon were employed [3].

Merigan [3] has observed tender erythematous skin reactions at the injection site when interferon was given subcutaneously. These skin reactions were limited in size (1-2 cm), appeared within the first day, and disappeared over 48-72 hr. Similar skin reactions have also been observed at the injection site of human fibroblast interferon [3]. Administering the daily dose of interferon in two divided doses appears to have decreased the incidence and severity of these skin reactions [3].

After receiving human leukocyte interferon for several days to weeks, patients exhibit an increasing effect on the hemopoietic system [66,78,79]. After some 3-5 days of therapy, polymorphonuclear leukocyte counts begin to fall, and this may be followed by a decrease in platelet and reticulocyte counts. These apparent bone marrow suppressive effects are reversible on discontinuing the interferon, since platelet, reticulocyte, and polymorphonuclear leukocyte levels return to pretreatment values.

Neonates with cytomegalovirus who received human leukocyte interferon developed an initial pyrogenic effect, decrease in weight gain, and elevated serum transaminase levels [80,81]. When the interferon was discontinued, the infants increased their food intake and gained weight.

To date, no evidence of transmission of hepatitis B virus by human leukocyte interferon has been reported. In addition, no apparent effect on renal function has been discovered. Whether the side effects observed in the clinical trials reported thus far will limit the usefulness and efficacy of exogenous interferon therapy must await further studies. Nevertheless, the observed hematopoietic suppression may be related to interferon's depressive effect on cell proliferation, since in vitro effects on bone marrow cultures of animals and humans have been demonstrated. This may pose special problems for long-term therapy [82,83]. Only additional studies with interferon preparations of increasing purity will determine if these side effects can be eliminated.

E. Conclusions

The studies of exogenously administered interferon in both animals and man have helped to define the variables influencing utilization of this anti-viral agent. Studies in animals demonstrated the basic pharmacokinetic principles found later to be operative in humans. Intravenously administered interferon was rapidly cleared from the serum regardless of the animal model employed. A half-life of a few minutes was found when one dose was given. Although the observed rapid clearance of intravenously administered interferon has been thought to be due to tissue binding, the reasons for the delayed disappearance or tailing effect are not so apparent.

The tailing effect may be due to different molecular forms with different clearance rates, to interferon reentering from tissue to serum, or to temporary saturation of organs responsible for removing interferon. Recent studies have suggested that the liver is responsible for clearing parenteral interferon and functions to remove the glycoprotein from the circulation.

Intramuscular or subcutaneous administration of interferon leads to a more sustained serum level that returns to low levels between 24 and 36 hr after a single dose. No significant accumulation of human leukocyte interferon has been observed after repeated intramuscular injections in animals and in humans. In both animal and human studies, interferon appears to distribute poorly into the respiratory tract, cerebrospinal fluid, eye [84], and across the placenta [85]. It penetrates poorly into interstitial fluids and is rarely recovered from the urine.

The presently available, partially purified human interferon preparations have not been without certain side effects when administered to patients. Constitutional symptoms and hematopoietic suppression have been very common with prolonged courses of therapy. Long-term evaluation of these treated patients has only begun; thus, presently unidentified problems may become significant in the future. It remains to be seen whether more purified or synthesized human interferon would have similar effects.

Although no major pharmacokinetic differences were found when crude and partially purified interferon preparations were compared in humans, studies will have to be repeated when a more purified or synthesized interferon preparation is available. Since the pharmacokinetic results of human leukocyte interferon in rabbits have been similar to those in humans, future pharmacokinetic information might more easily be obtained with a rabbit model.

The determinants of drug activity include a study of the distribution, metabolism, and excretion of the biological substance in the host animal. Past studies have defined the distribution and excretion of interferon, but little information is available on its metabolism in vivo. Although the antiviral effects of interferon are apparent for some time after it has disappeared, factors that could alter the pharmacokinetics of interferon may result in diminished or inconsistent antiviral activity [86]. To date, there is little or no information on the importance of such factors as nutritional state, age, race, sex, environmental factors, concurrent disease, and interferon-drug interactions in altering the pharmacokinetics of interferon. As additional clinical studies in humans are performed, the importance of each of these factors may become apparent.

ACKNOWLEDGMENTS

Our work on interferon has been supported by National Institutes of Health Contract No. AI-42530.

We gratefully acknowledge the excellent help of Linda Simmons in preparing this manuscript.

REFERENCES

1. M. Ho, in Interferons and Interferon Inducers (N. B. Finter, ed.), American Elsevier, New York, 1973, p. 241.
2. M. Ho and J. A. Armstrong, Ann. Rev. Microbiol. 29:131 (1975).
3. T. C. Merigan, Texas Repts. Biol. Med. 35:541 (1977).
4. K. Paucker, J. Immunol. 94:371 (1965).
5. J. S. Youngner and S. B. Salvin, J. Immunol. 111:1914 (1973).
6. K. Berg, C. A. Ogburn, K. Paucker, K. E. Mogensen, and K. Cantell, J. Immunol. 114:640 (1975).
7. J. Vilček, E. A. Havell, L. W. Mozes, and B. Berman, Proc. First Intersect. Congr. IAMS, Science Council of Japan, Tokyo 1975, Vol. 4, p. 65.

8. E. A. Havell, B. Berman, C. A. Ogburn, K. Berg, K. Paucker, and J. Vilček, Proc. Nat. Acad. Sci. U.S. 72:2185 (1975).
9. K. Paucker, B. J. Dalton, C. A. Ogburn, and E. Törmä, Proc. Nat. Acad. Sci. U.S. 72:4587 (1975).
10. J. Vilček, E. A. Havell, and S. Yamazaki, Ann. N.Y. Acad. Sci. 284: 703 (1977).
11. W. E. Stewart, II, and J. Desmyter, Virology 67:68 (1975).
12. J. Desmyter and W. E. Stewart, II, Virology 70:451 (1976).
13. K. Paucker, B. J. Dalton, E. T. Törmä, and C. A. Ogburn, J. Gen. Virol. 35:341 (1977).
14. S. Bose, D. Guarari-Rotman, U. T. Ruegg, L. Corley, and C. B. Anfinsen, J. Biol. Chem. 251:1659 (1976).
15. J. K. Chen, W. J. Jankowski, J. A. O'Malley, E. Sulkowski, and W. A. Carter, J. Virol. 19:425 (1976).
16. K. E. Mogensen, L. Pyhälä, E. Törmä, and K. Cantell, Acta Pathol. Microbiol. Scand., Sect. B 82:305 (1974).
17. E. Knight, Jr., Proc. Nat. Acad. Sci. U.S. 73:520 (1976).
18. C. B. Anfinsen, S. Bose, L. Corley, and D. Gurari-Rotman, Proc. Nat. Acad. Sci. U.S. 71:3139 (1974).
19. D. Stancek, M. Gressmerova, and K. Paucker, Virology 41:740 (1970).
20. L. W. Marshall, P. M. Pitha, and W. A. Carter, Virology 48:607 (1972).
21. T. C. Cesario, P. J. Schryer, and J. G. Tilles, Antimicrob. Agents Chemother. 11:291 (1977).
22. M. J. Valle, G. W. Jordan, S. Haahr, and T. C. Merigan, J. Immunol. 115:230 (1975).
23. P. DeSomer, M. Joniau, V. G. Edy, and A. Billiau, in The Production and Use of Interferon for the Treatment and Prevention of Human Virus Infections (C. Waymouth, ed.), Tissue Culture Assoc., Rockville, Md., 1974, p. 39.
24. E. A. Havell and J. Vilček, in The Production and Use of Interferon for the Treatment and Prevention of Human Virus Infections (C. Waymouth, ed.), Tissue Culture Assoc., Rockville, Md., 1974, p. 47
25. K. E. Mogensen and K. Cantell, Acta Pathol. Microbiol. Scand., Sect. B 81:382 (1973).
26. J. J. Sedmak and S. E. Grossberg, Texas Repts. Biol. Med. 35:198 (1978).
27. V. G. Edy, A. Billiau, M. Joniau, and P. DeSomer, Proc. Soc. Exp. Biol. Med. 148:249 (1974).
28. T. Cartwright, O. Senussi, and M. D. Grady, J. Gen. Virol. 36:317 (1977).
29. R. Jariwalla, S. E. Grossberg, and J. J. Sedmak, Arch. Virol. 49: 261 (1975).
30. R. J. Jariwalla, S. E. Grossberg, and J. J. Sedmak, J. Gen. Virol. 35:45 (1977).

31. J. J. Sedmak, P. Jameson, and S. E. Grossberg, in Human Interferon: Production and Clinical Use (W. Stinebring and P. J. Chapple, eds.), Plenum, New York,]978, p. 133.

32. K. E. Mogensen and K. Cantell, J. Gen. Virol. 22:95 (1974).

33. W. E. Stewart, II, P. DeSomer, V. G. Edy, K. Paucker, K. Berg, and C. A. Ogburn, J. Gen. Virol. 26:327 (1975).

34. D. Greiff and C. Greiff, Cryobiology 9:34 (1972).

35. V. G. Edy, J. Desmyter, A. Billiau, and P. DeSomer, Infec. Immun. 16:445 (1977).

36. T. Cartwright, O. Senussi, and M. D. Grady, J. Gen. Virol. 36:323 (1977).

37. C. Tanford, Advan. Protein Chem. 23:122 (1968).

38. J. Vilček and D. R. Lowy, Arch. Ges. Virusforsch. 21:253 (1967).

39. T. G. Rossman and J. Vilček, Arch. Ges. Virusforsch. 31:18 (1970).

40. T. Cesario and J. G. Tilles, J. Infec. Dis. 127:311 (1973).

41. T. C. Cesario, A. Mandell, and J. G. Tilles, Proc. Soc. Exp. Biol. Med. 144:1030 (1973).

42. M. W. Harmon, S. B. Greenberg, and R. B. Couch, Proc. Soc. Exp. Biol. Med. 152:598 (1976).

43. T. C. Cesario, Proc. Soc. Exp. Biol. Med. 155:583 (1977).

44. T. C. Merigan, E. DeClercq, and M. S. Finkelstein, Ann. N.Y. Acad. Sci. 173:746 (1970).

45. S. Baron, C. E. Buckler, R. V. McCloskey, and R. Kirschstein, J. Immunol. 96:12 (1966).

46. N. B. Finter, Brit. J. Exp. Pathol. 47:361 (1966).

47. I. Gresser, D. Fontaine, J. Coppey, R. Falcoff, and E. Falcoff, Proc. Soc. Exp. Biol. Med. 124:91 (1967).

48. T. P. Subrahmanyan and C. A. Mims, Brit. J. Exp. Pathol. 47:168 (1966).

49. M. R. Nuwer, E. DeClercq, and T. C. Merigan, J. Gen. Virol. 12:191 (1971).

50. T. W. Schafer, M. Lieberman, M. Cohen, and P. Came, Science 176:1326 (1972).

51. M. Ho and B. Postic, Nature 214:1230 (1967).

52. M. Ho and B. Postic, in First International Conference on Vaccines Against Viral and Rickettsial Disease of Man, Pan American Health Organization/WHO Publication no. 147 , 1967, p. 632.

53. L. Pyhälä and K. Cantell, Proc. Soc. Exp. Biol. Med. 146:394 (1974).

54. K. Cantell, S. Hirvonen, K. E. Mogensen, and L. Pyhälä, in The Production and Use of Interferon for the Treatment and Prevention of Human Virus Infections (C. Waymouth, ed.), Tissue Culture Assoc., Rockville, Md., 1974, p. 35.

55. K. Cantell and L. Pyhälä, J. Gen. Virol. 20:97 (1973).

56. K. Cantell and L. Pyhälä, J. Infec. Dis. 133:A6 (1976).

57. K. Cantell, L. Pyhälä, and H. Strander, J. Gen. Virol. 22:453 (1974).

58. V. G. Edy, A. Billiau, and P. DeSomer, J. Infec. Dis. 133:A18 (1976).
59. D. V. Habif, R. Lipton, and K. Cantell, Proc. Soc. Exp. Biol. Med. 149:287 (1975).
60. F. Skreko, I. Zajac, H. P. Bahnsen, R. F. Haff, and K. Cantell, Proc. Soc. Exp. Biol. Med. 142:946 (1973).
61. M. Ho, C. Nash, C. W. Morgan, J. A. Armstrong, R. G. Carroll, and B. Postic, Infec. Immun. 9:286 (1973).
62. T. C. Merigan, S. Reed, T. S. Hall, and D. A. J. Tyrrell, Lancet i: 563 (1973).
63. P. E. Johnson, S. B. Greenberg, M. W. Harmon, B. Alford, and R. B. Couch, J. Clin. Microbiol. 4:106 (1976).
64. H. B. Strander, K. Cantell, G. Carlstrom, and O. A. Jakobsson, J. Nat. Cancer Inst. 51:733 (1973).
65. G. Emodi, M. Just, R. Hernandez, and J. R. Hirt, J. Nat. Cancer Inst. 54:1045 (1975).
66. G. W. Jordan, R. P. Fried, and T. C. Merigan, J. Infec. Dis. 130: 56 (1974).
67. T. C. Merigan, K. H. Rand, R. B. Pollard, P. S. Abdallah, G. W. Jordan, and R. P. Fried, New Engl. J. Med. 298:981 (1978).
68. V. G. Edy, A. Billiau, and P. DeSomer, Lancet i:451 (1978).
69. G. M. Scott, S. E. Reed, T. Cartwright, and D. A. J. Tyrrell, paper submitted for publication in Interferon Scientific Memorandum.
70. S. B. Greenberg, M. W. Harmon, P. E. Johnson, and R. B. Couch, Antimicrob. Agents Chemother. 14:596 (1978).
71. E. DeClercq, V. G. Edy, H. DeVlieger, and P. DeSomer, J. Pediat. 86:736 (1975).
72. V. Bocci, A. Pacini, G. P. Pessina, V. Bargigli, and M. Russi, J. Gen. Virol. 35:525 (1977).
73. V. Bocci, A. Pacini, G. P. Pessina, V. Bargigli, and M. Russi, Experimentia 15:164 (1977).
74. V. Bocci, Texas Repts. Biol. Med. 34:436 (1977).
75. G. Ashwell and A. G. Morell, Advan. Enzymol. 41:99 (1974).
76. F. Dorner, M. Scriba, and R. Weil, Proc. Nat. Acad. Sci. U.S. 70: 1981 (1973).
77. S. Bose and J. Hickman, J. Biol. Chem. 252:8336 (1977).
78. H. B. Greenberg, R. B. Pollard, L. I. Lutwick, W. Robinson, and T. C. Merigan, New Engl. J. Med. 295:517 (1976).
79. S. J. Urbaniak, I. M. Halliday, G. W. Beveridge, and A. B. Kay, Lancet i:553 (1978).
80. A. Arvin, A. S. Yeager, and T. C. Merigan, J. Infec. Dis. 133:A205 (1976).
81. G. Emodi, R. O'Reilly, A. Miller, L. K. Eveson, U. Binswanger, and M. Just, J. Infec. Dis. 133:A199 (1976).
82. W. A. Fleming, T. A. McNeill, and K. Killon, Immunology 23:429 (1972).

83. P. L. Greenberg and S. A. Mosny, Cancer Res. 37:1794 (1977).

84. J. O. Oh and E. J. Gill, J. Bacteriol. 91:251 (1966).

85. J. C. Overall and L. A. Glasgow, Science 167:1139 (1970).

86. J. G. Wagner, Drug Metabolism and Drug Interactions (F. G. McMahon, ed.), Futura Publ., Mount Kisco, N.Y., 1974, p. 1.

87. J. Portnoy and T. C. Merigan, J. Infec. Dis. 124:545 (1971).

88. D. Neumann-Haefelin, B. Shrestha, and K. F. Manthey, J. Infec. Dis. 133:A211 (1976).

4

EXOGENOUS INTERFERON: USE IN HUMANS FOR TREATMENT OF MALIGNANCIES

Michio Ito and Rita F. Buffett
Roswell Park Memorial Institute
Buffalo, New York

I. INTRODUCTION

The inhibition of cell growth in L cells treated in vitro with interferon was first described by Paucker and his associates [1]. Their interesting finding did not attract much attention at that time, because interferon was considered not to have any effect on normal physiological functions. However, a number of years later, the antiproliferative function of interferon was studied extensively by Gresser and his co-workers [2,3]. Continuous

murine cell lines in suspension cultures, treated with interferon at relatively high concentrations, were found to multiply at a slower rate and to
reach a lower final cell density than untreated cells [1,4-6]. Slower growth
of cells was also observed in monolayer cultures of both normal and transformed cells [7-9]. The saturation densities of transformed cells were
lower in the presence of interferon than in untreated cultures, whereas the
densities of normal cells were not affected [8]. Colony formation by murine
L1210 tumor cells in soft agar was significantly reduced [10,11]. A variety
of methods have been used for the quantitation of the antiproliferative and
cell-regulatory activities of interferon; these include direct cell counting
[1,12-15], cell colony formation with [10] or without agar [16], macromolecular synthesis measured by incorporation of radioactive precursors
[9,17-19], etc. Whether the growth inhibitory effect is associated with
interferon itself or with other contaminants present in the preparations has
long been argued. Recently, several reports [8,16,20-22] appear to be in
good agreement that the antiproliferative effects are caused by the interferon molecules themselves. The mode of action of interferon in the inhibition of cell growth has been investigated. Evidence has been accumulated
that interferon exerts its effect on the G_1 and/or early S phase of the cell
multiplication cycle, resulting in elongation of the growth cycle and thus
subsequently in a decrease in the growth rate ([9,17,23]; M. Ito and R. F.
Buffett, unpublished data).

The antitumor effects of interferon in vivo have also been well documented [2,3]. Many of the early studies were carried out by Gresser and
his co-workers. They investigated the effect of interferon on viral carcinogenesis in the Friend and Rauscher murine leukemia virus systems. The
antitumor effect of interferon was observed only when interferon treatment
was continued in Swiss and DBA/2 mice for a long period of time [24-26],
and it was suggested that the continuous suppression of virus growth by
interferon was a prerequisite for the prevention of leukemogenesis in mice.
It was pointed out, however, that a direct action of interferon on the proliferation of virus-transformed cells could not be excluded. From these
series of experiments, Gresser and his colleagues first introduced a long-
range, large-dose administration scheme of interferon treatment for malignancies. The effect of interferon treatment on the development of spontaneous
leukemia, a virus-associated disease, in AKR mice was studied [27,28].
Daily exogenous interferon therapy from the time of birth was continued
for one year. The survival time of mice was considerably prolonged and
the incidence of leukemia was decreased from 95% in untreated controls to
63% in interferon-treated mice [22]. The development of mammary tumors
in C_3H mice (another instance of spontaneous virus-associated tumor) was
delayed by the repeated inoculation of interferon [29]. Of interest was that
there was no decrease in the amount of mammary tumor antigens in the
milk of interferon-treated mice, despite the clear-cut inhibitory effect of
interferon on tumor growth. In order to confirm the direct action of inter-

feron on neoplastic cells in vivo, Gresser and his co-workers also studied the efficacy of exogenous interferon therapy on the growth of various types of transplantable tumors. (Even though virus may not be implicated as an etiological agent in the development of some mouse tumors, the presence of virus cannot be totally excluded, since practically all mouse strains are notoriously recognized as carriers of both ecotropic and xenotropic endogenous viruses.) The repeated daily intraperitoneal administration of interferon prevented the growth of several ascitic tumors, including Ehrlich, RC19, EL-4, and L1210, in different strains of mice [30,31]. The most dramatic effect was observed in the Ehrlich ascites tumor-BALB/c mouse system [31]. The mean survival of BALB/c mice inoculated with 10^4 tumor cells was 18 days; and none of the untreated mice survived beyond 22 days, whereas 90% of interferon-treated mice survived more than six months without any evidence of tumor. From these experiments, several principles, important to the practical application of interferon therapy, have emerged: (1) the greatest antitumor effects were obtained when contact between interferon and tumor cells was maximal, i.e., when both interferon and tumor cells were inoculated intraperitoneally; (2) interferon treatment was ineffective when it was limited to the period preceding inoculation of tumor cells; and (3) interferon therapy was less effective in mice bearing solid tumor nodules than in mice which were inoculated with ascites tumor cells. However, it has been reported that daily intravenous inoculation of interferon resulted in suppression of the growth of a solid subcutaneous malignant tumor, Lewis lung carcinoma, in mice [32]. Also, the development of pulmonary metastasis was blocked. Even when the initiation of interferon therapy was delayed until six days after tumor inoculation and palpable nodules had already developed, the growth of both primary and metastatic tumors was inhibited.

Thus, the rationale for the application of human interferon therapy to human cancers is reinforced by the demonstration of effective antitumor activity against a variety of murine neoplasms.

II. RATIONALE FOR INTERFERON TREATMENT

A. Evidence from In Vitro Studies

In parallel with the results of investigations with murine interferon, evidence has been accumulated that human interferons also possess antiproliferative and cell-regulatory activities for both normal and neoplastic cells of humans. Growth inhibitory effects on a variety of human cells have been reported to date [18-22,33-46]. Adams et al. [37] tested several human lymphoblastoid cell lines, which were established from Burkitt's lymphomas, for susceptibility to the antiproliferative effect of interferon. Some cell lines were found to be quite sensitive to the effect of leukocyte interferon, whereas other cell lines were not. Hilfenhaus and his colleagues [18] used a sensitive lymphoblastoid cell line, Daudi, for studying the inhibition of growth of cells by interferon. They described a simple and quite sensitive assay for measuring the antiproliferative activity of interferon using incorporation of [14C]thymidine. By this method, approximately 15 U/ml of leukocyte interferon were found to be sufficient to reduce the uptake of radioactive precursor by 50%. It has been shown that human chromosome 21 is responsible for determining the susceptibility of human cells to the growth-inhibitory effect as well as to the antiviral activity of interferon [20]. A number of studies have reported a close correlation between antiviral and antiproliferative activity of interferon [16,18,20-22]. Dahl and Degré [38] claimed to have successfully separated these activities from human leukocyte interferon. However, evidence from many laboratories suggests that the cell growth-inhibitory effect is directly associated with the interferon molecule, and both antiviral and antiproliferative activities are inseparable [16,18,20-22].

In parallel with the first systematic trial of treatment of patients suffering from osteogenic sarcoma (see below), Strander and Einhorn [41] investigated the growth inhibitory effect of human leukocyte interferon in vitro on nine cell lines derived from osteosarcomas. All the tumor cell lines tested proved to be susceptible to the antiproliferative effect of leukocyte interferon. By long cultivation methods, i.e., treatment of cultures with interferon for 4-8 weeks, it was found that the growth rates of osteosarcoma cells were inhibited strongly in the presence of 10-100 U/ml of leukocyte interferon, while normal fibroblasts were not affected significantly.

In the authors' laboratory, cultured cell lines derived from various human neoplasms [47] have been tested for their susceptibility to the antiproliferative activity of purified human fibroblast interferon (specific activity 2×10^7 U/mg protein) using a method similar to that reported by Hilfenhaus et al. [18]. Diploid fibroblast cell strains initiated in our department [48] were used as normal cell controls. Incorporation of [3H]thymidine (TDR) was measured in the acid-insoluble fraction following labeling of both interferon-treated cells and untreated controls for 20-24 hr. The patterns of growth inhibition of tumor cells were distinct from those of nonmalignant fibroblasts. The inhibition by interferon was most prominent in normal fibroblasts when [3H]TDR uptake was measured during the initial 24-26 hr after subculturing and addition of interferon; this is comparable to results obtained from a mouse interferon-BALB/c fibroblast system (M. Ito and R. F. Buffett, unpublished data). However, a much stronger reduction in incorporation of TDR was observed in tumor cells between 72 and 96 hr after cell seeding and the addition of interferon than in the initial 24 hr. Table 1 summarizes the data obtained to date. Depending upon the levels of susceptibility to the antiproliferative effect of interferon, the malignant tumor cell lines could be divided readily into two groups; some cell lines were highly sensitive while others responded poorly.

TABLE 1. Antiproliferative Activity of Purified Human Fibroblast Interferon on a Variety of Cultured Human Neoplastic and Normal Cells in Vitro[a]

Cell line or strain	Origin	Cell type	Incorporation of [^{3}H]TDR[b]	
			50% inhibition endpoint (U/ml)[c]	Inhibition at maximum (%)[d]
Neoplastic cells				
RT-4	Carcinoma of urinary bladder	E[e]	28	96
SAOS-2	Osteosarcoma	F[f]	17	94
5959	Osteosarcoma	F	82	90
Daudi	Lymphoma	Ly[g]	130	91
HT-29	Colon carcinoma	E	>5000	40
MeWo	Melanoma	F	>5000	43
A204	Rhabdomyosarcoma	F	>5000	25
Nonmalignant cells				
HF604	Diploid foreskin fibroblast	F	53	82
BG-9	Diploid foreskin fibroblast	F	110	73
BG-10	Diploid foreskin fibroblast	F	130	61
BG-27	Diploid foreskin fibroblast	F	48	82

[a]Unpublished data from our laboratory. All the tumor cell lines employed, except A204, were kindly given by Dr. J. Fogh [47], Sloan-Kettering Memorial Institute; A204 cells were obtained from Dr. J. Whitman, Electro-Nucleotics Laboratories, Inc.

[b]Measured by the four-day assay: uptake of [^{3}H]TDR during 16–20 hr after 72–78 hr of cultivation with interferon was compared. The method described in our previous report [16] was employed with a change of time labelling.

[c]Expressed as concentration of interferon, international reference units per milliliter; mean value from two or more independent experiments.

[d]Percent inhibition at the maximum in the presence of up to 5000 U/ml of interferon.

[e]Epithelial.

[f]Fibroblastic.

[g]Lymphoblastoid.

When the interferon levels required for 50% inhibition of TDR uptake were compared, 17–130 U/ml of interferon were sufficient to reduce the uptake in the highly sensitive group, whereas 5000 U/ml failed to inhibit by 50% the poorly responding group (Figure 1). Maximum levels of inhibition by up to 5000 U/ml of interferon varied from one tumor cell line to another, even though a clear-cut difference was observed between the two groups. When tested by the same method, the susceptibility of normal diploid fibroblasts to human fibroblast interferon was intermediate between the two groups of neoplastic cell lines (Table 1). Figure 1 indicates the dose-response curves of seven tumor cell lines to the antiproliferative effect of purified fibroblast interferon. The two osteosarcoma cell lines studied in our laboratory were definitely sensitive to human fibroblast interferon, confirming and expanding earlier observations [41]. The high susceptibility of Daudi cells to the antiproliferative activity of interferon was also verified [18,37].

Our present studies imply a wide range of susceptibility to the antiproliferative activity of interferon among different types of human neoplasms. For this reason, the in vitro screening of neoplasms for degree of sensitivity of tumor cells to interferon can provide important information, prior to clinical application, for the selection of the types of human malignancies which may respond favorably to exogenous interferon treatment.

B. Evidence from In Vivo Studies (Nude Mice)

The nude mouse, because it is congenitally "athymic" and therefore severely immunodeficient, has become increasingly popular during the last decade as an animal model for the heterotransplantation of human tumors [49,50].

Tygaard and Povlsen [51] were the first to report the successful transplantation of a solid human tumor, a highly differentiated adenocarcinoma, in nude mice. This tumor grew rapidly and was carried in serial passage for more than 30 passages in nude mice [50]. Since then, a variety of solid human tumors have been grafted successfully in nude mice [52–59]. The percentage of successful "takes" from implants of individual human tumors obtained at surgery or autopsy may vary considerably, depending presumably upon grade of malignancy, size of inoculum, and variations in the tissue make-up of the graft. However, the implantation of cells from human tumors which have been successfully propagated in vitro appears to result quite consistently in successful "takes", which can then be carried in serial in vivo passage in nude mice [58,60–63]. Fogh et al. [47] have listed 127 individual cultured human tumor cell lines, 90% of which produce tumors within the first month after grafting and 10% within 2 to 5 months. The tumors grown in nude mice, whether from specimens obtained directly from the patient or cultured in vitro, maintain their human morphological and functional characteristics [53–64].

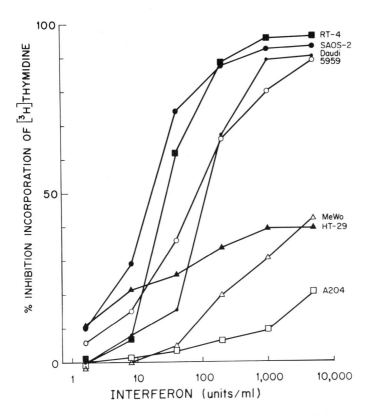

FIGURE 1. Dose-dependent inhibition of uptake of [³H]thymidine in various human tumor cell lines by human fibroblast interferon. The method employed is described in footnote b of Table 1. The inhibition curves were obtained from the experimental data of two or more independent assays.

The nude mouse system should be useful for the study of in vivo effects of chemotherapeutic agents on human tumors. The responses of a variety of tumors to drug therapy are being studied in a number of laboratories [65-68]. Although these studies have not been extensive to date, the results obtained thus far suggest that this animal model system is suitable for screening the sensitivity of individual human tumors to drug therapy. In general, the results obtained from the nude mouse resemble those from clinical reports, suggesting that the susceptibility of human tumors is retained after transplantation into the nude mouse. However, comparison of the responses of the same tumor in humans and nude mice has not as yet been made, undoubtedly because of the time required to establish the reproducible growth of the primary human tumor in the nude mouse.

In our department, a variety of established human tumor cell lines as well as primary tumors have been inoculated into nude mice, and studies on the in vivo antitumor activity of purified human fibroblast interferon have been initiated. Preliminary results indicate that the growth of human neoplastic cells, RT-4, which were established from carcinoma of the urinary bladder in vitro [47] and xenografted in nude mice, was inhibited markedly by daily administration of human fibroblast interferon [69]. Although these results are preliminary, there is no doubt about the efficacy of purified fibroblast interferon as an in vivo antineoplastic drug.

The nude mouse system is an excellent one for studying the effects of chemotherapeutic agents on human tumors, but it does not duplicate conditions that may influence the response of the cancer patient to the tumor or to treatment. If one considers, rather simplistically, that the antitumor activities of exogenous interferon may be expressed in two ways—(1) a direct (anticellular) effect on tumor cells, and (2) an indirect effect on host defense mechanisms (see Section IV)—then in the nude mouse system the direct effect on tumor cells can be demonstrated, but the indirect effect cannot.

C. Clinical Trials

More than 70 patients in Sweden have received intramuscular injections of human leukocyte interferon to date [70-74]. The concentrations of interferon that have been administered have varied from 2×10^6 to 2×10^7 U daily, or 2 to 3 times weekly. Some patients have received interferon for as long as $1\frac{1}{2}$ years. In the early stages, the interferon employed had a low specific activity, 10^4 U/mg protein, so that certain side effects such as transient fever, local pain, and mild allergic reactions were frequently observed. However, since the specific activity has been increased to 10^6 U/mg protein by improved methods of purification, almost all adverse reactions following the administration of interferon have been essentially eliminated. This is in sharp contrast to all other antineoplastic drugs, which are always associated with strong and undesirable side effects, because interferon is a physiological substance, naturally produced by cells.

The first systematic study of the effect of exogenous interferon treatment for malignancies in humans has been done by Strander and his colleagues [73-75]. Their clinical trial was begun at the Karolinska Hospital (Stockholm) in 1971, in which osteosarcoma patients received exogenous interferon therapy. To date, more than 28 patients have been treated with leukocyte interferon [73]. Strander's group selected osteosarcoma for the first trial for the following reasons: (1) its poor prognosis; (2) the capability of easy removal of tumors by surgery to decrease the tumor burden; and (3) the predictability of rapid development of metastasis within one year, which allowed them to set a fixed endpoint for the study. The

treatment consisted of injections of 3×10^6 U of leukocyte interferon intramuscularly daily for one month, during which time the patients stayed in
the hospital. During hospitalization, either exarticulation, amputation, or
resection was performed. After the first month, administration of interferon was continued three times weekly for an additional period of 17 months
(total 18 months, approximately 250 injections, and a total of 7.5×10^8 U
per patient). According to a recent review by Strander [73], life–table
analysis of the study reveals the following: (1) 64% of the interferon-treated
patients were free from metastasis at $2\frac{1}{2}$ years, whereas 30% of the concurrent control group consisting of 23 patients were free from metastasis;
(2) 73% of the interferon-treated group were surviving after $2\frac{1}{2}$ years, as
compared to 35% in the concurrent control group. The results obtained at
that time appeared so promising that the experimental groups were being
expanded. This first systematic trial of exogenous interferon treatment
was initiated without any knowledge of the susceptibility or resistance of
osteosarcoma cells to the growth-inhibitory activity of interferon. Soon,
however, it was found by Strander and Einhorn [41] that they had been lucky
enough to choose a neoplasm which was quite sensitive to interferon in in
vitro studies. Thus, the first clinical application of interferon therapy in
osteosarcoma has been successful with no adverse reactions. In addition,
the average incidence of symptoms considered to be typical of acute viral
infections (sore throat, cough, nausea, diarrhea, headache, fever, etc.)
in eight interferon-treated children and adolescents was compared with the
average incidence of these symptoms in 21 adult members of their immediate families [76]. All individuals were ambulatory and performing daily
duties. The interferon-treated patients remained symptom-free (at least
one symptom was scored) for five out of six months, whereas family members remained symptom-free for only one out of six months. Also, the
duration and severity of most persistent symptoms were less in the treated
patients. Therefore, treatment with exogenous interferon also appeared
to provide other benefits.

   Other studies have shown a temporary benefit from exogenous interferon therapy. Blomgren et al. [77] have reported on a case of Hodgkin's
disease (lymphocyte predominance, stage IV B). Partially purified leukocyte interferon was injected intramuscularly, $5-7 \times 10^6$ U daily for 7 months.
During interferon treatment, the peripheral lymph nodes decreased in size,
the general conditions of the patient improved, and symptoms disappeared.
However, the interferon therapy resulted in a remission of the disease that
lasted for six months only. A similar delay in the progression of disease
was observed in a case of multiple myeloma (in the review written by
Strander [73]). The patient, who suffered from far-advanced IgG-producing
myeloma, received 6×10^6 U of leukocyte interferon daily, and improvement in clinical symptoms as well as in laboratory parameters occurred
before the remission ended. At Roswell Park Memorial Institute, preliminary studies in which human fibroblast interferon was injected directly

TABLE 2. Clinical Trials of Exogenous Interferon Treatment for Human Neoplastic Diseases[a]

| Tumors | No. patients involved | Interferon therapy | | | Results | References |
		Source	Dose[b]	Duration		
Osteosarcoma	28	Leukocyte	3×10^6	~18 months	Increased survival	Strander [73]
Hodgkin's disease	1	Leukocyte	$5-7 \times 10^6$	7 months	Remission for 6 months	Blomgren et al. [77]
Multiple myeloma	1	Leukocyte	6×10^6	?	Clinical improve-ment	Strander [73]
Malignant melanoma (skin metastatic lesions)	2	Fibroblast	5×10^5 (local)	1 month	Disappearance of or reduction in size of skin tumors	Horoszewicz et al. [69]

[a]A number of other clinical trials have been done in various parts of the world (Belgium, Germany, Japan, the United States, Yugoslavia, etc.). Unfortunately, detailed information was not available at the time of writing. Therefore, these studies are omitted from the table.

[b]International reference units (U) per day per patient.

into metastatic cutaneous or subcutaneous lesions in two patients with malignant melanoma suggest that interferon may have antitumor potential [69]. Results obtained from trials to the time of writing are summarized briefly in Table 2.

D. Why Exogenous Interferon Treatment?

As described above, large amounts of interferon must be administered for a long period of time in the treatment of malignancies with exogenous interferon. The task of preparing large quantities of purified interferon is enormous.

An alternative approach, of course, is to apply inducers of endogenous interferon production. However, treatment with inducers has always been hampered by the appearance of a refractory phase in the response of host cells, during which interferon production becomes minimal even in the presence of adequate amounts of inducer. Furthermore, Stringfellow found a serum hyporesponsive factor to interferon production in leukemic mice that could transfer the hyporeactivity to interferon inducers to normal mouse cells in vitro [78]. A direct relationship was reported to exist between the concentration of the serum factor and the development of hyporesponsiveness to interferon induction in vivo. The discovery of this factor in leukemic animals appears not only to discourage attempting induction of endogenous interferon for treatment of malignancies, but also to reduce the potential therapeutic value of interferon inducers for neoplastic diseases. Another complication that must be considered when interferon inducers are used to stimulate the production of interferon endogenously is the toxicity that is always associated with administration of inducers [79,80]. Even after a single injection with poly I: poly C, a variety of side effects such as fever, mild elevation of liver enzymes, laboratory coagulation abnormalities, etc., were frequently observed [81].

Clinical trials for treatment of malignant diseases with poly I: poly C have been reported by a number of investigators [82-85]. Robinson et al. studied the therapeutic effect of poly I: poly C on malignant neoplasms [85]. They administered the inducer in multiple doses of $0.3-75$ mg/m^2 of body surface area to 37 patients with a variety of tumors, including 26 solid tumors, 9 acute leukemias, and 2 chronic myelogenic leukemias in blast crisis. Low levels of serum interferon, greater than 10 U/ml, were detectable following the first injection in 24 of 38 trials. It was reported that one of the patients experienced a favorable tumor response to the administration of poly I: poly C; progression of disease continued in most of them while they were receiving the drug.

From these results, the administration of exogenous interferon is considered definitely more promising than interferon inducers for the treatment of human malignancies, even though the preparation of adequate amounts

of purified interferon requires an extraordinary effort. However, most
recently, Stringfellow has reported that the co-administration of prostaglandins with four different interferon inducers prevented the appearance of
the refractory phase of interferon production in mice [86]. If the antagonis-
tic effect of prostaglandins on the hyporesponsiveness to interferon inducers
in tumor-bearing mice is confirmed, endogenous interferon therapy using
various interferon inducers will merit serious reconsideration for treatment of human malignancies.

III. PROBLEMS TO BE SOLVED

A. Large-Scale Production of Interferon

The future treatment of humans with exogenous interferon will depend
simply upon the successful mass production of interferon. To date, with
few exceptions [87], almost all clinical trials have been performed using
human leukocyte interferon, because pooled leukocytes from blood donors
are the most readily available source for the large-scale production of
human interferon. The technology for the production of a sufficient supply
of leukocyte interferon for the first systematic trial in humans was developed
by Cantell and his co-workers [88, 89].

     On the other hand, large-scale production of human fibroblast inter-
feron has been accomplished in our department [48], and an outline of our
production system (Figure 2 in Section III. C) will be discussed briefly. As
potential sources for interferon production, 15 new foreskin fibroblast
strains were isolated, cryopreserved, and characterized. The following
criteria were used for the selection of suitable cell strains: efficiency of
interferon production, saturation density, karyology, freedom from adventitious agents, and others that are listed in Figure 2. The cell cultures are
scaled up in large glass roller bottles with a 1585 cm^2 growth surface area.
The roller bottle cultures are superinduced by poly I: poly C (75 $\mu g/ml$)
with cycloheximide (60 $\mu g/ml$) and actinomycin D (0. 75 $\mu g/ml$). After washing three times, a "production" medium containing 5% human serum is
added, and cells are incubated for 22 hr at 34° C. Approximately 2×10^6
U of interferon are obtained per bottle. The crude interferon from a number
of bottles is pooled, clarified by centrifugation, and stored at -90° C for
purification later.

     Most recently, attempts have been made to mass produce interferon
with a lymphoblastoid cell line, Namalva; this cell line has been selected
from more than 100 similar cell lines and does not produce Epstein-Barr
virus [90-93]. Since the cells can be propagated in tank cultures, this
method appears extremely promising for the industrialization of human
interferon production. Interferon produced by Namalva cells resembles
leukocyte interferon [94].

B. Purification of Interferon

Human fibroblast interferon has been purified in our department on several ligands: macroligands (bovine serum albumin, concanavalin A) and microligands (hydrocarbons, Cibacron Blue F3GA, aromatic amino acids, etc.) [95-99]. Currently, purification of large quantities of human fibroblast interferon involves utilization of concanavalin A-Sepharose [95] and phenyl-Sepharose CL-4B column chromatography (A. J. Mikulski, J. S. Horoszewicz, E. Sulkowski, and W. A. Carter, personal communication, Interferon Scientific Memoranda, October, 1976). By direct combination of the two columns, a highly purified preparation is eluted from the second column in a very narrow and highly concentrated fraction (specific activity approximately 2×10^7 U/mg protein).

In contrast, purification of leukocyte interferon is more difficult to achieve and awaits the development of new simple technology.

C. Quality Control of Interferon for Clinical Use

The safety and potency of interferon, a biological product, should be certified for administration to humans by extensive tests under an established quality control scheme. The scheme might differ slightly depending upon the purpose for which the drug is to be used, i.e., for treatment of viral diseases of children and for administration to patients with far-advanced malignant neoplasms. Unfortunately, federal regulations controlling interferon products are not available to date. We prepared a quality control scheme for production of human fibroblast interferon, adapted from U.S. Food and Drug Administration (FDA) and British Medical Council (BMC) guidelines for vaccine production as well as of human diploid fibroblasts (Figure 2) [48]. It identified specific steps during production, purification, and lyophilization of interferon at which the product is evaluated for potency and other features and is designed for the general use of fibroblast interferon. Since the quality control procedure accommodates both safety as well as the new technology for production and purification of interferon, it may be a valuable prototype for future establishment of formal regulations controlling different types of interferon products.

D. Development of a Simple, Reliable Test for Determining
   the Susceptibility of Tumor Cells to Interferon

Our recent results, described earlier (Section II.A) indicate that the susceptibility of neoplastic cells to the antiproliferative effect of fibroblast interferon differs from one tumor cell type to another. As repeatedly emphasized, the exogenous interferon treatment for malignancies requires enormous amounts of purified interferon, and not only is its supply limited

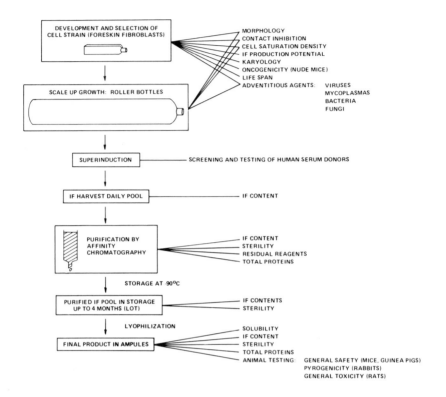

FIGURE 2. Scheme of quality control of human fibroblast interferon based on FDA and BMC regulations. (Reprinted from Ref. 48, p. 724, by courtesy of American Society for Microbiology.)

but its production is expensive as well. From a practical point of view, therefore, each malignant neoplasm (or type of neoplasm) should be screened carefully for its sensitivity to interferon prior to initiation of treatment of tumor-bearing patients. The development of a simple in vitro screening test using clinical specimens (or established tumor cell lines) would be of tremendous value in the selection of patients for clinical trials. While the model system of use of xenografts in nude mice has its value, it is not an ideal one because of the long time and large amounts of interferon that are required for definitive screening tests. Also, as noted previously, it has been reported that the rate of tumor "takes" in nude mice is not very high following heterotransplantation of clinical materials, and establishment of the transplantability of a tumor, therefore, becomes a major prerequisite for studies in this in vivo model system. In vitro assays, similar to the methods for cultured cells described earlier (Section II.A), appear to be a feasible approach for screening the susceptibility of tumors to the antiproliferative activity, particularly since there is some indication that in vivo and in vitro results of the effect of interferon are comparable ([41, 73]; unpublished data from our department). Bech-Hansen et al. [100] have described a similar method, using incorporation of radioactive precursors, for measuring drug sensitivity of tumor cells. They used neoplastic cells collected directly from pleural and abdominal perfusions of cancer patients. A simple, reliable in vitro test for determining the susceptibility to interferon of tumor cells from clinical specimens is still in the developmental stage.

E. Fibroblast Interferon vs. Leukocyte Interferon

Einhorn and Strander [44] were the first to notice that fibroblast interferon inhibited the growth of fibroblastic osteosarcoma cell lines to a much greater degree than leukocyte interferon. The reverse was true in the case of lymphoblastoid cell lines. Accordingly, they concluded that interferon might have tissue-type specificity. The results indicate new biological properties of interferon and are of important significance for selection of the type of interferon that may be useful in clinical applications. However, more extensive studies are needed before drawing definite conclusions on the significance of this phenomenon, because crude fibroblast interferon that was prepared by the superinduction method using actinomycin D was employed. Recently, our group discovered that crude superinduced interferon contained actinomycin D-like nonspecific inhibitor(s) for cell growth; but after purification, this activity could not be detected (S. S. Leong, J. S. Horoszewicz, and W. A. Carter, unpublished data).

Future experiments should be done using purified preparations. Our preliminary results indicate that both purified fibroblast and leukocyte interferons are capable of reducing the growth of normal fibroblasts equally well. Unfortunately, at present, additional data are not available on the tissue-type specificity of purified interferons.

In addition to fibroblast and leukocyte interferons, there is another type of interferon, i.e., type II or immune interferon, which is produced by lymphocytes following stimulation with either antigens or mitogens [101-110]. To the best of our knowledge, there have been no reports of experimental studies on the antiproliferative activity of immune interferon. Also, the combined effect of two or more different types of interferon on cell growth inhibition has not been described as yet.

From the practical point of view, fibroblast interferon is prepared using monolayer cultures of selected strains of human fibroblasts, whereas leukocyte interferon is induced by pooled peripheral leukocytes from blood donors. Fibroblast cell strains can, therefore, be characterized prior to their use for interferon production and for this reason are considered to be safer than peripheral leukocytes. The purification of fibroblast interferon is easily accomplished by column chromatography with various affinity ligands, as described earlier (Section II.B). Considering that the source of cells for induction of leukocyte interferon is limited, and considering the magnitude of the effort required for induction of fibroblast interferon, production systems for either type of interferon may not be adequate to produce sufficient quantities of the drug for large-scale clinical applications.

IV. DISCUSSION

In early studies on interferon therapy in animal systems, the effects of treatment on established virus-induced tumors as well as on the progression of viral carcinogenesis in animal systems, i.e., antiviral activity, were emphasized and provided a strong background for the rationale of interferon therapy. Now, it has been clearly demonstrated that interferon itself is a growth-regulatory substance produced by cells and that it affects cells directly, without any apparent involvement of viruses. It should be stressed that interferon is a normal physiological substance with little if any toxic effect on normal cell functions. It is, therefore, quite unique among many anticancer drugs, which are always associated with strong toxicity causing severe side effects. To pursue exogenous interferon treatment, preparation of large quantities of purified interferon is a prerequisite. This is the most critical step to be overcome for the clinical application of interferon to become a practical mode of therapy. At present, leukocyte interferon is produced using pooled materials of peripheral leukocytes from blood donors, and fibroblast interferon is prepared by the superinduction procedure with poly I:poly C in diploid human fibroblast cultures. The methodology developed thus far is inadequate for the production of the massive amounts of interferon required for large-scale clinical application. For this reason, the development of new technology for the mass production of interferon is critical for the future of exogenous interferon in the treatment of malignancies.

It has been noted that the efficacy of interferon treatment depends mainly upon the tumor load in each patient [2, 78]. Accordingly, the tumor burden must be minimized by other treatments such as surgical ablation. From the practical point of view, one can speculate that interferon therapy alone might not be powerful enough to cure certain malignant neoplasms in humans. The development of modalities of treatment combining the use of interferon with other methods of treatment, such as chemotherapy, immunotherapy, endocrine therapy, radiation therapy, etc., should be pursued urgently in animal model systems. To our knowledge, there are very few reports in the literature concerned with this approach. Chirigos and Pearson [111] studied the effect on LSTRA leukemia in mice of combining treatment with interferon and the chemotherapeutic agent bischloroethylnitrosourea (BCNU). It has been known that BCNU was capable of arresting this systemic leukemia in CDF-1 mice temporarily, with 70-80% of the treated mice showing relapse following 2-3 weeks remission in the progression of their disease. When interferon treatment was combined with BCNU treatment, the survival rate of the leukemic mice improved considerably from 25% to more than 90%. We have to emphasize that, in this pioneering study, interferon treatment alone had no effect at all on this systemic leukemia in mice. Most recently, the efficacy of combined therapy of interferon with cyclophosphamide has been reported [112]. Female AKR mice developed palpable lymphomas prior to initiating treatment. The mean survival time of treated AKR mice, which received a single injection of cyclophosphamide intraperitoneally, was 25-29 days, whereas it was 17 days for untreated animals. The survival time was further elongated to 53 days in the case of combining chemotherapy with interferon treatment (daily administration of 3.2×10^6 U of mouse interferon). The antiproliferative effect of human leukocyte interferon in vitro has been reported to be enhanced with the treatment of cells with chemicals such as ouabain, cycloheximide, and puromycin [45,46].

Surprisingly enough, there are no references available in the literature regarding combination of the modalities of interferon with immunotherapy. Several interesting observations, however, have been described that imply a significant role of the immune systems of the tumor-bearing host receiving interferon therapy [113]. Interferon increased phagocytosis of carbon particles by macrophages [114,115]. It has been reported that phagocytosis of tumor cells by peritoneal macrophages was observed toward the sixth day following inoculation of Ehrlich ascites or RC19 tumor cells in interferon-treated mice, but not in untreated mice [31]. Furthermore, surviving interferon-treated mice showed an enhanced specific resistance to reinjection of tumor cells. Other important findings suggest that the antitumor action of interferon might be mediated in part by host factors [116,117]. A clone of interferon-resistant cells was isolated from murine leukemia L1210 cells by prolonged cultivation in an interferon-containing medium. Interferon was unable to inhibit the multiplication of these resistant cells in vitro. However, mice inoculated with the resistant cells were protected against neoplastic disease by daily administration of interferon. Since these resistant cells did not revert to interferon sensitivity in vivo, the results were interpreted as evidence that the antitumor effect of interferon in this system was mediated by the host rather than by a direct action on tumor cell growth.

Evidence has accumulated that interferon is capable of modulating host immune mechanisms, involving activation of macrophages and a variety of lymphocytes (see Chapter 11). Interferon may activate syngeneic or allogeneic, sensitized or nonsensitized lymphocytes, subsequently enhance the lysis of tumor cells, and thereby suppress tumor growth [118,119]. Recent studies revealed that macrophages played an important role on cell-mediated immunity as well as host-defense mechanisms for malignant diseases [120]. It is well known that, following inoculation of certain bacteria, such as BCG and products derived from them, the reticuloendothelial system is stimulated, resulting in intense hypertrophy of spleen and liver. Animals treated in this way are subsequently more resistant to challenge with microorganisms as well as tumor cells. This nonspecific immunotherapy for malignant neoplasms has been extensively studied in recent years [121]. On the other hand, the view that specific immunological reactions play an important role in modifying, or even controlling, neoplastic diseases, has now gained wide acceptance. Many experimental tumors, including those induced by viruses and chemical carcinogens, and those of unknown etiology elicit immune-rejection responses against tumor cells [122]. Animals previously immunized against tumor cells are found to reject a subsequent challenge with the same tumor. Therefore, investigation of the combination of specific and nonspecific immunotherapy with interferon therapy for human malignancies merits serious consideration. Results obtained from such studies should provide more effective and more powerful ways to apply exogenous interferon in the treatment of human neoplastic diseases.

V. SUMMARY

Interferon is a physiological substance, produced by cells, which does not cause strong side effects. Interferon is also a promising new antitumor drug. This is supported by the results of numerous studies on the antiproliferative activity of interferon in vitro, as well as its antitumor activity in vivo. Evidence has been obtained by in vitro studies that the susceptibility of human neoplastic cells to interferon differ from one tumor to another. Results obtained from a clinical test with osteosarcoma argue for the increase of therapeutic trials on a variety of neoplasms in humans. Exogenous interferon treatment consists of frequent long-term, large-dose administrations of the drug. Lack of a practical method for efficient mass production of interferon has thus far prevented sufficiently large-scale clinical trials. Thus, a new technology for pursuing the mass production of interferon is essential and of first priority. Simple and practical procedures for large-scale purification of human fibroblast interferon have been developed in our department, whereas simple purification methods for leukocyte interferon are not described yet. The development of a simple screening test using clinical specimens for determining the susceptibility to interferon would be of tremendous value in the selection of patients for clinical trials. Studies on combining modalities of interferon treatment with other antineoplastic therapies are warranted in order to investigate the capabilities of increasing the efficacy of exogenous interferon treatment of human malignancies.

ACKNOWLEDGMENTS

The authors thank the staff of the interferon production unit in our department (headed by Dr. J. S. Horoszewicz) for supplying purified human fibroblast interferon. They also express their appreciation to Dr. J. S. Horoszewicz for providing normal and neoplastic cell cultures.

REFERENCES

1. K. Paucker, K. Cantell, and W. Henle, Virology 17:324 (1962).
2. I. Gresser, Advan. Cancer Res. 16:97 (1972).
3. I. Gresser, in Chemotherapy Cancer: A Comprehensive Treatise (F. F. Becker, ed.), Vol. 5, Plenum Press, New York 521, 1977.
4. I. Gresser, D. Brouty-Boyé, M. T. Thomas, and A. Macieira-Coelho, Proc. Nat. Acad. Sci. U.S. 66:1052 (1970).
5. I. Gresser, D. Broute-Boyé, M. T. Thomas, and A. Macieira-Coelho, J. Nat. Cancer Inst. 45:1145 (1970).
6. I. Gresser, M. Thomas, and D. Brouty-Boyé, Nature 231:20 (1971).
7. P. Lindahl-Magnusson, P. Leary, and I. Gresser, Proc. Soc. Exp. Biol. Med. 138:1044 (1971).
8. E. Knight, Jr., J. Cell Biol. 56:846 (1973).
9. M. V. O'Shaughnessy, K. B. Easterbrook, S. H. S. Lee, L. J. Katz, and K. R. Rozee, J. Nat. Cancer Inst. 53:1687 (1974).
10. I. Gresser, M. T. Thomas, D. Brouty-Boyé, and A. Macieira-Coelho, Proc. Soc. Exp. Biol. Med. 137:1258 (1971).
11. I. Gresser, M. Bandu, and D. Brouty-Boyé, J. Nat. Cancer Inst. 52:553 (1974).
12. M. Ohwaki and Y. Kawade, Acta Virol. 16:477 (1972).
13. T. Matsuzawa and Y. Kawade, Acta Virol. 18:383 (1974).
14. L. Borecký, N. Fuchsberger, and V. Hajnická, Intervirology 3:369 (1974).
15. N. Fuchsberger, V. Hajnická, and L. Borecký, Acta Virol. 19:59 (1975).
16. R. F. Buffett, M. Ito, A. M. Cairo, and W. A. Carter, J. Nat. Cancer Inst. 60:243 (1978).
17. M. Tovey, D. Brouty-Boyé, and I. Gresser, Proc. Nat. Acad. Sci. U.S. 72:2265 (1975).
18. J. Hilfenhaus, H. Damm, H. E. Karges, and K. F. Manthey, Arch. Virol. 51:87 (1976).
19. A. Fuse and T. Kuwata, J. Gen. Virol. 33:17 (1976).
20. Y. H. Tan, Nature 260:141 (1976).
21. W. E. Stewart, II, I. Gresser, M. G. Tovey, M. Bandu, and S. L. Goff, Nature 262:300 (1976).
22. E. Knight, Jr., Nature 262:302 (1976).

23. M. Collyn d'Hooghe, D. Brouty-Boyé, E. P. Malaise, and I. Gresser, Exp. Cell Res. 105:73 (1977).
24. I. Gresser, J. Coppey, E. Falcoff, and D. Fontaine, Proc. Soc. Exp. Biol. Med. 124:84 (1967).
25. I. Gresser, J. Coppey, D. Fontaine-Brouty-Boyé, and R. Falcoff, Nature 215:174 (1967).
26. I. Gresser, R. Falcoff, D. Fontaine-Brouty-Boyé, F. Zajdela, J. Coppey, and E. Falcoff, Proc. Soc. Exp. Biol. Med. 126:791 (1967).
27. I. Gresser, J. Coppey, and C. Bourali, J. Nat. Cancer Inst. 43:1083 (1969).
28. S. Graff, R. Kassel, and O. Kastner, Trans. N.Y. Acad. Sci. 32:545 (1970).
29. P. E. Came and D. H. Moore, J. Nat. Cancer Inst. 48:1151 (1972).
30. I. Gresser, C. Bourali, J. P. Levy, D. Fontaine-Brouty-Boyé, and M. T. Thomas, Proc. Nat. Acad. Sci. U.S. 63:51 (1969).
31. I. Gresser and C. Bourali, J. Nat. Cancer Inst. 45:365 (1970).
32. I. Gresser and C. Bourali-Maury, Nature [New Biol.] 236:78 (1972).
33. K. Cantell, Ann. N.Y. Acad. Sci. 173:160 (1970).
34. S. H. S. Lee, M. V. O'Shaughnessy, and K. R. Rozee, Proc. Soc. Exp. Biol. Med. 139:1438 (1972).
35. E. V. Gaffney, P. T. Picciano, and C. A. Grant, J. Nat. Cancer Inst. 50:871 (1973).
36. J. Hilfenhaus and H. E. Karges, Z. Naturforsch. 29c:618 (1974).
37. A. Adams, H. Strander, and K. Cantell, J. Gen. Virol. 28:207 (1975).
38. H. Dahl and M. Degré, Nature 257:799 (1975).
39. T. Kuwata, A. Fuse, and N. Morinaga, J. Gen. Virol. 33:7 (1976).
40. H. Dahl and M. Degré, Acta Pathol. Microbiol. Scand., Sect. B 84:285 (1976).
41. H. Strander and S. Einhorn, Int. J. Cancer 19:468 (1977).
42. J. Hilfenhaus, H. Damm, and R. Johannsen, Arch. Virol. 54:271 (1977).
43. H. Dahl, Acta Pathol. Microbiol. Scand., Sect. B 85:54 (1977).
44. S. Einhorn and H. Strander, J. Gen. Virol. 35:573 (1977).
45. T. Kuwata, A. Fuse, and N. Morinaga, J. Gen. Virol. 34:537 (1977).
46. T. Kuwata, A. Fuse, and N. Morinaga, J. Gen. Virol. 37:195 (1977).
47. J. Fogh, J. M. Fogh, and T. Orfeo, J. Nat. Cancer Inst. 59:221 (1977).
48. J. S. Horoszewicz, S. S. Leong, M. Ito, L. A. DiBerardino, and W. A. Carter, Infec. Immun. 19:720 (1978).
49. S. P. Flanagan, Genet. Res. (Cambridge) 8:295 (1966).
50. J. Rygaard, Thymus and Self: Immunobiology of the Mouse Mutant Nude, Wiley, New York, 1973.
51. J. Rygaard and C. O. Povlsen, Acta Pathol. Microbiol. Scand. 77:146 (1969).

52. C. O. Povlsen and J. Rygaard, Acta Pathol. Microbiol. Scand., Sect. A 79: 159 (1971).
53. B. Sordat, R. Fritsche, J. P. Mach, S. Carrel, L. Ozzello, and J. C. Cerottini, Proc. First Internat. Workshop on Nude Mice, Fischer, Stuttgart, Germany, 1974, p. 269.
54. Y. Shimosato, T. Kameya, K. Nagai, S. Hirohashi, T. Koide, H. Hayashi, and T. Nomura, J. Nat. Cancer Inst. 56: 1251 (1976).
55. H. Maguire, Jr., H. C. Outzen, R. P. Custer, and R. T. Prehn, J. Nat. Cancer Inst. 57: 439 (1976).
56. J. Visfeldt, C. O. Povlsen, and J. Rygaard, Acta Pathol. Microbiol. Scand., Sect. A 80: 169 (1972).
57. C. O. Povlsen and J. Rygaard, Acta Pathol. Microbiol. Scand., Sect. A 80: 713 (1972).
58. B. C. Giovanella, J. S. Stehlin, and L. J. Williams, Jr., J. Nat. Cancer Inst. 52: 921 (1974).
59. C. O. Povlsen, P. J. Fialkow, E. Klein, G. Klein, J. Rygaard, and F. Wiener, Int. J. Cancer 11: 30 (1973).
60. B. C. Giovanella, S. O. Yim, J. S. Stehlin, and L. J. Williams, Jr., J. Nat. Cancer Inst. 48: 1531 (1972).
61. B. C. Giovanella, S. D. Yim, A. C. Morgan, J. S. Stehlin, and L. J. Williams, Jr., J. Nat. Cancer Inst. 50: 1051 (1973).
62. T. Kameya, Y. Shimosato, M. Tumuraya, N. Ohsawa, and T. Nomura, J. Nat. Cancer Inst. 56: 325 (1976).
63. H. R. Schlesinger, J. M. Gerson, P. S. Moorhead, H. Maguire, and K. Hummeler, Cancer Res. 36: 3094 (1976).
64. S. Carrel, B. Sordat, and C. Merenda, Cancer Res. 36: 3978 (1976).
65. C. O. Povlsen and G. K. Jacobsen, Cancer Res. 35: 2790 (1975).
66. D. Houchens, A. Ovejera, R. Johnson, A. Bogden, and G. Neil, Proc. Amer. Assoc. Cancer Res. 19: 40 (1978).
67. W. R. Cobb, Proc. Amer. Assoc. Cancer Res. 19: 41 (1978).
68. W. Shapiro, G. Basler, B. Horten, N. Chernik, and J. Posner, Proc. Amer. Assoc. Cancer Res. 19: 153 (1978).
69. J. S. Horoszewicz, S. S. Leong, M. Ito, R. F. Buffett, C. Karakousis, E. Holyoke, L. Job, J. G. Dolen, and W. A. Carter, Cancer Treatment Repts. 62: 1899 (1978).
70. H. Strander and K. Cantell, In Vitro Monograph 3: 49 (1974).
71. H. Strander, K. Cantell, G. Carlström, and P. Å. Jakobsson, J. Nat. Cancer Inst. 51: 733 (1973).
72. L. Åhström, A. Dohlwitz, H. Strander, G. Carlström, and K. Cantell, Lancet i: 166 (1974).
73. H. Strander, Blut 35: 277 (1977).
74. H. Strander, K. Cantell, P. Å. Jakobsson, U. Nilsonne, and G. Söderberg, Acta Orthop. Scand. 45: 958 (1974).
75. H. Strander, K. Cantell, S. Ingimarsson, P. Å. Jakobsson, U. Nilsonne, and G. Söderberg, Fogarty Int. Center Proc. (Washington, D.C.) 28: 377 (1977).

76. H. Strander, K. Cantell, G. Carström, S. Ingimarsson, P. Å. Jakobsson, and U. Nilsonne, J. Infec. Dis. 133 (Suppl. A):245 (1976).

77. H. Blomgren, K. Cantell, B. Johansson, C. Lagergren, U. Ringborg, and H. Strander, Acta Med. Scand. 199:527 (1976).

78. D. A. Stringfellow, Infec. Immun. 13:392 (1976).

79. W. A. Carter and E. De Clercq, Science 186:1172 (1974).

80. P. F. Torrence and E. De Clercq, Pharmacol. Therap. 2A:1 (1977).

81. A. I. Freeman, N. Al-Bussam, J. A. O'Malley, L. Stutzman, S. Bjornsson, and W. A. Carter, J. Med. Virol. 1:79 (1977).

82. C. W. Young, Med. Clinics N. Amer. 55:721 (1971).

83. A. K. Field, in Selective Inhibitors of Viral Function (W. A. Carter, ed.), CRC Press, Cleveland, 1973.

84. T. C. Merigan, Cancer Chemother. Repts. 58:571 (1974).

85. R. A. Robinson, V. T. DeVita, H. B. Levy, S. Baron, S. P. Hubbard, and A. A. Levine, J. Natl. Cancer Inst. 57:599 (1976).

86. D. A. Stringfellow, Science 201:376 (1978).

87. J. Desmyter, M. B. Ray, J. DeGroote, A. F. Bradburne, V. J. Desmet, V. G. Edy, A. Billiau, P. DeSomer, and J. Mortelmans, Lancet ii: 645 (1976).

88. K. Cantell, S. Hirvonen, K. E. Mogensen, and L. Pyhälä, In Vitro Monograph 3:35 (1973).

89. K. E. Mogensen and K. Cantell, Pharmacol. Therapeutics A1:369 (1977).

90. G. Klein, L. Dombos, and B. Gothoskar, Int. J. Cancer 10:44 (1972).

91. H. Strander, K. E. Mogensen, and K. Cantell, J. Clin. Microbiol. 1:116 (1975).

92. P. J. Bridgen, C. B. Anfinsen, L. Corley, S. Base, K. C. Zoon, U. T. Rüegg, and C. E. Bucker, J. Biol. Chem. 252:6585 (1977).

93. K. C. Zoon, C. E. Buckler, P. J. Bridgen, and D. Gurari-Rotman, J. Clin. Microbiol. 7:44 (1978).

94. E. A. Havell, Y. K. Yip, and J. Vilček, J. Gen. Virol. 38:51 (1978).

95. M. W. Davey, E. Sulkowski, and W. A. Carter, Biochemistry 15:704 (1976).

96. E. Sulkowski, M. W. Davey, and W. A. Carter, J. Biol. Chem. 251:5381 (1976).

97. W. J. Jankowski, W. von Muenchhausen, E. Sulkowski, and W. A. Carter, Biochemistry 15:5182 (1976).

98. M. W. Davey, E. Sulkowski, and W. A. Carter, J. Biol. Chem. 251:7620 (1976).

99. J. K. Chen, W. J. Jankowski, J. A. O'Malley, E. Sulkowski, and W. A. Carter, J. Virol. 19:425 (1976).

100. N. T. Bech-Hansen, F. Sarangi, D. J. A. Sutherland, and V. Ling, J. Nat. Cancer Inst. 59:21 (1977).

101. E. F. Wheelock, Science 149:310 (1965).

102. H. M. Friedman, A. G. Johnson, and P. Pan, Proc. Soc. Exp. Biol. Med. 132: 916 (1967).
103. J. A. Green, S. R. Cooperband, and S. Kibrick, Science 164: 1415 (1969).
104. L. B. Epstein, M. J. Cline, and T. C. Merigan, J. Clin. Invest. 50: 744 (1971).
105. G. E. Gifford, A. Tibor, and D. L. Peavy, Infec. Immun. 3: 164 (1971).
106. R. Falcoff, J. Gen. Virol. 16: 251 (1972).
107. J. S. Youngner and S. B. Salvin, J. Immunol. 111: 1914 (1973).
108. W. C. Wallen, J. H. Dean, and D. O. Lucas, Cell Immunol. 6: 110 (1973).
109. J. Stobo, I. Green, L. Jackson, and S. Barron, J. Immunol. 112: 1589 (1974).
110. G. R. Klimpel, K. D. Day, and D. O. Lucas, Cell Immunol. 20: 187 (1975).
111. M. A. Chirigos and J. W. Pearson, J. Nat. Cancer Inst. 51: 1367 (1973).
112. I. Gresser, C. Maury, and M. Tovey, Eur. J. Cancer 14: 97 (1978).
113. I. Gresser, Cell Immunol. 34: 406 (1977).
114. K. Y. Huang, R. M. Donahoe, B. F. Goldon, and H. R. Dressler, Infec. Immun. 4: 581 (1971).
115. J. Imanishi, Y. Yokota, T. Kishida, T. Mukainaka, and A. Matsuo, Acta Virol. 19: 52 (1975).
116. I. Gresser, C. Bourali, I. Chouroulinkov, D. Fontaine-Brouty-Boyé, and M. T. Thomas, Ann. N.Y. Acad. Sci. 173: 694 (1970).
117. P. Lindahl, P. Leary, and I. Gresser, Proc. Nat. Acad. Sci. U.S. 69: 721 (1972).
118. G. J. Svet-Moldavsky and I. Y. Chernyakhovskaya, Nature 215: 1299 (1967).
119. I. Y. Chernyakhovskaya, E. G. Slavina, and G. J. Svet-Moldavsky, Nature 228: 71 (1970).
120. P. Alexander, Ann. Rev. Med. 26: 207 (1976).
121. J. F. Lancius, A. J. Bodurtha, M. J. Mastrangelo, and R. H. Creech, J. Reticuloendothelial Soc. 16: 347 (1974).
122. R. W. Baldwin, F. R. C. Path, and M. R. Price, Ann. Rev. Med. 26: 151 (1976).

5

CLINICAL USE OF INTERFERONS IN VIRAL INFECTIONS

Alfons Billiau and Piet De Somer

Rega Institute
University of Leuven
Leuven, Belgium

I. INTRODUCTION

It has often been said and written that the clinical application of interferon
has so far not materialized because sufficient amounts of purified and concentrated preparations have not been available to perform adequate clinical
trials. In the last five years sizable quantities of both leukocyte and fibroblast interferons have become available. This has confronted interferon-
ologists with the choice of one or more viral diseases for their clinical
experiments. This choice has not been an easy one, especially since initial
pilot experiments have not yielded the spectacular results one had hoped
for. The older workers in the interferon community have nostalgically
recalled the era of the first antibiotic, penicillin, the clinical potential of
which was convincingly demonstrated by the spectacular improvement in
just a few patients suffering from severe bacterial infections. One should
recognize that, in spite of its broad antiviral spectrum in vitro, the clinical
spectrum of interferon is a narrow one, a situation embodied by the epi-
gram "Interferon is a drug looking for a disease."
        Most virus infections in humans, such as rhinovirus and enterovirus,
are self-limited and cause only minor symptomatology. The few that
are life-threatening or invalidating, e.g., poliomyelitis and variola, have
been mastered by effective vaccinations that are inexpensive and easy to
implement. Until recently it was thought that, on a logical basis, the
clinical application of interferon (except for its potentialities in oncology)
would be limited to two kinds of diseases:

1. Respiratory and eye infections, both extremely common diseases
    which have eluded the vaccination approach

2. Rare life-threatening conditions such as rabies, Ebola, Marburg,
    or Lassa fever, herpes B (HB) virus infection, extensive varicella
    or zoster

The rather poor results of the 1975 controlled trial with respiratory infections [1] reduced hopes for a broad application of interferon and temporarily
reoriented the attention to the application in malignancy and in viral complications of malignancy, such as extensive varicella or zoster. A sudden
revival occurred recently when it was found that systemic interferon
administration, rather unexpectedly, affected viral parameters in chronic
HB virus infections [2,3]. Again, with this disease, the interferon community is confronted with a rather peculiar dilemma. As will be shown,
large amounts of interferon—indeed much larger ones than those currently
available—will be needed to establish whether or not interferon therapy
can eradicate the HB virus infection from chronic carriers with or without
signs of disease. For this, large financial efforts will have to be made,
while it is becoming increasingly clear that efficient vaccines for HB virus

infection will become available in a not-to-distant future. One might therefore argue that current efforts in interferon carry the risk of only serving
the purpose of saving the honor of interferon, rather than to open a broad
market.

In reviewing the available evidence we will try to demonstrate that the
efforts currently put into clinical trials are worthwhile and may indeed be
of benefit to a large group of patients.

II. RATIONALES FOR INTERFERON APPLICATION
IN VIRAL DISEASES

Interferons are biomolecules evolved by natural selection to serve a certain
purpose. It is logical to derive their clinical potentialities from the function
they exert in a natural situation. Therefore, it is important to know which
role interferon plays in spontaneous recovery from virus infections. Excellent reviews exist on this matter [4,5], and we will limit ourselves to
restate the general consensus in this respect. The organism possesses
two important defense mechanisms against viral infection: the interferon
mechanism and the immune response, cellular as well as humoral. These
mechanisms are complementary to each other. Interferon is produced in
loco by any cell, immediately after virus infection; in contrast, the immune
response is generated by specialized cells at a site distant from the viral
infection and requires several days to become active. Interferon acts on
cells and delays virus replication especially in cells adjacent to those already infected; the immune response, on the other hand, kills extracellular
virus particles at any site in the organism. Certain immune active cells
are even attracted to the site of virus replication. It thus seems that the
essential task of interferon consists in delaying the progress of viral invasion, allowing the immune response to be mounted and to become effective.
It is known that in some virus infections the immune response may do more
harm than good [6]; therefore a possible role of interferon may be to limit
the production of viral components which constitute targets for immune
attack, and thus to alleviate the immune-mediated inflammatory responses.

In designing the interferon molecule, nature has apparently been confronted with the same problem as biochemists currently involved in designing
antiviral agents: It is extremely difficult to interfere with virus replication
without damaging the host. The fact that the interferon mechanism is
switched off in between virus infections suggests that interferons have
undesirable effects on cellular or organ physiology. In fact, it seems not
improbable that some of the unexplained symptoms of acute virus diseases
are caused by interferons. In this context it is worthwhile to note that no
interferon seems to be produced during chronic viral infections such as
the HB virus carrier state.

In applying exogenous interferon in clinical situations, one should not expect it to achieve more than what is achieved by the interferon spontaneously produced during virus infections, i.e., a delay in virus replication and virus spread and an alleviation of symptoms. Also, after systemic administration, one might expect undesired side effects, most likely resembling some of the symptoms occurring during virus infections. Furthermore, one can only expect a beneficial effect from exogenous interferon if one can reach local concentrations exceeding those resulting from spontaneous interferon production. Local concentrations in infected tissues are extremely high, due to the fact that all the interferon is concentrated in the narrow intercellular spaces [8]. Concentrations reached at distant sites are mainly determined by the blood levels. In those cases where interferon can be applied topically to the site to be protected, it may be quite possible to reach tissue levels superior to those resulting from the virus infection itself. For systemic administration to be effective, the doses of interferon must necessarily be at least an order of magnitude larger than the total amount of endogenous interferon. Currently available preparations are not always potent enough to achieve this goal.

III. RELEVANT ANIMAL MODEL SYSTEMS

Various animal studies have been undertaken to demonstrate prophylactic or therapeutic effects of exogenous interferon. In these studies one has attempted to answer questions of principle. Can interferon act in vivo? Does it act only when given before the virus or also when the virus has already replicated? One has also asked questions of a more practical nature. What is the dose necessary? What is the best sequence if repeated dosages are given? Finally, some workers have attempted to use animal systems which faithfully reflect defined human diseases.

It is of obvious clinical importance to know whether exogenous interferon therapy can exert a beneficial effect when started after the virus has already multiplied in the target organ. This question has been dealt with in studies involving topical as well as systemic application of interferon. In earlier studies, as reviewed by Finter [9], it appeared that systemic administration of interferon can afford protection against various acute experimental viral infections. In mice infected with Semliki Forest virus (SFV) or encephalomyocarditis (EMC) virus, judiciously chosen regimens of interferon treatment could increase survival rates when started shortly after virus inoculation. This is not strictly to say that interferon treatment was effective when virus replication had already occurred. More recently the question has been reevaluated using higher doses of interferon and different animal systems. Olsen et al. [10] found that daily doses of 40,000 to 200,000 U could protect mice against intranasal or intraperitoneal challenge with EMC virus when started 1 hr after inoculation. When started

24 hr after inoculation, the treatment was effective against intranasal but not against intraperitoneal challenge. Conceivably, seeding of the target organ occurred earlier after intraperitoneal than after intranasal challenge. Worthington et al. [11] found that interferon did not alter mortality in mice when treatment was initiated two days after infection with SFV. De Clercq and De Somer [12] and Gresser et al. [13] used intranasal challenge of mice with vesicular stomatitis virus (VSV). Repeated intraperitoneal injections of surprisingly small doses of interferon (300 arbitrary units) were found to increase the survival rates even when the treatment was started five days after virus challenge [12]. Similar results, although with higher doses of interferon, were described by Gresser et al. [13], when the treatment was started at day 4 after virus challenge. These investigators also determined the time of onset of virus replication in the brain, and they concluded that interferon still had an effect when given at a time when virus replication had already occurred. However, about 30% of the mice had no evidence of virus replication in the brain at day 4, and it is logical to suppose that those mice would preferentially be protected by late interferon therapy. It seems safe to conclude that interferon therapy does have an effect when given in time to inhibit replication at the portal of entry; the important question whether it can also protect when the virus is already replicating in the brain remains essentially unsettled. However, it must be remarked that, of all organs, the brain is probably the most difficult one to reach with exogenous interferon.

The same basic question, i.e., whether interferon has therapeutic potentiality, was approached by using topical application. Ho et al. [14] were unsuccessful in attempting to protect rabbits against rabies virus infection by intraventricular administration of interferon. In contrast Hilfenhaus et al. [15] reported partial protection against lethal rabies in monkeys receiving intramuscular or intralumbar injections of human interferon starting ≥24 hr after inoculation. Rabies virus replicates and spreads slowly. Hence the effect seen in this study should be considered as prophylactic rather than therapeutic. Significantly the surviving monkeys, which had received intramuscular injections of interferon, failed to develop antibody, indicating that peripheral virus replication had been inhibited; intralumbar interferon therapy did not prevent the antibody response, indicating that only the target organ was protected.

Experimental eye infections are particularly relevant to the clinical applicability of interferon in humans. Recurrent herpes is a problem of major importance in ophthalmology. Both rabbit and monkey model systems have been used to study the effect of ocular application of interferon. Regular treatment started shortly before, but not after, herpes simplex virus (HSV) inoculation is able to protect the eyes of monkeys against ulceration [16]. Human fibroblast and leukocyte interferons were found to be essentially equivalent in the monkey model [17]. Of especial interest is a rabbit recurrence used by Sugar et al. [18]: 70 survivors out of 200

HSV-inoculated rabbits were treated with placebo or rabbit interferon and observed for recurrence of the ocular lesions. No significant effect was seen, despite the use of a rather potent interferon preparation. The investigators pointed out, however, that interferon also had no effect on primary infection in rabbits, while good results were obtained in monkeys. McGill et al. [18a] studied the effect of human leukocyte interferon on primary herpetic keratitis in rabbits and found a reduction in the infectivity of the inoculum which was dependent on the concentrations of interferon in the drops but not on the total dose administered.

So far we have discussed experimental models in which the disease (or death) of the animal is due to rather sudden replication of virus in a target organ and to the resulting acute inflammatory response. It is surprising to note how little attention has been paid in these studies to the question of whether endogenous interferon was produced as a result of the virus challenge. It is known that some of the viruses used as a challenge in protection experiments, e.g., EMC virus, can induce circulating interferon. Perhaps late interferon therapy is ineffective because it has little to add to the interferon which is already present.

In recent years it has become increasingly clear that some pathological conditions in humans are due to persistent, often low-grade, replication of certain viruses. The tissue damage occurring in these persistent viral infections is often ascribed to the everlasting immune attack on the viruses and the virus-infected cells, rather than to the cytopathic effect of the viruses themselves [6, 7]. Various animal model systems exist in which chronic viral infections lead to tissue damage and early death. The effect of interferon in chronic infection of mice with murine leukemia viruses (MLV) was studied by several groups, as reviewed by Oxman [19]. No endogenous interferon is produced in these animals. Long-term administration of large amounts of exogenous interferon delayed the development of disease but did not cure the animals, all of which eventually died of their leukemia. It is not clear whether the delay in disease development was to be attributed to a suppressive effect of interferon on virus replication or of tumor cell growth.

Another chronic persistent infection in mice is that by lactic dehydrogenase virus (LDV). Circulating interferon was detected for 48 hr after inoculation of the virus [20]. When exogenous interferon was given from days 5 to 8 after inoculation, the blood titers of LDV were lowered. Arrest of interferon treatment resulted in a rise to control titers. This seems to indicate that interferon treatment can inhibit the production of virus by noncytolytically infected cells in vivo. This may be relevant to the clinical potentialities of interferon. Reduced production of viral antigens may alleviate the immune-mediated inflammatory responses to the persistent infection. However, in considering this possibility, one should be extremely cautious in that a reduction in infectious titers is not necessarily due to a reduction in the synthesis of viral components. It has amply been shown, in vitro, that interferon does not affect the synthesis rate of the major viral proteins in cells chronically infected with MLV, although it reduces the number of virus particles released by these cells [21-24].

A classical model of viral persistence is the so-called persistent tolerant infection (PTI) of mice with lymphocytic choriomeningitis (LCM) virus. The role of interferon in this model has not been studied to any great extent. Wagner and Snyder [25] failed to detect interferon in mice acutely or persistently infected with LCM virus. In contrast, Rivière et al. [26] did find interferon during acute infection. The effect of interferon on the development of renal involvement occurring late during PTI has, to our knowledge, not been studied. Scrapie is the animal model system for the so-called "subacute spongiform virus encephalopathies," of which Creutzfeldt-Jakob disease and kuru are the human representatives. No interferon was found in serum, spleen, or brains of mice affected with scrapie, and long-term administration of interferon did not affect the progression of scrapie in mice [27,28].

In considering the rationales underlying interferon therapy, we mentioned that the organism possesses a mechanism to switch off interferon synthesis in between virus infections, thereby implying that interferons may have undesired effects on cell or organ physiology. The harmful effects of interferon (and/or associated molecules) are exemplified in two animal model systems. Gresser et al. [29] found that high doses of exogenous interferon caused liver cell degeneration and death in newborn mice. When interferon treatment was limited to the first week of life, most mice recovered. However, in ensuing months several of these survivors developed a progressive glomerulonephritis resembling immune complex nephritis [30]. The disease symptoms in newborn mice resembled those occurring after infection with LCM virus. Therefore the investigators hypothesized that endogenous interferon is responsible for part or all of the symptoms of an acute LCM virus infection in newborn mice [28]. Their hypothesis was supported by the observation that high levels of interferon were being produced during acute LCM virus infection and that specific anti-interferon antibody could alleviate the symptoms and reduce the mortality in LCM virus infected suckling mice. In other experimental infections, e.g., EMC in mice, treatment of newborn or adult mice with anti-interferon serum enhanced the evolution, attesting to the importance of interferon in the resistance of the host [31,32]. Thus the obnoxious effect of interferon(s) or associated molecules seems to be most pronounced in very young animals. To further test this hypothesis, fertilized mouse eggs were treated with interferon in order to detect a possible effect on the blastula formation. However, no effect was seen (H. Alexander, A. Billiau, and P. DeSomer, unpublished data).

So far no undesirable effects of interferon treatment have been reported in adult animals, except for one study, by Heremans' group [32a], in which NZB or NZB/NZW-F$_1$ mice were treated for several months with high doses of interferon. NZB and NZB/NZW-F_1 mice spontaneously develop an auto-immune disease some aspects of which resemble systemic lupus erythematosus (SLE) in humans. One hypothesis is that an endogenous oncornavirus may be involved in the pathogenesis of the disease. Treatment with interferon might inhibit the replication of this virus and thereby delay the development of the disease. However, in contrast to this expectation, both NZB and NZB/NZW-F_1 mice developed disease symptoms faster when they were treated with interferon than when a mock preparation or plain saline was given. In this regard it is perhaps worthwhile to mention a hypothesis holding that the pathogenesis of SLE in mice and humans is primarily due to an imbalance in prostaglandin (PG) metabolism [33]. It has recently been found that interferon stimulates the synthesis of prostaglandin (PG)E [34]. It will be interesting to find out whether the toxic effects of interferon in young and adult mice are mediated by the prostaglandin system.

IV. TOPICAL APPLICATION OF INTERFERON
     IN HUMANS

A. Dermatological Affections

Although topical application to the skin constituted the first attempt to demonstrate a protective effect of interferon in man, this approach has not been followed up by many investigators. Early studies, as reviewed by Finter [35] and Merigan et al. [36], showed that intracutaneous injection of monkey interferon prevented the development of vaccinia lesions in the injected area. An attempt to treat a single case of vaccinia gangrenosa failed. These early studies were done with interferon preparations of low potency and were not repeated using higher dosages. In any case, the injection of interferon in the skin is inpracticable for controlling extended viral lesions of the skin. Topical application in the form of an ointment was attempted by Ikic and his co-workers for a number of viral skin lesions. In an uncontrolled study they treated 11 patients with persistent ulcers after revaccination with vaccinia virus [37]. Treatment was started around day 42 after vaccination; improvement was seen around day 4 of the treatment, and healing was complete around day 12. Another uncontrolled study involved 69 patients with recurrent labial herpes and 69 with recurrent genital herpes [38]. The general impression from this study was that the development of blisters could be aborted by early application and that the healing of existing lesions was accelerated and the intervals between recurrences were prolonged. The same authors also attempted to cure condylomata accuminata (genital warts) [39]. It is generally assumed that these benign, but potentially malignant, tumors are caused by a papillomavirus. They can persist for months or years but eventually regress spontaneously. The usual surgical and chemical treatments do not always yield satisfactory

results and are in fact impossible for some localizations. Papillomatosis
of the larynx is more frequently found in children born to mothers who had
genital warts at the time of delivery. In a double-blind, placebo-controlled
study on 20 patients, Ikic et al. found regression of the tumor (in 4 to 12
weeks) in all 10 patients treated with interferon-containing ointment. Regression occurred only in 3 out of 10 placebo-treated patients [39].

  These results should encourage further investigation. In view of the
unpredictable clinical course of the skin lesions, the need for double-blind,
placebo-controlled studies is evident.

B. Eye Infections

Instillation of interferon in the eye has been used by several groups to treat
viral infections of the cornea or the conjunctiva. Earlier studies, as reviewed by Merigan et al. [36], yielded favorable impressions for herpetic
or vaccinal keratitis. In a double-blind, placebo-controlled study involving
95 patients, Kaufman et al. [40] did not find a prophylactic effect of leukocyte interferon (potency 64,000 U/ml) on the recurrence of herpetic keratitis. Jones et al. [41] treated 38 patients with mechanical débridement
and either leukocyte interferon or placebo to see whether the addition of
interferon would reduce the recurrence rate. Although the potency of the
interferon preparation in this study was high, i.e., 10 million units (MU)/ml,
the recurrence rate was not significantly reduced. Sundmacher et al. [42-
45] did similar studies comparing the effect of débridement only, with
débridement plus interferon, and with interferon only. In a first study [42],
interferon (potency 62,000 U/ml) was found to have no effect. In later
studies [43-45] these authors found that leukocyte or fibroblast interferons
of higher potency ($\geq$1 MU/ml) significantly accelerated healing and inhibited
shedding when given topically in addition to débridement.

  Interferon instillation has also been used in a trial with keratoconjunctivitis by adenovirus [46]. During an epidemic in Zagreb (Yugoslavia), 70
patients were given leukocyte interferon while 72 received a conventional
treatment. When the treatment was started in the early phase of disease,
accelerated healing was observed. During the same epidemic, three cases
occurred in an eye clinic; prophylactic instillation of interferon was given
to all 28 contacts, four of which seroconverted but did not develop clinical
disease. These results need confirmation in a controlled double-blind or
randomized trial, especially since a rather weak preparation (4000 U per
gram of suspension) was used.

C. Stomatological Affections

Topical application on the oral mucosa has been used in a controlled study,
involving 34 children, to demonstrate a beneficial effect on the course of
primary herpetic gingivotomatitis [47]. The authors claimed a statistically

significant acceleration in the healing of the lesions in children receiving 12 daily doses of 2000 U of lyophilized interferon for 4-6 days.

D. Respiratory Affections

Attempts to control respiratory tract infections by inhalation of aerosolized interferon were discontinued after a decisive volunteer trial [1] was completed at the Common Cold Unit of the British Medical Research Council. This and earlier clinical trials have been reviewed elsewhere [35,36]. In summary, a single day of pre-exposure treatment (16 doses of 50,000 U of leukocyte interferon) did not reduce the severity of an influenza virus B infection. By using a greater daily dosage and by combining one day of pre-exposure with three days of post-exposure treatment (total of 14 MU per patient), a statistically significant reduction in clinical symptoms and virus shedding was achieved in volunteers challenged with rhinovirus 4.

This demonstration of a beneficial effect of interferon on a frequent, distressing, and economically important disease has, to our knowledge, not been put into practice; nor have any attempts to further improve the treatment schedule been made. The reasons for this are obvious. First, the treatment schedule is tedious, requiring 10 applications per day. Second, the treatment would have to be started before exposure to the virus. Since, in nature, exposure at any particular time cannot be foreseen, the treatment would have to be given during the whole autumn and winter period, when respiratory infections are most frequent. Third, at 10 MU per exposure, each exposure would cost about $500; a six-month continuous treatment would cost an unrealistic $30,000. The most optimistic perspective would be that the costs of interferon can be drastically (at least 100-fold) reduced and that a suitable vehicle can be developed which will allow interferon to be kept in permanent contact with the nasal mucosa using only one or two inhalations per day. Only on these terms can one expect interferon to become a broadly used prophylactic against common cold or other respiratory infections.

V. SYSTEMIC APPLICATION

A. Therapeutic Studies

The idea that systemic application of interferon might be useful in the therapy of a generalized viral disease stems from the concept that, during a natural virus infection, interferon is released early at one site of virus replication with the "purpose" of protecting secondary sites of viral invasion and replication. Exogenous interferon given at an early phase of a virus disease, i.e., before invasion of a critical target organ, may therefore delay the invasion of that organ by several days, allowing the organism to develop an immune response and to eradicate the virus before extensive tissue damage has occurred. This reasoning is limited by several considerations:

1. The amount of exogenous interferon should be larger by an order of magnitude than the amount of endogenous interferon generated as a result of the infection.

2. The exogenous interferon should reach the target organ in due time. The shorter the time interval between the first signs of disease (symptoms resulting from infection of the portal of entry) and interferon administration, the better the effect may be.

3. The exogenous administration of interferon should result in sufficiently high tissue levels in the target organ. Some organs, such as the central nervous system, may not be reached at all by interferon injected intravenously or intramuscularly.

Studies on the systemic use of interferon in the therapy of viral diseases have been confined to varicella zoster and hepatitis B virus infections. Patients with other virus infection have been treated sporadically.

Varicella Zoster Studies

At Stanford University a large trial was conducted to evaluate the usefulness of systemic interferon administration in varicella zoster infections in immunosuppressed patients. In a preliminary study done mainly to evaluate tolerance and pharmakokinetics, the experimenters were encouraged by the finding that rather high blood interferon levels could be realized [48]. However, the interferon did not penetrate in the vesicle fluids. Subsequent placebo-controlled, double-blind trials [49,50] involved three groups of patients:

1. Early disseminated zoster in malignancy (first two days). These patients were treated intramuscularly for three days with either 0.04, 0.17, or 0.51 MU/kg/day. No benefit was noted with the lowest dose. With the middle and highest dosage schedules there was significant reduction in disease progression as measured by number of patients and number of days.

2. Early localized zoster in malignancy (45 interferon-treated and 45 placebo-treated patients, mostly lymphoma, first 7 days [50]). These patients received the same treatment schedules as the first group. With the highest dose no distal cutaneous dissemination occurred; with the middle dose level the incidence of dissemination was reduced. Patients receiving the highest dose also had a shorter

course of new vesicle formations in the primary dermatome. The incidence of visceral complications totalled one out of 45 in the interferon-recipient groups against six out of 45 in the placebo groups. Postherpetic neuralgia appeared reduced in the group receiving the middle and higher dosage schedules.

3. Early varicella (first three days) in children with malignant disease mostly leukemia) received either of the two lower dosage levels for three days [49]. Visceral complications were reduced from six out of nine to two out of nine. The numbers were too small to distinguish differences between the low and high dose interferon groups.

An open placebo-controlled study by Emödi et al. [51] involved 37 patients with herpes zoster, six of which had a confirmed tumor. Interferon was given to 28 patients intramuscularly in one daily dose of 1 MU for 5-8 days. Interferon was detectable in the skin lesions (vesicle fluid) before the injections; 1 hr after the injections the titers were increased approximately 10-fold. In the interferon-treated group the duration of pain was shortened and the lesion seemed to heal more quickly.

Studies on Viral Hepatitis

In a small number of infected patients, hepatitis B virus (HB virus) persists in the liver cells in an as-yet-undefined form. Its activity is manifested by the presence of large amounts of viral surface antigen (HB_SAg) in the blood and sometimes by the presence of virion-associated DNA polymerase. In some patients the virus persistence leads to chronic active liver disease (CALD). This condition ultimately leads to portal cirrhosis of the liver. Children born from mothers who carry infectious HB virus during pregnancy are invariably infected and develop a chronic carrier state. The prognosis of this condition is not fully known as yet, except that a small percentage of such children develop hepatoma.

The idea to treat these patients with interferon stems from three considerations:

1. Although active virus replication takes place in DNA polymerase positive patients, no endogenous interferon seems to be produced. Under these conditions, exogenous interferon is more likely to be beneficial than in acute infections where sizable amounts of endogenous interferon are generated by the infection itself.

2. In some chronically infected cells interferon inhibits virus replication despite the fact that the viral genome is integrated in that of the cell. Specifically, cells which are chronically infected with Retroviridae show a reduced release of virus particles after treat-

ment with small amounts of interferon [21,22]. However, more recent investigations have shown that the synthesis of the major viral proteins and of viral RNA is not inhibited [22,23,24]. The inhibition of particle release is thought to result from minor disturbances in terminal processing of viral components.

3. The presence of HB_SAg and of DNA polymerase in the serum enables one to quickly detect an inhibitory effect of interferon therapy on viral functions.

Studies involving the administration of interferon to patients with positive HB-viral parameters are in progress in several centers. We here summarize the evidence available through publications and formal or informal meetings as well. When this book appears, some of this information and possibly more will have been published. The conclusions of this survey will necessarily be tentative.

The first, and so far most convincing, evidence of an effect of interferon on viral activity in chronic HB virus infection has come from workers at Stanford University. Greenberg et al. [3] treated four CALD patients with leukocyte interferon. Three of them had constant and high levels of particle-associated DNA polymerase in the serum. Doses of 0.3 to 3 MU/day were associated with a rapid and reproducible fall in DNA polymerase activity, HB-core antigen (HB_CAg), and Dane-particle-associated DNA in the serum. The effect was transient when the interferon was given for 10 days or less but appeared to be more permanent when the interferon administration was prolonged for one month or more. In further studies, the same group of investigators (T. C. Merigan, personal communication) found that DNA-particle-positive CALD patients treated for several months with doses in the order of magnitude of 3 MU/day (e.g., 800 MU over a period of 8 months) responded in three possible ways. Out of 11 patients six showed a reversible, partial reduction in the number of Dane particles in the blood with no change in HB_SAg levels. Three showed a permanent disappearance of detectable Dane particles and a partial reduction in HB_SAg levels. Finally, two out of the 11 patients showed permanent disappearance of detectable Dane particles and HB_SAg. Scullard and his co-investigators [51a] reported on five patients with active HB virus infection (three with CALD and two with e-antigen positive persistent infection) whom they treated for five weeks with approximately 3.5 MU of leukocyte interferon. Transient decreases occurred in the number of circulating Dane particles, in the levels of DNA polymerase, and of e-antigen.

So far two research groups have used fibroblast interferon to treat CALD patients. As of this writing nine CALD patients have received fibroblast interferon prepared at our Institute (Table 1). Four of these patients (Nos. 017, 018, 019, and 020) were followed by Weimar et al. [52-54] at the Dijkzigt Hospital (Erasmus University, Rotterdam, The Netherlands)

TABLE 1. Viral and Disease Parameters in Nine Patients with CALD, Treated with Interferon

| Patient code No. | Consecutive treatments[a] | Concurrent favorable evolution of | | | Follow-up |
		Polymerase levels	Transaminase levels	HB_cAg in hepatocytes	
031	F_a	$-^b$	No	Yes	Normalized transaminases; permanent decrease in hepatocyte HB_cAg
003	F_b	Yes	Yes	Yes	Polymerase remains undetectable; transaminases normalized; arthritis
019	F_c and L_d	Yes (L)	Yes (F/L)	?	Polymerase lowered during interim period (F_c, L_d), remaining undetectable in follow-up
018	F_e, F_c, and L_d	Yes (F/L)	Yes (F)	?	Improvement transient
020	F_c and L_d	Yes (F/L)	Yes (F)	?	Improvement transient
033	F_f	Yes	No	?	Improvement transient
034	F_f	No	Yes	?	Improvement transient
002	F_g, F_h, and L_f	No	No	?	Polymerase lowered 10–fold during interim period (F_g, F_h); no change during follow–up
017	F_e	No	No	?	No change

^{a}F = fibroblast interferon; L = leukocyte interferon; F_a = 7×10 MU in 2 weeks; F_b = daily injections for 4 weeks, 7×0.1 MU, 7×0.3 MU, 7×1 MU, and 7×3 MU; F_c = 14×2.2 MU (2 weeks); L_d = 14×3 MU (2 weeks); F_e = 3×2 MU, 3×4 MU, and 3×8 MU in 3 consecutive weeks; F_f, L_f = 7×3 MU in 1 week; F_g = daily injections for 3 weeks, 7×0.3 MU, 7×1 MU, and 7×3 MU; F_h = daily injections for 2 weeks, 7×3 MU and 7×10 MU.
^{b}e–Antigen undetectable before treatment.

and five (Nos. 002, 003, 031, 033, and 034) by Desmyter et al. [2; also paper in preparation] at the Academic Hospital of the University of Leuven. Some of the patients received more than one treatment course, including leukocyte interferon for comparison. In two out of the nine patients, no changes occurred in the disease parameters; in seven out of nine, a favorable evolution of viral or disease parameters occurred during or shortly after one of the treatment courses; in three of these seven patients, the improvement was permanent for the time of follow-up. The evolution of patient No. 031 has been described in detail elsewhere [2]. During and shortly after the treatment a decrease in HB_CAg staining of hepatocytes was observed. Over three years following treatment this patient has evolved into a chronic HB_SAg carrier; at the time of this writing no HB_CAg was detectable in the hepatocytes, and serum transaminase levels were normalized.

Patient No. 003, a 50-year-old man, had suffered from chronic active liver disease for 2 years before interferon treatment. Serum transaminases were elevated [glutamic oxaloacetic transaminase (GOT), ~80 U/liter; glutamic pyruvic transaminase (GPT), ~70 U/liter] with two episodes of aggressive disease (five and 15 months before treatment with interferon) characterized by peaks in serum transaminase levels up to 1500 (GPT) and 2000 (GOT) U/liter. For this the patient was being treated with prednisone (15-30 mg/day). The decision to administer interferon was taken on the basis of a high particle-associated DNA polymerase level in the serum. Increasing doses (Figure 1) were given over a period of 4 weeks, and serum samples were taken daily. All samples were assayed simultaneously. It appeared that DNA polymerase levels had already been decreasing before the treatment was started. During the first three weeks of treatment (0.1 to 1 MU/day) no further decrease was seen. However, in the last week of treatment (3 MU/day) DNA polymerase became undetectable. Simultaneously, an increase in HB_CAg level was observed. HB_SAg levels were increasing steadily as were the levels of serum transaminases. In the follow-up period (seven months, at the time of this writing) DNA polymerase remained undetectable, HB_CAg decreased, and transaminases normalized. It may be important to note that a nondestructive arthritis developed in the course of this period.

The third patient (code No. 019), in whom a favorable evolution occurred during interferon treatment, was a 35-year-old woman with confirmed CALD for five years. She received 14 daily injections of 2.2 MU of fibroblast interferon and 14 daily injections of 3 MU of leukocyte interferon, with an interval of two months. During the treatment with fibroblast interferon the DNA polymerase level did not change, but the transaminase levels were transiently decreased. In the interval between the two treatments the DNA polymerase levels decreased and e-antigen became undetectable. During the second treatment course (leukocyte interferon) DNA polymerase levels remained low and transaminases decreased. Shortly after the treatment

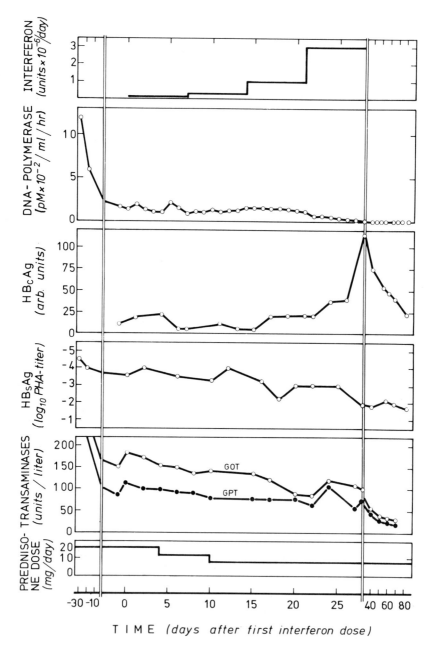

FIGURE 1. Evolution of viral and clinical parameters in a patient with
CALD (code No. 003) during and after greatment with fibroblast interferon.

DNA polymerase became undetectable and transaminases continued to nor-malize. At the time of this writing (three months after the last interferon dose) transaminase levels were normal.

In four patients (Nos. 018, 020, 033, and 034) the changes in viral and liver function parameters were ambiguous. A transient decrease in trans-aminase levels occurred in three out of the four patients during treatment with fibroblast but not with leukocyte interferon. Also in three out of the four patients the DNA polymerase levels showed a transient and unconvincing decrease.

Finally, in two patients (Nos. 002 and 017) fibroblast interferon had no effect on polymerase or transaminase levels. One of these refractory patients (002) also received leukocyte interferon without effect.

Fibroblast interferon has also been used by Kingham et al. [55] to treat two patients with documented CALD. The patients received 10 MU daily for two weeks. Both patients were e-antigen negative before treat-ment. The $HB_S Ag$ levels showed a transient decrease during treatment. The most striking finding was a 64-fold fall in antibody against $HB_C Ag$, occurring during treatment and being maintained during the follow-up period. Furthermore, the transaminase level normalized in one patient.

It is impossible to say whether the favorable evolution seen in some of the patients was an effect of interferon treatment. Too little is known about the spontaneous evolution of DNA polymerase levels in CALD patients to exclude the possibility that the negativation occurred spontaneously rather than as a result of the interferon administration. However, the available results suffice to justify a large-scale, double-blind, placebo-controlled trial. It also appears that fibroblast interferon is probably as effective (or as ineffective) as leukocyte interferon; future trials should therefore include both interferons. One could save time and effort by concerting the trials using a single placebo group.

Pilot Studies in Various Acute Viral Infections

Drug trials involving relatively large numbers of patients are usually preceded by pilot tests with single patients. Undoubtedly, a number of patients with various affections have received interferon, but they were never reported in the literature because no effect was seen. Leukocyte interferon was used to treat congenital or acquired cytomegalovirus infec-tions [56,57]. These uncontrolled trials yielded encouraging results in that viral and disease parameters evolved favorably. As fibroblast inter-feron became available in large quantities, we have treated a few patients with various diseases of viral or presumed viral origin. The purpose of these studies was to obtain preliminary indications which could orient us to concentrate more efforts on one or another disease. The results of these investigations are summarized in Table 2. The diseases treated included acute and fulminant hepatitis by HB virus infection; cutaneous, laryngeal, and venereal pipillomas; and one patient with multiple sclerosis.

TABLE 2. Pilot Trials with Fibroblast Interferon in Patients with Various Diseases of Proven or Presumed Viral Etiology

Patient code No.	Age (yr)	Sex	Diagnosis	Interferon treatment			Outcome
				No. of injections	Avg. dose (MU)	Duration (days)	
025	43	F	Acute hepatitis	14	2.0	14	Recovery as expected, HB_sAg positive for $\pm$ 3 months
026	40	F	Acute hepatitis	14	2.0	14	Recovery as expected, HB_sAg positive for 3 months
027	48	F	Acute hepatitis	14	2.0	14	Recovery as expected, HB_sAg positive for 2 months
024	20	M	Fulminant hepatitis	10	3.5	15	Recovery, HB_sAg positive for 3 months
028	40	F	Fulminant hepatitis	6	6.0	6	Died on day 7
029	25	F	Fulminant hepatitis	6	3.5	6	Recovery
030	31	F	Fulminant hepatitis	5	4.4	5	Died on day 5
032	45	F	Papilloma of larynx	13	3.5	18	Partial regression, followed by rejection
005	35	F	Multiple warts in renal transplant carrier	14	5.9	24	Regression of small verrucae planae, not of large warts
037	25	M	Multiple warts	8	3.5	14	No effect
038	18	F	Multiple plantar warts	8	3.5	14	No effect
035	23	F	Condyloma accuminatum	8	3.5	14	No effect
036	80	F	Condyloma accuminatum	8	3.5	14	No effect
001	40	M	Osteosarcoma	15	3.5	15	No effect
006	13	M	Osteosarcoma	42	3.5	90	Transient delay in progression (?)
007	3	F	Neuroblastoma	18	1.7	28	No effect

No spectacular changes were seen in any of these conditions. We were encouraged, however, by the regression of the small verrucae planae in a renal transplant carrier (patient No. 005) with multiple cutaneous warts and by the partial regression and subsequent necrosis of a laryngeal papilloma (patient No. 032), which had been recurring after repeated surgical resections.

B. Prophylactic Studies

Interferon is designed by nature to protect uninfected cells against exogenous virus. For this reason, it is more logical to use interferon as a prophylactic than as a therapeutic agent against virus infection. However, very few clinical situations are such that the exact time of a viral infection can be predicted. One such situation occurs in patients receiving immunosuppressive therapy for organ transplantations. About 84% of all renal transplant patients show a seroconversion against one or more viruses within three months after transplantation. More than half of these seroconversions are against HSV or cytomegalovirus (CMV). Both of these are thought to result from activation of latent infection, existing since early lifetime. The pathogenesis of this activation is not known. Cellular immunity rather than circulating antibody seems to be the most important factor keeping latent infection in check. It is not known in which cells the viruses are residing during latency; in animal models HSV can be reactivated from the sensory ganglia. Finally it is not known whether interferon can prevent activation of HSV in latently infected cells. In any case it seems safe to assume that the situation of herpetic infections in renal transplant patients differs from that occurring in the animal model systems where the prophylactic effect of interferon on exogenous virus infection has been demonstrated.

A double-blind clinical trial employing fibroblast interferon in renal transplant patients has recently been completed by Weimar et al. [58] at the Erasmus University of Rotterdam (The Netherlands). A similar trial using leukocyte interferon is being conducted by Dr. M. S. Hirsch (Harvard Medical School, Boston, Mass.). The Rotterdam renal transplant trial was started in February 1976 and included 16 non-diabetic, HB_SAg negative patients between 18 and 45 years of age receiving a cadaver kidney at the Dijkzigt Academic Hospital. The immunosuppressive regimen consisted of prednisone (35 mg daily) and azathioprine (1-2 mg/kg daily). The study was set up in a double-blind, placebo-controlled fashion in consecutive pairs to allow early detection of possible side effects of the interferon therapy. In each pair the patients received either placebo or fibroblast interferon (3 MU, twice weekly) for three months, starting 1-2 hr before transplantation. The patients were observed for six months. Hematological and liver function parameters of interferon-treated patients did not differ from those of placebos. The virological observations are summarized in Table 3. No differences were seen between interferon- and placebo-treated

TABLE 3. Viral Infections in Renal Transplant Patients Treated
Prophylactically with Fibroblast Interferon[a]

	Treatment	
	Mock-interferon	Interferon
Number of patients in group	8	8
Proven viral infections		
Clinical	4	4
Seroconversion	9	10
Patients with proven viral infections		
Clinical	4	4
Seroconversion	6	6
Life-threatening viral infections	0	2 (CMV and rubella)
Patients with herpes virus infections		
Clinical	3 (severe)	1 (minor)
Seroconversion	4	1

[a]Double-blind, placebo-controlled trial performed by Weimar et al. [58];
serology done for HSV, CMV, rubella virus, influenza virus, respiratory
syncytial virus, and varicella zoster virus. Treatment regimen: 3 MU
of AS-concentrated fibroblast interferon, twice weekly, intramuscularly
for 6 weeks, starting on the day of transplantation. Follow-up period:
6 months.

patients in the total number of clinically apparent viral infections nor in
the total number of seroconversions. Two life-threatening infections
occurred in the interferon-treated group, none in the group receiving
placebo. The only indication for a beneficial effect of interferon was in
the occurrence of HSV infections. In the interferon-treated group seroconversions occurred in four out of eight interferon-treated patients; three
of these had severe orofacial eruptions. Of the eight patients who received
placebo, only one showed a seroconversion; this was accompanied by a
minor fever blister. In interpreting these results one should take into
account the relatively small dose of interferon. It is possible that better
results might have been obtained had the dose been increased 3- to 10-fold.
Furthermore all viral infections occurred within a period of 3 weeks, starting the third week after transplantation. Hence, in future trials one might
consider the possibility of limiting the interferon treatment to this period.

Convincing results were obtained [59] in the prophylaxis of HSV activation following surgical treatment of a condition called "tic douloureux," a neuralgia resulting from compression of the ganglion nervi trigemini. The patients were given intramuscular injections of either placebo or 5 MU of leukocyte interferon on days -1, 0, 1, 2, and 3 after operation. Ten out of 11 placebo-treated patients showed reactivation (cold sores or virus shedding or both); only five out of 12 interferon-treated patients showed signs of reactivation.

VI. NONTRIVIALITY OF SIDE EFFECTS

A. Fever and Malaise

Fever and malaise occurring shortly after each injection were reported in studies [3,48,60-62] involving systemic administration of leukocyte interferon in humans. These reactions were thought to be rather aspecific and were assigned to trivial impurities in the interferon preparations; as purer preparations became available, less fever and malaise seemed to occur. Recently it has become clear that fever does occur with relatively pure preparations of leukocyte interferon [36] and with fibroblast interferon as well [63].

From a group of 27 patients who received intramuscular injections of fibroblast interferon (≥ 2 MU per injection), 11 developed fever peaks exceeding 38.0°C (see Table 4). This interferon was prepared at our Institute and purified by absorption and elution from controlled pore glass (CPG method) [64]. Interferon preparations which underwent an additional purification using affinity chromatography on zinc iminodiacetate Sepharose (An method) [65] were less pyrogenic. This indicates that the pyrogenic effect is not due to interferon itself but to molecule(s) of a similar chemical nature. If this is so, it would be unjustified to consider fever as an aspecific and trivial side reaction of interferon therapy; interferon may be one of a family of molecules which may be responsible for some of the unexplained systemic symptoms of acute virus infections, e.g., fever, muscle pains, headache, malaise, and others.

B. Hematological Side Effects

Interferon has been shown to inhibit the proliferation of bone marrow cells in vitro [66-69]. However, in the majority of patients who have been treated with leukocyte or fibroblast interferon, no gross signs of bone marrow suppression have been observed. In two patients receiving interferon for a CMV infection complicating bone marrow transplantation, no suppression of bone marrow engraftment was observed [58]. In animal systems inter-

TABLE 4. Fever Reaction in Patients Given Intramuscular
Injections of Fibroblast Interferon

Patient code No.	Age (yr)	Sex	Diagnosis[a]	Purification method[b]	Number of injections	Avg. dose (MU)	Fever[c]
					Interferon treatment		
031	42	M	CALD	AS	7	10.0	+
009	35	M	Renal transplant	AS	26	3.0	−
010	31	M	Renal transplant	AS	26	3.0	−
011	24	F	Renal transplant	AS	26	3.0	−
012	37	M	Renal transplant	AS	26	3.0	−
013	37	F	Renal transplant	AS	26	3.0	+
014	26	F	Renal transplant	AS	26	3.0	−
015	34	F	Renal transplant	AS	26	3.0	+
016	19	M	Renal transplant	AS	26	3.0	−
017	57	F	CALD	CPG	9	4.6	−
018	21	F	CALD	CPG	16	4.5	−
002	36	M	CALD	CPG	37	3.6	+
003	50	M	CALD	CPG	28	1.2	−
019	35	F	CALD	CPG	14	2.2	−
020	39	M	CALD	CPG	14	2.2	+
025	43	F	Acute hepatitis	CPG	14	2.0	−
026	48	F	Acute hepatitis	CPG	14	2.0	−
027	40	F	Acute hepatitis	CPG	14	2.0	−
024	20	M	Fulminant hepatitis	CPG	10	3.5	−
023	36	M	Renal transplant	CPG	26	3.0	−
001	40	M	Osteosarcoma	CPG	15	3.5	+
006	13	M	Osteosarcoma	CPG	42	3.5	+
005	35	F	Multiple warts	CPG	14	5.9	+
004	30	F	Multiple sclerosis	CPG	7	4.7	−
008	6	M	Avian tuberculosis	CPG	37	1.5	+
022	9	M	SSPE	CPG	12	4.6	+
007	3	F	Neuroblastoma	CPG	18	1.7	+

[a]CALD = chronic active liver disease; SSPE = subacute sclerosing panencephalitis.
[b]AS = zinc iminodiacetate Sepharose method; CPG = controlled pore glass method.
[c]Peaks exceeding 38.0°C.

feron has been shown to modulate immune phenomena (see Chapter 11). In patients treated with interferon, parameters of cellular immune responsiveness have not been extensively studied. Emödi et al. reported suppression of lymphocyte response to phytohemagglutinin in two patients (out of an undetermined number studied) who received leukocyte interferon for CMV infection [57]. It would be important to know whether this is a generalized finding in interferon-treated patients. Failure of interferon to act prophylactically against CMV and HSV infections in renal transplant patients may be due to the cumulative immunosuppressive effects of interferon and azathioprine-prednisone therapy.

In patients receiving intramuscular injection of fibroblast interferon we observed an increase in the percentage of granylocytes and a decrease in the percentage of lymphocytes, most pronounced 4-8 hr after each injection. The blood formula restored to normal within 24 hr. The relative numbers of B and T cells, as determined by rosette assay, remained unaltered. One CALD patient (Table 1, No. 018) developed overall leukopenia after each injection of either fibroblast (2.2 MU) or leukocyte interferon (3 MU). With the latter, the total white blood cell count decreased to ≤ 3000 cells/mm^3, necessitating arrest of treatment. Since the reaction occurred with both fibroblast and leukocyte interferon, it seems highly probable that it was due to interferon.

C. Skin Reactivity

Intracutaneous injection of fibroblast interferon preparations ($\geq 20,000$ U in 0.1 to 2.0 ml) was found to provoke erythema and induration at the site of injection [63, 70, 71]. The reaction is painless. Anatomopathologically it resembles a delayed type hypersensitivity response, being characterized by the presence of a mononuclear infiltrate especially around the blood vessels, few polynuclear cells, very little edema, and absence of vascular lesions. The reaction peaks at 12-16 hr after injection and subsides in 26 to 48 hr. The size of the reaction is remarkably constant within single test persons but varies from one individual to another. Patients with depressed cellular immunity react as normal persons. It is not known with certainty whether the reaction is caused by interferon itself or by associated molecules. Fibroblast interferon purified by the Zn-chelate method was less reactive than that purified by the CPG method. Leukocyte interferon was also less active in provoking the skin reaction. On the basis of these findings we proposed [71] that the skin reaction is caused by molecules resembling interferon, rather than by interferon itself.

VII. DIFFERENCES IN PHARMACOKINETICS OF LEUKOCYTE AND FIBROBLAST INTERFERONS

Recently it has become apparent that there are differences in the pharmaco-kinetic behavior of leukocyte and fibroblast interferons. Patients injected with leukocyte interferon at dosages of >10,000 U/kg show measurable levels of interferon activity in the blood (>50 U/ml) [3]. In contrast, patients injected with as much as 40,000 U/kg of fibroblast interferon failed to demon-strate detectable serum levels (<10 U/ml) [72]. Although earlier informa-tion [73,74,75] obtained in rabbits suggested that the pharmacokinetics of fibroblast and leukocyte interferon would be similar, more recent work [71] confirmed that intramuscular injection of fibroblast interferon in rabbits resulted in lower serum titers than those obtained with similar doses of leukocyte interferon. In monkeys the difference was also present but less pronounced [77]. Experiments with intravenously injected rabbits [71] failed to support the concept that fibroblast interferon was removed more rapidly from the circulation. Rapid destruction at the site of injection remains a possibility.

VIII. RECENT STUDIES

The following recent information has become available. Scott et al. [78] showed protection of human volunteers against vaccinia virus scarification by prophylactic intradermal administration of human fibroblast interferon. Similar experiments were done in rhesus monkeys [77]: intramuscular doses of leukocyte as well as fibroblast interferons provided protection against vaccinia virus scarification. The interferon was given daily for 7 days starting on the day of scarification. A dose of 0.4 MU/kg of fibroblast interferon was about as effective as 0.1 MU/kg of leukocyte interferon. The protection obtained in this model cannot be explained by the direct antiviral effect of interferon since vaccinia virus replication was found not to be inhibited by either interferon in monkey cells in vitro [79]. It was suggested that the protection is mediated by activation of aspecific resistance on the level of the immune system.

 Additional uncontrolled studies on chronic HB-virus infection were done by Dolen et al. [80,81]. Fibroblast interferon was administered at daily doses of 1 MU intramuscularly for periods up to 82 days. In 2 out of 3 patients, a rapid and apparently permanent decline in viral markers was observed. In another uncontrolled study [82] leukocyte interferon was used in conjunction with adenine arabinoside over periods varying from 4 to 6 months. Complete loss of viral markers was seen in 1 out of 6 patients while in the 5 others a decrease occurred. Clinical parameters also tended to improve. A double-blind placebo-controlled study was done by Weimar et al. [83]. Leukocyte interferon treatment was given for 6 weeks, 12 MU per day in the first week, 6 MU in the second week, and so on. A rapid decrease occurred in particle-associated DNA polymerase levels in the serum. Otherwise all other viral and clinical parameters were not significantly different from those in the control group. Since polymerase levels increased again in spite of high daily doses of interferon, the authors expressed doubts as to whether the effect on polymerase was to be ascribed to interferon rather than to impurities causing aspecific reactions such as fever. On the basis of their results they also pleaded against implementation of long-term interferon therapeutic trials in patients with chronic hepatitis. This, however, remains a matter of judgment rather than of solid logic.

A. Romane, M. Revel, D. Gurari-Rotman, M. Blummenthal, M. Sokolovsky, and R. Stein (personal communication) performed a controlled trial on a group of 50 patients with adenovirus conjunctivitis and reported significant shortening of disease and reduction in the incidence of corneal involvement.

Cheeseman et al. [84] completed their double-blind placebo-controlled trial on renal transplant patients and reported a reduction in cytomegalovirus shedding. As there was no apparent clinical benefit from this effect, the practical conclusion from this trial agreed with that from the trial with fibroblast interferon [58] mentioned earlier.

IX. DISCUSSION AND CONCLUSIONS

Clinical trials with any drug are necessarily preceded by animal studies to test efficacy and safety. In the case of interferon the number of animal studies preceding clinical application is remarkably small when compared to drugs used in other areas of medicine. We can see several explanations for this. First, there are only a few model systems involving small laboratory animals that faithfully reflect those human viral infections that one would like to treat with interferon. Thus, there are no good model systems for viral hepatitis, for acute respiratory diseases, for recurrent herpes, or for CMV recurrence. Second, for each animal species one needs the homologous interferon, which is expensive to produce. Therefore one is limited to the use of only a few animal species, preferentially small ones. Safety assessments in animals have not been done to any great extent because it has been postulated that interferon would by definition have no toxic side effects. Recent animal and clinical studies have provided ample evidence to the contrary.

The efficacy studies in animals irrefutably prove that interferon given before virus inoculation can favorably influence the evolution of several acute viral infections. It would seem that in well-defined conditions interferon can still act when given at a time when viral replication in the target organ has already begun. Probably this important question will have to be reevaluated for each type of viral infection. It is clear, however, that for one particular model, higher doses of interferon are necessary and results are less favorable when the treatment is started later during the course of infection. The effect of systemic administration on viral parameters, in established chronic virus infection in animals such as persistent tolerant LCM virus infection, LDH, or MLV virus infections, has not been extensively studied. Yet studies of this type would seem extremely worthwhile in view of current interest in the effect of interferon in chronic active hepatitis and other chronic diseases of proven or suspected viral origin. Finally, topical application of interferon in animal model systems of herpetic keratitis has yielded rather discouraging results. Possibly the doses used in animals were too small. In clinical trials, topical application of interferon following mechanical débridement of corneal herpes lesions accelerated healing and inhibited virus shedding. In contrast, even high doses of interferon did not prevent recurrence. Possibly this failure was due to the inability of interferon to penetrate into the deeper layers of the cornea.

A controlled trial in upper respiratory disease established a prophylactic but not therpeutic effect of topical interferon. However, the doses needed were so high that practical application of interferon for the prevention of common colds must be held in abeyance until better techniques for the production of interferon become available.

Encouraging results were obtained in a controlled study involving application of an interferon-containing ointment in condyloma acuminatum.

A controlled study using systemic interferon administration in humans was done in renal transplant recipients in an attempt to demonstrate a prophylactic effect on the occurrence of viral infections due to immunosuppressive therapy. In view of the small number of patients included in this study, the results could hardly be expected to be significant. Its main merit was to prove the feasibility of double-blind, placebo-controlled studies in renal transplant patients and to provide orienting indications for further trials of this kind. From the results it would appear that little effect is to be expected on CMV infections; HSV infection, on the contrary, might be reduced by interferon treatment.

Treatment with leukocyte interferon was shown to reduce the incidence of herpes virus reactivation in patients operated on for a condition called "tic douloureux."

Another controlled study demonstrated that cancer patients treated with interferon had less dissemination and complications with herpes zoster, as well as less postherpetic neuralgia, than controls. Leukemic children with early varicella also could be protected against visceral complications.

All other trials done so far have been essentially uncontrolled. The most significant ones are perhaps those on chronic HB virus infection, because it is possible to study the effect of interferon administration on the evolution of viral activity in time. Base levels of viral activity can first be established, and changes occurring after interferon administration can then be studied. Such studies are currently in progress in several laboratories. From those reviewed in this paper, it would appear that about two-thirds of the patients react favorably to one or another regimen of treatment.

Clearly, some patients are resistant to treatment; less clearly, some are responsive. The interpretation of these studies suffers heavily from the fact that the study of viral parameters in chronic HB virus infection has only recently become possible and, hence, that very little background information on this subject is available as yet. Perhaps the merit of the clinical trials done so far will have been to provide some of that background and to orient investigators toward the establishment of a suitable treatment protocol with which double-blind, placebo-controlled studies can be undertaken.

Systemic administration of interferon has been attempted to treat sporadic cases of several other viral infections, including acquired or congenital CMV infection and acute and fulminant hepatitis. The performance of such sporadic tests can be criticized on the basis that they are a waste of time, effort, and money which would be better spent if concentrated on one properly controlled trial in one particular disease. However, both the choice of a particular disease to be studied and the choice of a particular treatment protocol to be used must be decided on the basis of preliminary pilot experiments. If one were to make these choices on a merely arbitrary basis, a single controlled trial would certainly be useless and would at the same time consume more effort than a number of individual pilot trials. Interferon is no exception in this regard; controlled trials with any drug are preceded by pilot trials on individual cases. However, with rather inexpensive drugs these preliminary tests are never brought to the attention of the scientific community, for the simple reason that the ensuing controlled trials can be performed without delay. In the case of interferon the decision to start a controlled trial is painstaking because it does involve an enormous financial effort. In the meantime it is useful to collect and carefully study all the fragmentary evidence from uncontrolled trials done in several centers, in order to make as educated a decision as possible.

While the clinical trials were being performed, it became clear that current interferon preparations exert some unexplained side effects: fever and malaise, transient lymphopenia, and skin reactivity. The question whether these effects are due to the interferon molecule or to some impurities remains unresolved. We favor the view that they are due to molecules that resemble and hence tend to copurify with interferon. These molecules might be as relevant as interferon to explain some of the beneficial efforts seen in vivo, e.g., the antitumor effect. An important task will be to find animal model systems to study these side effects and then to isolate and identify the substances responsible for these effects.

Finally, while in the past leukocyte and fibroblast interferons were merely seen as alternative technologies for preparing the same drug, it has now become clear that these interferons have quite different physicochemical, serological, biological, and pharmacokinetic properties. Perhaps each of them will also turn out to have its own place in the prophylaxis or therapy of human disease.

ACKNOWLEDGMENTS

The studies from the authors' laboratory, commented upon in this paper, were made possible by grants from the Belgian A.S.L.K. (General Savings and Retirement Fund) and from the Belgian Ministries of Economic Affairs and of Science Administration (O.O.A.).

The authors are indebted to many colleagues from St. Rafaël Academic Hospital (Leuven, Belgium), Academic Hospital (Ghent, Belgium), and Dijkzigt Hospital (Rotterdam, The Netherlands), who cooperated in the clinical trials.

Editorial help of Christiane Callebaut is gratefully acknowledged.

REFERENCES

1. T. C. Merigan, S. E. Reed, T. S. Hall, and D. A. Tyrrell, Lancet i: 563 (1973).
2. J. Desmyter, M. B. Ray, J. De Groote, A. F. Bradburne, V. J. Desmet, V. G. Edy, A. Billiau, and P. De Somer, Lancet ii: 645 (1976).
3. H. B. Greenberg, R. B. Pollard, L. I. Lutwick, P. B. Gregory, W. S. Robinson, and T. C. Merigan, New Engl. J. Med. 295: 517 (1976).
4. S. Baron, in Interferons and Interferon Inducers (N. B. Finter, ed.), American Elsevier, New York, 1973, p. 267.
5. L. A. Glasgow, in Interferons, Proc. Symp. New York Heart Association, 1970, p. 212.
6. D. Gilden, in Viruses and Immunity (C. Koprowski and H. Koprowski, eds.), Academic Press, New York, 1975, p. 83.
7. A. D. Steinberg, in Viruses and Immunity (C. Koprowski and H. Koprowski, eds.), Academic Press, New York, 1975, p. 95.
8. F. Dianzani and S. Baron, Nature 257: 682 (1975).
9. N. B. Finter, in Interferons and Interferon Inducers (N. B. Finter, ed.), American Elsevier, New York, 1973, p. 295.
10. G. A. Olsen, E. R. Kern, L. A. Glasgow, and J. C. Overall, Jr., Antimicrob. Agents Chemother. 10: 669 (1976).
11. M. Worthington, H. Levy, and J. Rice, Proc. Soc. Exp. Biol. Med. 143: 638 (1973).
12. E. De Clercq and P. De Somer, Proc. Soc. Exp. Biol. Med. 138: 301 (1971).
13. I. Gresser, M. G. Tovey, and C. Bourali-Maury, J. Gen. Virol. 27: 395 (1975).
14. M. Ho, C. Nash, C. W. Morgan, J. A. Armstrong, R. G. Carrol, and B. Postic, Infec. Immun. 9: 286 (1974).
15. J. Hilfenhaus, E. Weinman, M. Majer, R. Barth, and O. Jaeger, J. Infec. Dis. 135: 846 (1977).

16. R. Sundmacher, D. Neumann-Haefelin, and B. Shrestha, Albrecht v. Graefes Arch. Klin. Exp. Ophthalmol. 195:263 (1975).

17. D. Neumann-Haefelin, R. Sundmacher, R. Skoda, and K. Cantell, Infec. Immun. 17:468 (1977).

18. J. Sugar, H. E. Kaufman, and E. Varnell, Invest. Ophthalmol. 12: 378 (1973).

18a. J. I. McGill, P. Collins, K. Cantell, B. R. Jones, and N. B. Finter, J. Infec. Dis. 133:A13 (1976).

19. M. N. Oxman, in Interferons and Interferon Inducers (N. B. Finter, ed.), American Elsevier, New York, 1973, p. 391.

20. H. Dubuy, S. Baron, C. Uhlendorf, and M. L. Johnson, Infec. Immun. 8:977 (1973).

21. A. Billiau, V. G. Edy, H. Sobis, and P. De Somer, Int. J. Cancer 14:335 (1974).

22. R. M. Friedman, E. H. Chang, J. M. Ramseur, and M. W. Meyers, J. Virol. 16:569 (1975).

23. A. Billiau, H. Heremans, P. T. Allen, J. De Maeyer-Guignard, and P. De Somer, Virology 73:537 (1976).

24. S. Z. Shapiro, M. Strand, and A. Billiau, Infec. Immun. 16:742 (1977).

25. R. R. Wagner and R. M. Snyder, Nature 196:393 (1962).

26. Y. Rivière, I. Gresser, J. C. Cuillon, and M. G. Tovey, Proc. Nat. Acad. Sci. U.S. 74:2135 (1977).

27. E. J. Field, G. Joyce, and A. Keith, J. Gen. Virol. 5:149 (1969).

28. M. Worthington, Infec. Immun. 6:643 (1972).

29. I. Gresser, M. G. Tovey, C. Maury, and I. Chouroulinkov, Nature 258:76 (1975).

30. I. Gresser, C. Maury, M. Tovey, L. Morel-Maroger, and F. Pontillon, Nature 263:420 (1976).

31. I. Gresser, M. Tovey, M. T. Bandu, C. Maury, and D. Brouty-Boyé, J. Exp. Med. 144:1305 (1976).

32. I. Gresser, M. Tovey, C. Maury, and M. T. Bandu, J. Exp. Med. 144:1316 (1976).

32a. H. Heremans, A. Billiau, A. Colombatti, J. Hilgers, and P. De Somer, Infec. Immun. 21:925 (1978).

33. D. F. Horrobin, R. A. Karmali, M. S. Manku, A. I. Ally, M. Kamazyn, R. O. Morgan, A. Swift, and H. Zinner, IRCS J. Med. Sci. 5:547 (1978).

34. M. Yaron, I. Yaron, D. Gurari-Rotman, M. Revel, H. R. Lindner, and V. Zor, Nature 267:457 (1977).

35. N. B. Finter, in Interferons and Interferon Inducers (N. B. Finter, ed.), American Elsevier, New York, 1973, p. 363.

36. T. C. Merigan, G. W. Jordan, and R. P. Fried, in Perspectives in Virology (M. Pollard, ed.), Vol. 9, Academic Press, New York, 1975, p.

37. D. Ikic, I. Petricevic, K. Cupak, D. Trajer, I. Soldo, E. Soos,
    D. Jusic, and S. Smerdel, in Proc. Symp. Clinical Use of Interferon
    (D. Ikic, ed.), Yugoslav Acad. Sci. and Arts, Zagreb, 1975, p. 207.
38. D. Ikic, S. Smerdel, M. Rajninger-Miholic, E. Soos, and D. Jusic,
    in Proc. Symp. Clinical Use of Interferon (D. Ikic, ed.), Yugoslav
    Acad. Sci. and Arts, Zagreb, 1975, p. 195.
39. D. Ikic, N. Bosnic, S. Smerdel, D. Jusic, E. Soos, and N. Delimar,
    in Proc. Symp. Clinical Use of Interferon (D. Ikic, ed.), Yugoslav
    Acad. Sci. and Arts, Zagreb, 1975, p. 229.
40. H. E. Kaufman, R. F. Meyer, P. R. Laibson, S. R. Waltman,
    A. B. Nesburn, and J. J. Shuster, J. Infec. Dis. 133: A165 (1976).
41. B. R. Jones, D. J. Coster, M. G. Falcon, and K. Cantell, J. Infec.
    Dis. 133: A169 (1976).
42. R. Sundmacher, D. Neumann-Haefelin, K. F. Manthey, and O. Müller,
    J. Infec. Dis. 133: A160 (1976).
43. R. Sundmacher, D. Neumann-Haefelin, and K. Cantell, Albrecht v.
    Graefes Arch. Klin. Exp. Ophthalmol. 201: 39 (1976).
44. R. Sundmacher, D. Neumann-Haefelin, and K. Cantell, Lancet i: 1406
    (1976).
45. R. Sundmacher, K. Cantell, R. Skoda, C. Hallermann, and
    D. Neumann-Haefelin, Albrecht v. Graefes Arch. Klin. Exp. Opthalmol.
    208, 229 (1978).
46. D. Ikic, K. Cupak, D. Trajer, E. Soos, D. Jusic, and S. Smerdel,
    in Proc. Symp. Clinical Use of Interferon (D. Ikic, ed.), Yugoslav
    Acad. Sci. and Arts, Zagreb, 1975, p. 189.
47. D. Ikic, M. Prazic, S. Smerdel, D. Jusic, N. Delimar, and E. Soos,
    in Proc. Symp. Clinical Use of Interferon (D. Ikic, ed.), Yugoslav
    Acad. Sci. and Arts, Zagreb, 1975, p. 203.
48. G. W. Jordan, R. P. Fried, and T. C. Merigan, J. Infec. Dis. 130:
    56 (1974).
49. T. C. Merigan, K. H. Rand, R. B. Pollard, P. S. Abdallah,
    G. W. Jordan, and R. P. Fried, New Engl. J. Med. 18: 981 (1978).
50. A. N. Arvin, S. Feldman, and T. C. Merigan, Antimicrob. Agents
    Chemother. 13: 605 (1978).
51a. G. H. Scullard, A. Alberti, M. H. Wansborough-Jones, C. R. Howard,
    A. L. W. F. Eddleston, A. J. Zuckerman, K. Cantell, and R. Williams,
    Clin. Lab. Immunol. in press.
52. W. Weimar, R. A. Heijtink, S. W. Schalm, and H. Schellekens,
    Gastroenterology 74: 1150 (1978).
53. W. Weimar, R. A. Heijtink, S. W. Schalm, M. van Blankenstein,
    H. Schellekens, N. Masurel, V. G. Edy, A. Billiau, and P. De Somer,
    Lancet ii: 1282 (1977).
54. W. Weimar, R. A. Heijtink, S. W. Schalm, and H. Schellekens, Eur.
    J. Clin. Invest. 9: 151 (1979).

55. J. G. Kingham, N. K. Ganguly, Z. D. Shari, R. Mendelson, T. Cartwright, G. M. Scott, B. M. Richards, and R. Wright, Gut 18: A952 (1978).

56. R. J. O'Reilly, L. K. Everson, G. Emödi, J. Hansen, E. M. Smithwick, E. Grimes, S. Pahwa, R. Pahwa, S. Schwartz, D. Armstrong, F. P. Siegal, S. Gupta, B. Dupont, and R. A. Good, Clin. Immunol. Immunopathol. 6: 51 (1976).

57. G. Emödi, R. O'Reilly, A. Müller, L. K. Everson, U. Binswanger, and M. Just, J. Infec. Dis. 133: A199 (1976).

58. W. Weimar, H. Schellekens, L. D. F. Lameijer, N. Masurel, V. G. Edy, A. Billiau, and P. De Somer, Eur. J. Clin. Invest. 8: 255 (1978).

59. G. J. Pazin, J. A. Armstrong, M. T. Lam, G. C. Tarr, P. J. Janetta, and M. Ho, New Engl. J. Med. 301: 225 (1979).

60. L. Ahström, A. Dohlwitz, H. Strander, G. Carlström, and K. Cantell, Lancet i: 166 (1974).

61. G. Emödi, M. Just, R. Hernandez, and H. R. Hirt, J. Nat. Cancer Inst. 54: 1045 (1975).

62. H. Strander, K. Cantell, G. Carlström, and P. A. Jakobsson, J. Nat. Cancer Inst. 51: 733 (1973).

63. P. De Somer, V. G. Edy, and A. Billiau, Lancet ii: 47 (1977).

64. V. G. Edy, I. A. Braude, E. De Clercq, A. Billiau, and P. De Somer, J. Gen. Virol. 33: 517 (1976).

65. V. G. Edy, A. Billiau, and P. De Somer, J. Biol. Chem. 252: 5934 (1977).

66. T. A. McNeill and I. Gresser, Nature [New Biol.] 244: 173 (1973).

67. P. L. Greenberg and S. A. Mosny, Cancer Res. 37: 1794 (1977).

68. C. Nissen, B. Speck, G. Emödi, and N. N. Iscove, Lancet ii: 203 (1977).

69. E. Van 't Hull, H. Schellekens, B. Löwenberg, and M. J. de Vries, Cancer Res. 38, 911 (1978).

70. G. M. Scott, J. K. Butler, T. Cartwright, B. M. Richards, J. G. Kingham, R. Wright, and D. A. J. Tyrrell, Lancet ii: 402 (1977).

71. A. Billiau, P. De Somer, V. G. Edy, E. De Clercq, and H. Heremans, Antimicrob. Agents Chemother. 16: 56 (1979).

72. V. G. Edy, A. Billiau, and P. De Somer, Lancet i: 451 (1978).

73. V. G. Edy, A. Billiau, and P. De Somer, J. Infec. Dis. 133: A18 (1976).

74. K. Cantell and L. Pyhälä, J. Gen. Virol. 20: 97 (1973).

75. K. Cantell and L. Pyhälä, J. Infec. Dis. 133: A6 (1976).

76. T. C. Cesario, Proc. Soc. Exp. Biol. Med. 155: 583 (1977).

77. W. Weimar, A. Billiau, K. Cantell, L. Stitz, and H. Schellekens, J. Gen. Virol. in press (1980).

78. G. M. Scott, T. Cartwright, G. Le Du, and D. Dicker, J. Biol. Standardization 6: 73 (1978).

79. H. Schellekens, W. Weimar, K. Cantell, and L. Stitz, Nature 278: 742 (1979).

80. J. G. Dolen, W. A. Carter, J. S. Horoszewicz, A. O. Vladutiu, A. I. Leibowitz, and J. P. Nolan, Amer. J. Med. 67:127 (1979).

81. J. G. Dolen, S. S. Leong, A. O. Vladutiu, A. I. Leibowitz, and J. S. Horoszewicz, J. Clin. Haematol. Oncol. 9:63 (Abstr.) (1979).

82. G. Scullard, A. Makal, S. Sacks, P. Gregory, W. Robinson, and T. Merigan, J. Clin. Haematol. Oncol. 9:58 (Abstr.) (1979).

83. W. Weimar, R. A. Heijtink, K. Cantell, F. J. P. ten Kate, S. W. Schalm, N. Masurel, and H. Schellekens, Lancet in press (1979).

84. S. H. Cheeseman, R. H. Rubin, J. A. Stewart, N. E. Tolkoff-Rubin, A. B. Cosimi, K. Cantell, J. Gilbert, S. Winkle, J. T. Herrin, P. H. Black, P. S. Russell, and M. S. Hirsch, New Engl. J. Med. 300:1345 (1979).

6

INTERFERON INDUCERS: THEORY AND EXPERIMENTAL APPLICATION

Dale A. Stringfellow

The Upjohn Company
Kalamazoo, Michigan

I. INTRODUCTION

Following the discovery of interferon a great deal of speculation has centered around its use as an effective antiviral and antineoplastic agent and, more recently, as a modulator of the immune response. Essentially two approaches had been taken toward the development of this agent. The first, as described in the preceding portion of this book, involved mass production of enough interferon for the direct treatment of virus-infected individuals or those bearing various types of malignancies. At present, this approach has as a major limitation the amount of interferon which can be produced. Currently available methods do not appear sufficient for the successful production of enough interferon for routine clinical use. This situation may obviously be reversed if interferon or an active component of the interferon molecule can be synthesized synthetically or if the inter-

feron gene can be transferred to procaryotic cells that can then produce it.
The theory behind a second approach to the use of the interferon system
has, therefore, centered around the identification and development of agents
capable of stimulating the host's own cells to produce interferon, thereby
circumventing the necessity of producing large quantities of exogenous interferon.

Over the past several years a variety of agents have been found capable
of stimulating interferon production both in vivo and in vitro. Besides most
types of viruses, many bacteria, and bacterial cell wall extracts, synthetic
and naturally occurring nucleic acids (i.e., double-stranded RNA), protozoa,
mytogens, antigens, and a variety of high- and low-molecular-weight compounds with diverse chemical structures have been found to be effective
interferon inducers in the appropriate cell (in vitro) or animal (in vivo) systems (Table 1 [1-19]). The number of agents which have been found to be
effective interferon inducers increases each year, yet at present none have
been successfully employed as clinically useful antiviral agents; however,
only a very few (three or four) have been evaluated in humans. This area is
in its infancy, and the purpose of this and the next few chapters is to identify

TABLE 1. Major Classes of Agents That Induce Interferon

Class	Example	Reference
Naturally occurring		
Viruses, RNA	Influenza	1
Viruses, DNA	Vaccinia	2
Bacteria	Brucella abortus	3
Bacterial extracts	B. abortus	4
Rickettsia	Rickettsia tsutsugamushi	5
Protozoa	Taxoplasma gondii	6,7
Endotoxin (LPS)	Escherichia coli	8,9
Mitogens	Phytohemagglutinin	10
	Poke weed	11
Antigens	Viral	12
	Bacterial (BCG)	13
Synthetic		
Polynucleotides	Poly I: poly C	14
Polycarboxylates	Pyran copolymer	15
Low molecular weight	Tilorone	16
	Propanediamine	17
	Acradines	18
	Pyrimidines	19

TABLE 2. Minimal Requirements an Interferon-Inducing Agent
Should Meet To Be Considered for Clinical Use

---

1. Safe; nontoxic and not irritating

2. Rapidly cleared from the animal; does not accumulate

3. Prophylactically, and preferably therapeutically, active

4. Able to induce interferon in the animal species to be treated

5. Effective by a practical route of administration

6. Free of adventitious agents

7. Relatively inexpensive to prepare

---

the progress so far achieved and the problems being encountered in the
development of effective interferon-inducing, antiviral agents.

An inducer must meet certain minimal criteria to be considered for
human use (Table 2). It must be relatively nontoxic for the treatment of
life-threatening diseases and entirely safe if it is to be used in the treatment of what are considered to be benign self-limiting infections. It must
be effective prophylactically and preferably therapeutically, must be able
to induce interferon in humans or the animal species in which it is to be
used, and should be relatively inexpensive as well as effective by practical
routes of administration. It should be relatively nonirritating, should be
cleared from the animal fairly rapidly, and not contain any adventitious
agents. Certain of the agents to be considered in this and later chapters
possess many but not all of these characteristics, while others have not
been tested clinically; thus, many of the answers are not yet available.

II. CHEMICAL REQUIREMENTS

The chemical structures of molecules that can induce interferon are diverse.
Various double-stranded RNAs [14], lipopolysaccharides (endotoxins) [8,9],
polycarboxylates [15], anthraquinones [20], fluoronones [16], propanedi-
amines [17], pyrimidines [19], etc., are able to induce high serum interferon levels in the appropriate animal species. In general, however, it
seems that minor modification of the structure of various low-molecular-
weight compounds disrupts the antiviral activity [21,22]. For example,
a series of isocytosine interferon inducers clearly demonstrate (Table 3)
that minor alterations in structure drastically affect biological activity.
As illustrated in Table 3, occupation of the 2-position (R_1) with amino and
the 4-position (R_2) with hydroxy were essential for antiviral activity. If

TABLE 3. Effect of Structural Alterations on Ability of Pyrimidine
Molecules to Protect Mice Against a Lethal Encephalomyocarditis
(EMC) Virus Infection

R_1	R_2	R_3	R_4	MPD[a]
H	OH	Br	CH_3	—
$NHCH_3$	OH	Br	CH_3	—
NH_2	OH	Br	CH_3	250
NH_2	CH_3	Br	CH_3	—
NH_2	NH_2	Br	CH_3	—
NH_2	OH	I	CH_3	200
NH_2	OH	Cl	CH_3	—
NH_2	OH	CH_3	CH_3	—
NH_2	OH	H	CH_3	—
NH_2	OH	Br	CH_2CH_3	500
NH_2	OH	Br	$CH_2CH_2CH_3$	—
NH_2	OH	Br	$CH(CH_3)_2$	—
NH_2	OH	I	CH_2CH_3	400
NH_2	OH	I	$CH_2CH_2CH_3$	1000
NH_2	OH	I	$CH(CH_3)_2$	—
NH_2	OH	I	$CH_2C_6H_5$	800

[a]Minimum dose (mg/kg, i.p.) needed to protect mice against EMC virus
infection. Drugs were administered 18 hr prior to infection.

either was altered or substituted, antiviral and interferon-inducing activity was lost. Likewise the 5-position (R_3) had to be occupied by a halogen (preferably chlorine, bromine, or iodine) while as the 6-position (R_4) alkyl side chain was lengthened, antiviral activity progressively decreased. This type of selective activity of specific structures appears to be the rule rather than the exception for inducers in general. At present a precise definition of structural characteristics an inducer requires is not available. A slightly better predictability is available for polynucleotides with regard to how structural and physical alterations affect biological activity [23-29].

III. SPECIES-TO-SPECIES VARIABILITY

Not only are inducers difficult to predict in terms of activity of specific structures, but it is very difficult to predict if a compound capable of inducing interferon in, for example, mice will also be active in other animal species. For example, tilorone hydrochloride (Chapter 8) induces very high levels of serum interferon in mice but is not active in chickens, cats, dogs, rabbits, and apparently not in humans ([30,31]; see also Chapter 8). Similar results in terms of inability to induce interferon in humans have been reported with a few other inducers, although not many have yet been tested clinically. Some inducers however, do have a broad species range. For example, poly I:poly C induces high levels of interferon in a variety of cells (in vitro) and animals, including humans and nonhuman primates ([32-34]; see Chapter 7). A new polynucleotide complex, poly ICLC, developed at the National Institutes of Health (Chapter 7), appears to be an effective interferon inducer in humans and protected monkeys against an otherwise lethal virus infection [35]. Likewise, a pyrimidine interferon inducer 2-amino-5-bromo-6-methyl-4-pyrimidinol (ABMP) can induce high levels of interferon in mice and is a very good interferon inducer in cats [36]. We have therefore been interested in developing a system in which we can predict whether such agents will be able to induce interferon in humans. In preliminary studies we evaluated the rhesus monkey as such a model system. During these studies a variety of viruses [Newcastle disease virus (NDV)], polynucleotides (poly I:poly C), and low-molecular-weight compounds were evaluated without success. This raised the question of whether the monkey was a good species to use as a predictor of human activity. To try to answer this question, as well as possibly develop a better system, we turned to evaluating the ability of human tissues cultured in vitro to respond to various compounds and agents previously found to be active in rodents. Since several different cell types appear to be involved in the in vivo induction process [37-40], a mixture of several cell types cultured together in vitro seemed to be a better simulation of in vivo conditions and a more predictive system than single types of cells cultured

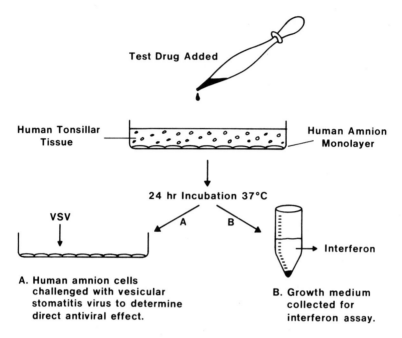

Test Drug Added

Human Tonsillar
Tissue

Human Amnion
Monolayer

24 hr Incubation 37°C

VSV

A   B

Interferon

A. Human amnion cells
   challenged with vesicular
   stomatitis virus to determine
   direct antiviral effect.

B. Growth medium
   collected for
   interferon assay.

FIGURE 1. In vitro system to determine the ability of compounds to induce
interferon or antiviral resistance in human cells as a predictive tool for
future evaluation in humans.

alone. Since the lympho-reticuloendothelial system has been implicated
as a major contributor in the induction process with low-molecular-weight
compounds [37-38], a system consisting of human tonsillar or splenic
tissue cultured alone or with a monolayer of human cells was investigated.
After several unsuccessful attempts to induce interferon, it was found that
human tonsillar tissue minsed in small pieces and incubated over a confluent
monolayer of human amnion cells (Figure 1) was a consistently good re-
sponder to poly I:poly C and NDV, yet it appeared to be selective to induction by various low-molecular-weight molecules. Also, using this system,
both direct antiviral activity (on amnion cells) and ability to induce interferon could be measured. In this system ABMP induced antiviral resistance
at 50 μg/ml and stimulated moderate (50-100 U/ml) levels of interferon.
NDV and poly I:poly C were also very active and tilorone was inactive.
Presently it is not known if this system is predictive of activity in humans.
We obviously will not know until more compounds have been evaluated clinically. It does not seem unreasonable, however, to assume that an agent
that induces interferon and antiviral resistance in human cells in vitro will

stand a better chance of being active in humans than a compound that had activity only in mice or other experimental animals. The predictability of compounds, therefore, remains one key unanswered question in the search for agents that will be effective, clinically useful interferon inducers.

IV. HOW MUCH INTERFERON IS ENOUGH?

Problems raised in the previous section are even more complicated than they might first appear. Even if an inducer can stimulate interferon production in humans, the questions remain as to how much is needed for in vivo antiviral activity and whether serum interferon levels are a reflection of antiviral activity. Dianzani and Baron [41,42] and Dianzani et al. [43] have addressed this problem using cell culture systems that simulated in vivo conditions. Their data suggest that extremely high interferon levels are achieved in extracellular spaces in various tissues after induction and that in many cases serum interferon levels are misleading in terms of the actual concentration that cells are exposed to. In some cases the serum interferon titers might be higher than the concentration in certain tissues such as the central nervous system, and the reverse might also be true where cells in the immediate vicinity of the site of interferon production might be exposed to much higher levels of interferon than can be detected systemically in serum. Also, cells only needed to be exposed to interferon for a very short period of time (30 min) for development of full antiviral resistance. Using mice infected with either Semliki Forest virus (SFV) or encephalomyocarditis (EMC) virus, we have addressed this question; and our data would suggest that there is a rough correlation between circulating interferon levels and protection against these neurotropic diseases (Table 4). Concentrations of inducers that stimulated peak interferon levels of greater than 50-100 U of interferon/ml of serum protected animals against SFV and EMC virus infection. Less than 50 U/ml did not seem to be protective. Whether the same correlation will be observed in humans is not yet answered (Chapter 5 deals more with this question). Also, local administration of inducer at the site of infection may stimulate high enough local interferon titers to be protective without a need for a systemic (serum) response. The important point to be made is that inducers apparently do not have to stimulate serum interferon titers of 5000-10,000 U/ml for extended periods of time to be protective but that lower titers of 50-100 U/ml of short duration may be sufficient. In the future, instead of searching for agents that stimulate more total interferon, a more practical approach might be to search for compounds that are more active at lower concentrations and treatment regimens that provide a constant antiviral state for an extended time.

TABLE 4. Comparison of the Minimum Dose of Inducer That
Stimulates Interferon Production and Antiviral Resistance in Mice

Inducer[a]	Dosage (mg/kg)	Maximum interferon response (U/ml)	Antiviral protection	
			SFV	EMC
Tilorone	200	6500	+	+
	100	1300	+	+
	50	500	+	+
	25	120	+	+
	12	25	−	−
ABMP	1000	7300	+	+
	500	1500	+	+
	250	70	+	+
	120	< 10	−	−
	60	< 10	−	−
Poly I: poly C	5	5500	+	+
	1	4000	+	+
	0.5	510	+	+
	0.1	80	+	±
	0.05	< 10	−	−

[a]Tilorone (p.o.), ABMP (p.o.), and poly I: poly C (i.p.) were administered
18 hr prior to infection with EMC or SFV. Serum was collected for interferon assay 4 hr after poly I: poly C, 6 hr after ABMP, or 18 hr after
tilorone administration.

V. HYPOREACTIVITY

One of the main problems confronting the development of inducers has been
that animals progressively lose their ability to respond to various compounds
following repeated administration [3,44,45]. For example, the serum
interferon response of mice to inducers given once a day for five consecutive
days is illustrated in Figure 2 [55]. In each case, the ability of mice to
respond by producing serum interferon levels progressively decreases.
The rate of onset of the hyporeactive state was, however, inducer dependent.
That is, mice were hyporeactive to a second dose of tilorone on the second
day but were still responsive to ABMP or poly I: poly C through the third
dose of compound. Others have also reported that the rate and severity
of the hyporeactive state depends upon the inducer, dose, and route of
administration [46-49]. A small initial dose of an inducer caused a moder-

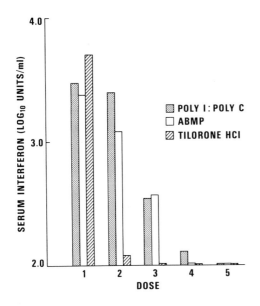

FIGURE 2. Development of hyporeactivity in mice following daily doses of poly I: poly C (100 µg/mouse, i.p.), ABMP (500 mg/kg, p.o.), or tilorone (250 mg/kg, p.o.). (Reprinted from Ref. 55 with permission of the American Society for Microbiology.)

ate suppression in responsiveness, whereas larger doses increased the severity of the hyporeactive state. These data suggest that judicious selection of inducers and treatment regimens may be extremely important in controlling the development of hyporeactivity. This was in fact found to be the case in children given various dosage regimens of poly I: poly C [39]. Another approach around the same problem concerns whether alteration between different inducers can avoid development of hyporeactivity. In early studies it was found that in general once the hyporeactive state had been established, the response to other inducers was also inhibited [45,50]. More recently, however, it has been demonstrated that alteration of inducers in some cases completely avoided the development of hyporeactivity [51-53]. As illustrated in Table 5, mice given an initial dose of an inducer, for example, ABMP, progressively became less responsive (decreased with each injection) to induction by the same inducer, but they remained responsive to other unrelated compounds. Likewise, mice rendered hyporeactive with an anthraquinone interferon inducer were hyporeactive to the same or a related compound (tilorone) but remained responsive to ABMP. These data suggest that proper selection of treatment regimens may be critical in developing the most effective methods of using such agents.

TABLE 5. Development of Hyporeactivity to Interferon Induction
in Mice Given Daily Doses of the Same or Another Inducer[a]

Dose 1	Interferon (U/ml)	Dose 2	Interferon (U/ml)	Dose 3	Interferon (U/ml)	Dose 4	Interferon (U/ml)
ABMP	1200						
ABMP		ABMP	500				
ABMP		Tilorone	4600				
ABMP		BAA	4500				
ABMP		PBS	<50				
ABMP		ABMP		ABMP	300		
ABMP		ABMP		Tilorone	4100		
ABMP		ABMP		BAA	3100		
ABMP		ABMP		PBS	<50		
ABMP		ABMP		ABMP		ABMP	<50
ABMP		ABMP		ABMP		Tilorone	4000
ABMP		ABMP		ABMP		BAA	2500
ABMP		ABMP		ABMP		PBS	<50
BAA	3500						
BAA		BAA	400				
BAA		ABMP	5000				
BAA		Tilorone	50				
BAA		BAA		BAA	550		
BAA		BAA		ABMP	730		
BAA		BAA		Tilorone	<50		
BAA		BAA		BAA		BAA	<50
BAA		BAA		BAA		ABMP	900
BAA		BAA		BAA		Tilorone	<50

[a]ABMP = 2-amino-5-bromo-6-methyl-4-pyrimidinol; BAA = 1,5-bis[(3-morpholinopropyl)amino]anthraquinone.

Part of this same question revolves around how fast animals recover
their ability to respond to inducers after onset of a hyporeactive state. In
other words, how often can inducers be given without loss of responsiveness.
With most inducers (Figure 3) four to six days between injection of the same
inducer were required before animals (or humans) were fully responsive to
the next dose of compound [34,49,54,55]. Based upon these data we have
evaluated the ability of cats to respond to compounds which were given on

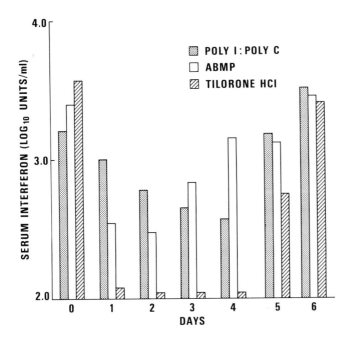

FIGURE 3. Recovery of interferon responsiveness in mice that received
a single dose of ABMP (500 mg/kg, p.o.), poly I:poly C (100 µg/mouse,
i.p.), or tilorone (250 mg/kg, p.o.) on day 0 and a second dose of the
same inducer either 1, 2, 3, 4, 5, or 6 days later. (Reprinted from Ref.
55 with permission of the American Society for Microbiology.)

a weekly or biweekly basis [36]. As summarized in Table 6, ABMP was
given on a biweekly basis to cats over an 18-week period. Animals remained
fully responsive to each subsequent injection of inducer. Since ABMP and
other inducers can create an antiviral state that persists for up to several
days [55], the possibility exists that giving such compounds on a weekly
basis could maintain a high nonspecific, antiviral state for an extended
period of time.

   Animals also develop hyporeactivity to interferon induction as a consequence of viral infections. Mice infected with one of several viruses have
been found to have a suppressed ability to respond to interferon inducers
[56-60]. In Table 7 the ability of virus-infected mice to respond to a
battery of inducers is summarized [55]. In general, as the infection pro-
gressed the ability of mice to respond to interferon inducers decreased.
Again the development of hyporeactivity created by virus infection was
inducer-dependent. For example, animals remained quite responsive to
poly I:poly C for longer time-periods than to inducers such as tilorone
hydrochloride. Development of such a hyporeactive state could severely

TABLE 6. Circulating Interferon Response of Cats Orally Given
ABMP (200 mg/kg) Every Other Week

Cat No.	Weight (kg)	Experimental week	Hours after inducer was given				
			0	6	12	24	48
1	3.0	0	$< 10^a$	2560	80	10	< 10
	3.2	2	< 10	1280	40	< 10	< 10
	3.3	4	10	5120	640	20	< 10
	3.2	6	10	2560	160	40	< 10
	3.3	10	10	1280	160	20	< 10
	3.2	12	10	2560	320	20	< 10
	3.2	14	20	2560	160	10	< 10
	3.2	16	10	1280	80	40	< 10
	3.2	18	< 10	2560	160	< 10	< 10
2	3.0	0	< 10	320	20	< 10	< 10
	3.5	2	< 10	40	20	< 10	< 10
	4.1	4	< 10	320	20	< 10	< 10
	4.3	5	< 10	160	40	< 10	< 10
	4.9	10	< 10	320	80	10	< 10
	4.9	12	< 10	640	40	10	< 10
	4.9	14	10	80	40	40	20
	5.0	16	< 10	1280	40	10	< 10
	5.0	18	< 10	640	160	10	< 10

[a]Serum interferon titers (U/3 ml).

restrict the use of interferon inducers as therapeutically active antiviral
agents, since in many cases virus-infected mice developed hyporeactivity
before symptoms of illness were observed. In a series of studies designed
to determine why animals developed hyporeactivity, it was found that cells
from virus-infected mice (peritoneal cells) were functionally normal except
in their ability to respond to interferon inducers (Table 8). This suggested
that a specific control process was operating and that the hyporeactive state
might be reversible. In a series of studies it was found that the only consistently observed difference between normal and hyporeactive cells (cells
from virus-infected mice) was that hyporeactive cells consistently had
lower membrane-associated adenylate cyclase levels and intracellular
cyclic AMP levels than did normal cells (Table 8). If cyclic AMP suppression was modulating the hyporeactive condition, then stimulating cyclic
AMP might be able to restore the interferon response of hyporeactive cells.
Catecholamines, theophylline, and other agents that had the ability to increase intracellular cyclic AMP levels, however, in general did not affect
the response of normal or hyporeactive cells. Prostaglandins, on the

TABLE 7. Serum Interferon Levels Induced by Poly I:poly C
(100 μg, i.p.), ABMP (1000 mg/kg, p.o.), or Tilorone HCl
(250 mg/kg, p.o.) in EMC- or SFV-Infected or Uninfected
Control Mice[a]

Inducer	Days Post-infection	Serum interferon response (U/ml)		
		Uninfected control	EMC infected (%)[b]	SFV infected (%)[b]
Poly I:poly C	1	3,500	9,500 (270)	5,000 (140)
	2	4,300	4,300 (100)	2,100 (49)
	3	2,100	850 (40)	720 (34)
	4	2,900	270 (9)	300 (10)
ABMP	1	5,500	9,500 (170)	4,200 (76)
	2	4,300	4,500 (104)	1,500 (35)
	3	3,700	1,100 (30)	900 (24)
	4	4,800	120 (2)	250 (5)
Tilorone HCl	1	10,000	1,500 (15)	1,200 (12)
	2	6,500	350 (5)	190 (3)
	3	7,000	150 (2)	100 (<1)
	4	6,500	100 (1.5)	100 (<1)
PBS	1	<50	150	350
	2	<50	100	100
	3	<50	<50	<50
	4	<50	<50	<50

[a]Animals received a single injection of inducer 24, 48, 72, or 96 hr after
infection. Blood and subsequent serum samples were collected 4 hr after
poly I:poly C, 6 hr after ABMP or phosphate-buffered saline (PBS), and
18 hr after tilorone HCl.
[b]Number in parentheses is percentage of uninfected control response.
Source: Reprinted from Ref. 55 with permission of the American Society
for Microbiology.

other hand, could increase the interferon response of hyporeactive cells
or animals but had little or no effect on the responsiveness of normal cells
or animals (Figures 4 and 5) [61]. The prostaglandin restoration phenomena
appeared to be ubiquitous in that animals infected with any of several viruses
including EMC, SFV, A$_2$ influenza virus, and Friend leukemia virus were
restored in their ability to respond to a variety of interferon inducers.
These results are particularly important, since they suggest that prostaglandins may be able to significantly enhance therapeutic efficacy of interferon
inducers as antiviral agents. At present, a firm correlation does not exist
between the state of hyporeactivity that develops as a consequence of multiple

TABLE 8. Comparison of Hyporeactive and Normal
Interferon-Producing Cells[a]

Macromolecular synthesis	
DNA	same
RNA	same
Protein	same
Morphology (SEM)	same
Inducer uptake	
NDV	same
CV	same
Doubling time	same
Adenylate cyclase	Hyporeactive cells (lower ($< 70\%$ of normal)
cyclic AMP	Hyporeactive cells (20–25% of normal)

[a]Hyporeactive cells were peritoneal cells from EMC-virus-infected mice
(96 hr) or mouse embryo cells incubated with serum from EMC-virus-
infected mice. Normal cells were from uninfected mice or cells incubated
with normal mouse serum.

doses of inducer and prostaglandins. Preliminary evidence indicates that
prostaglandins can, in specific instances, restore the ability of mice
rendered hyporeactive by multiple doses of poly I:poly C to respond to a
second dose of the same or another inducer, for example, tilorone hydrochloride. Prostaglandins have not, however, consistently been able to
increase responsiveness. This may indicate that other mechanisms may
be involved in the development of hyporeactivity following multiple doses
of inducer. Development of hyporeactivity may be a reflection of several
mechanisms, including the ability of animals to clear compounds from the
circulation and the reticuloendothelial system. For example, many
low-molecular-weight inducers, such as anthraquinones and tilorone
hydrochloride, are not rapidly cleared by the animal and persist in the
reticuloendothelial system for extended periods of time (Chapter 7). Animals dosed with such agents are not amenable to prostaglandin restoration
of interferon responsiveness, whereas poly I:poly C is rapidly cleared and
animals injected with it appear to be the most sensitive in their ability to
be restored by prostaglandin administration. At present, evidence indicates
that prostaglandins can restore the response of hyporeactive animals and
may be able to significantly improve the therapeutic efficacy of interferon
inducers in experimental viral infections or neoplastic diseases.

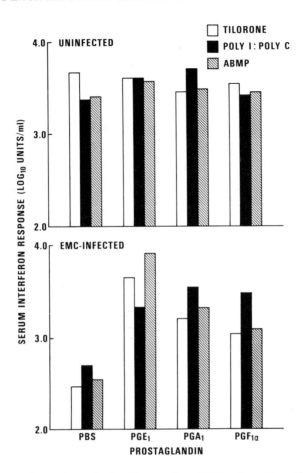

FIGURE 4. Effect of prostaglandins on the ability of peritoneal cells from normal or hyporeactive (EMC–virus–infected) mice to respond to interferon inducers in vitro. Prostaglandins were added to cells 30 min after inducer (Newcastle disease virus, NDV). Growth medium was collected 24 hr after the addition of inducer and was assayed for interferon.

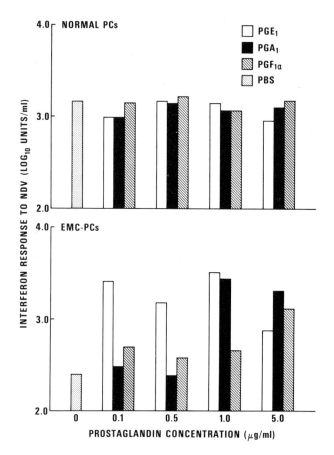

FIGURE 5. Prostaglandin enhancement of the serum interferon response
of hyporeactive (EMC-virus-infected) but not normal uninfected mice.
Inducers were injected 96 hr after infection, and prostaglandins (1 mg/kg,
i.p.) were administered 30 min later.

VI. TOXICITY

Another problem facing the development of most of the presently known
interferon inducers is toxic side effects associated with drug administration.
Only a few inducers have been given to humans. The chief side effects
observed in animals have included, depending upon the inducer, inability
of the animal to clear the compound from its system and toxic manifestations such as leukopenia, fever, headache, nausea, lethargy, insomnia,
and changes in hematopoietic and liver function ([31-34,62]; see also

Chapters 7, 8, and 10). Data from experimental animals firmly suggest that many of the presently known interferon inducers have too many undesirable side effects. For example, tilorone caused many of the toxic manifestations listed above in dogs and cats, and the drug was apparently deposited in various tissues for extended periods of time ([63]; see also Chapter 8). Poly I:poly C, likewise, has caused many of the side effects listed above in experimental animals. It had a maximum tolerated dose of less than 4 mg/kg (i.v.) in cats [64]; yet it appeared to be well tolerated at low doses in children, with little toxicity being observed [34], although only low levels of interferon were induced at the doses given. A series of pyrimidine molecules that we have been developing have a toxic manifestation that appears to be due to insolubility. As reported by Levine [65] and confirmed in our own laboratories (J. Gray, unpublished results), following systemic or oral administration of fairly large doses of 2-amino-5-bromo-6-methyl-4-pyrimidinol (ABMP, 300 mg/kg), the drug crystallized in the kidneys of rats, causing tubular obstruction. The rat appears to be very sensitive to development of this side effect, since rabbits, cats, and dogs maintained on similar treatment regimens did not develop tubular obstruction even though in some cases slight crystallization was observed in kidneys and urine. Not all members of this group of inducers caused this side effect, and specific analogs have been identified that have the same or greater antiviral activity yet do not crystallize in kidneys [66-67].

New inducing molecules—or analogs of currently known inducers with less toxicity and fewer side effects—need to be developed if these agents are to be used in the treatment of mild, self-limiting infections such as the common cold. Side effects that have been reported with most inducers probably would be acceptable if they were being used in treatment of gravely ill persons with various life-threatening viral infections or neoplasias.

VII. EFFECT OF INDUCERS ON IMMUNE SYSTEMS

A great deal of attention has recently been focused on interferon as a key regulator of the immune response. As might be expected, inducers likewise appear to affect the immune response and appear to have actions separable from those mediated specifically by interferon (see Chapters 10 and 11). Inducers appear to affect the humoral and cellular immune response and also macrophage function, either enhancing or depressing activity depending on dosage or route of administration with regard to immunogen and the parameter being investigated. The fact that inducers can mediate macrophage function is particularly interesting with the current interest in immune modulators. The development of an agent that could have at least three modes of action that could account for the antiviral and antitumor activity may not be unrealistic. The agent could induce interferon, have direct antiviral activity, and modulate the immune response. The potential of inducers in treating transplant patients may be particularly important to investigate, if a compound could be identified that depresses T-cell function while inducing interferon or having other antiviral activity.

VIII. OUTLOOK

The future for the development of interferon inducers appears to be bright, particularly if molecules can be identified that are devoid of the problems currently being encountered. Toxicity must be decreased without markedly reducing, and hopefully increasing, the antiviral activity of such agents. This may be particularly difficult to do, since minor changes of the structure of most interferon-inducing molecules markedly affects (generally depresses) antiviral activity. This is further complicated by the fact that simply because interferon inducers are effective in mice is no guarantee that the same compound will have equivalent activity in humans. A system for predicting the ability of molecules to induce interferon in humans therefore needs to be established, and then not until enough inducers have been evaluated in humans will it be known whether the system is accurate. Development of hyporeactivity due to infection or multiple doses of an inducer would appear to be an avoidable and reversible event. By proper selection of treatment regimens, inducers can be given in combination with other inducing agents or in a proper time sequence that will allow avoidance of the hyporeactive state. The recent observation that prostaglandins can restore the interferon responsiveness of hyporeactive virus-infected animals suggests that the therapeutic efficacy of inducers may be significantly enhanced by co-administration of prostaglandins with inducing agents. Reports that interferon and its inducers modulate immune responsiveness have significantly broadened the horizon of inducer development. They suggest that in the future inducers should be developed not only for their ability to stimulate interferon production or conversely mediate antiviral activity, but that their ability to enhance macrophage activity and suppress or enhance the cellular or humoral immune response may be just as critical to consider. Answers to many of the remaining questions should be forthcoming in the next few years as compounds at various stages of preclinical development advance toward clinical evaluations.

REFERENCES

1. A. Isaacs and J. Lindenmann, Proc. Roy. Soc., Ser. B 147: 258 (1957).
2. Y. Nagano and Y. Kujima, C. R. Soc. Biol. 154: 2172 (1958).
3. J. S. Youngner and W. R. Stinebring, Science 144: 1022 (1964).

4. P. De Somer, E. DeClercq, C. Cocito, and A. Billiau, Ann. N.Y. Acad. Sci. 173:274 (1970).
5. H. E. Hopps, S. Kohno, M. Kohno, and S. E. Smadel, Bacteriol. Proc. 115:92 (1964).
6. M. W. Rytel and T. C. Jones, Proc. Soc. Exp. Biol. Med. 123:859 (1966).
7. M. M. Freshman, T. C. Merigan, J. S. Remington, and I. E. Brownlee, Proc. Soc. Exp. Biol. Med. 123:862 (1966).
8. W. R. Stinebring and J. S. Youngner, Nature 204:712 (1964).
9. M. Ho, Science 146:1472 (1964).
10. E. F. Wheelock, Science 149:310 (1965).
11. R. M. Friedman and H. L. Cooper, Proc. Soc. Exp. Biol. Med. 125:901 (1967).
12. L. A. Glasgow, J. Bacteriol. 91:2185 (1966).
13. J. A. Green, S. R. Cooperband, and S. Kibrick, Science 164:1415 (1969).
14. A. K. Field, A. A. Tytell, G. P. Lampson, and M. R. Hilleman, Proc. Nat. Acad. Sci. U.S. 58:1004 (1967).
15. T. C. Merigan, Nature 214:416 (1967).
16. G. D. Mayer and R. F. Krueger, Science 169:1214 (1970).
17. W. W. Hoffman, J. J. Korst, J. F. Niblack, and T. H. Cronin, Antimicrob. Agents. Chemother. 3:498 (1973).
18. E. T. Glaz, E. Szolgay, I. Stoger, and M. Talas, Antimicrob. Agents Chemother. 3:537 (1973).
19. F. R. Nichol, S. D. Weed, and G. E. Underwood, Antimicrob. Agents Chemother. 9:433 (1976).
20. J. M. Grisar, K. R. Hickey, R. W. Fleming, and G. D. Mayer, Biochem. Biophys. Res. Commun. 73:149 (1976).
21. A. A. Carr, J. F. Gunwell, A. D. Sill, D. R. Meyer, F. W. Sweet, B. J. Schweve, J. M. Grisnar, R. W. Fleming, and G. D. Mayer, J. Med. Chem. 19:1142 (1976).
22. P. Chandra and M. Woltersdorf, FEBS Lett. 41:169 (1974).
23. C. Colby and M. J. Chamberlin, Proc. Nat. Acad. Sci. U.S. 63:160 (1969).
24. E. DeClercq, F. Eckstein, and T. C. Merigan, Ann. N.Y. Acad. Sci. 173:444 (1970).
25. E. DeClercq and T. C. Merigan, Nature 222:1148 (1969).
26. P. F. Torrence and B. Witkop, Proteins, Nucleic Acids and Enzymes 21:536 (1976).
27. P. F. Torrence and E. DeClercq, Biochemistry 16:1039 (1977).
28. P. F. Torrence and E. DeClercq, Pharmacol. Therapeut. 2:1 (1977).
29. W. A. Carter, P. M. Pitha, L. W. Marshall, I. Tazawa, S. Tazawa, and P. O. P. Ts'o, J. Mol. Biol. 70:567 (1972).
30. J. Portnoy and T. C. Merigan, J. Infec. Dis. 124:545 (1971).

31. H. E. Kaufman, Y. M. Centifanto, E. D. Ellison, and D. C. Brown, Proc. Soc. Exp. Biol. Med. 137:357 (1971).

32. A. K. Field, C. W. Young, I. H. Krakoff, A. A. Tyteh, G. P. Lampson, M. M. Nemes, and M. R. Hilleman, Proc. Soc. Exp. Biol. Med. 136:1180 (1971).

33. A. K. Field, A. A. Tytell, E. Piperno, G. P. Lampson, M. M. Nemes, and M. R. Hilleman, Medicine 51:169 (1972).

34. M. A. Guggenheim and S. Baron, J. Infec. Dis. 136:50 (1977).

35. H. B. Levy, W. London, D. A. Fucillo, S. Baron, and J. Rice, J. Infec. Dis. 133:A256 (1975).

36. D. A. Stringfellow and S. D. Weed, Amer. J. Vet. Res. 38:1963 (1977).

37. D. A. Stringfellow and L. A. Glasgow, Antimicrob. Agents Chemother. 2:73 (1972).

38. P. Siminoff, J. Infec. Dis. 133A:37 (1976).

39. Y. Ito, I. Nagata and A. Kunji, Virology 52:439 (1973).

40. M. Ho, M. C. Breinig and N. Maehara, J. Infec. Dis. 133A:30 (1976).

41. F. Dianzani and S. Baron, Nature 257:682 (1975).

42. F. Dianzani and S. Baron, Proc. Soc. Exp. Biol. Med. 155:562 (1977).

43. F. Dianzani, I. Viano, M. Santiano, M. Zucca, and S. Baron, Proc. Soc. Exp. Biol. Med. 155:445 (1977).

44. M. Ho and Y. Kono, J. Clin. Invest. 44:1059 (1965).

45. M. Ho, Y. Kono, and M. K. Brening, Proc. Soc. Exp. Biol. Med. 119:1227 (1965).

46. C. E. Buckler, H. G. DuBuy, M. L. Johnson, and S. Baron, Proc. Soc. Exp. Biol. Med. 136:394 (1971).

47. H. G. DuBuy, M. L. Johnson, C. E. Buckler, and S. Baron, Proc. Soc. Exp. Biol. Med. 135:340 (1970).

48. E. DeClercq, Proc. Soc. Exp. Biol. Med. 141:340 (1971).

49. M. C. Breinig, J. A. Armstrong, and M. Ho, J. Gen. Virol. 26: 149 (1975).

50. G. H. Bansek and T. C. Merigan, Proc. Soc. Exp. Biol. Med. 134: 672 (1970).

51. E. T. Glaz and M. Talas, Arch. Virol. 48:375 (1975).

52. F. I. Yershov, E. B. Tazulakhov, and A. S. Novokhatsky, Acta Virol. 20:15 (1976).

53. D. A. Stringfellow, S. D. Weed, and G. E. Underwood, Antimicrob. Agents Chemother. 15:111 (1979).

54. D. J. Giron, J. P. Schmidt, F. F. Pindak, and J. E. Connell, Acta Virol. 17:209 (1973).

55. D. A. Stringfellow, Antimicrob. Agents Chemother. 11:984 (1977).

56. J. DeMaeyer-Guignard, Science 177:797 (1972).

57. D. A. Holtermann and E. A. Havell, J. Gen. Virol. 9:101 (1970).

58. D. A. Stringfellow and L. A. Glasgow, Infec. Immun. 6:743 (1972).

59. J. E. Osborn and D. N. Medearis, Proc. Soc. Exp. Biol. Med. 124: 347 (1967).

60. D. A. Stringfellow, E. R. Kern, D. K. Kelsey, and L. A. Glasgow, J. Infec. Dis. 135:540 (1977).
61. D. A. Stringfellow, Science 201:376 (1978).
62. P. O. P. Ts'o, J. L. Alderfer, J. Levy, L. W. Marshall, J. O'Malley, J. S. Horoszewicz, and W. A. Carter, Mol. Pharmacol. 12:299 (1976).
63. M. W. Rohovsky, J. W. Newberne, and J. P. Gibson, Toxicol. Appl. Pharmacol. 17:556 (1970).
64. B. McCullough, J. Infec. Dis. 125:174 (1972).
65. S. Levine and R. Sowinski, Toxicol. Appl. Pharmacol. 42:603 (1977).
66. D. A. Stringfellow and S. D. Weed, J. Clin. Hematol. Oncol. in press (1980).
67. D. A. Stringfellow, H. C. Vanderberg, and S. D. Weed, Curr. Chemother. Infec. Dis. in press (1980).

7

INDUCTION OF INTERFERON
BY POLYNUCLEOTIDES

Hilton B. Levy

National Institute of Allergy and Infectious Diseases
Bethesda, Maryland

I. INTRODUCTION

Interferon was first named in 1957 by Isaacs and Lindenman [1]. At about the same time Nagano and Kojina [2] and Chany [3] were reporting analogous findings. While many were skeptical about the existence of interferon, it was realized by some that interferon potentially represented a broadspectrum antiviral agent that could have widespread clinical application. The realization of this potential has been painfully slow. The difficulty of preparing large quantities of interferon has kept the supply at a very low level and the price very high. It has been estimated that a mouse might make about $1-2 \times 10^6$ units (U) of interferon in response to a virus infection. If one wanted to treat the infected mouse with interferon, the slope of the dose-response curve would suggest that perhaps $2\text{-}6 \times 10^6$ additional units of interferon should be given to augment significantly the antiviral effect. Until recently this represented several liters of mouse interferon. With humans, the situation would be even more dramatic. Recently, as a result of the work of many laboratories, the situation has become a good deal better, and very limited, very costly experiments in humans are beginning. Even now, for the foreseeable future, the use of interferon itself in human disease will be severely limited by cost and availability.

II. EARLY STUDIES

Attention was turned, therefore, to finding nonviral inducers that would cause the host to synthesize large quantities of its own interferon, and a number of such materials were found. The types are tabulated in Table 1.

Of the several inducer types, some are active both in tissue culture and in vivo, and others are effective primarily in vivo. The latter, in some instances, have been shown to induce interferon in cultures of leukocytes, macrophages, or spleen cells.

By far the most effective nonviral interferon inducers have been the double-stranded ribonucleic acids (RNA). Two series of experiments led to their discovery. Isaacs [4] postulated that interferon production is the cell's response to the presence of foreign nucleic acid. He presented some data that indeed indicated that treatment of tissue culture cells with nucleic acids extracted from heterologous cells induced the formation of interferon. Even chemical modification of homologous nucleic acids with nitrous acid was sufficient to make the nucleic acid an interferon inducer. However, the amount of interferon induced was very small, the experiments were hard to reproduce, and the question of nucleic acid induction of interferon was held in abeyance. More direct evidence leading to the development of

TABLE 1. Nonviral Inducers of Interferon

1. Endotoxins	7. Fungal viruses
2. Bacteria	8. Natural and synthetic nucleic acids
3. Trachoma-inclusion conjunctivitis agents	9. Synthetic polymers and other chemicals
4. Mycoplasmas	10. Mitogens
5. Protozoa	11. Polysaccharides
6. Rickettsiae	12. Antibiotics

the double-stranded RNAs came from work with helenine [5], a crude
material found in cultures of Penicillium funiculosum, which shows antiviral activity [6]. Helenine contains a ribonucleoprotein [7] that stimulates
tissue culture cells and mice to make interferon [8]. When helenine was
extracted with phenol and the resulting product partially purified, a double-
stranded RNA was obtained which was able to induce interferon [9]. It was
later shown that the double-stranded RNA was derived from a virus that
infected the P. funiculosum [10].

III. DOUBLE-STRANDED RNA: EARLY WORK

A series of papers from workers at Merck, Sharp and Dohme [11-15]
showed that a variety of both natural and synthetic double-stranded RNAs
were effective interferon inducers in tissue cultures and in rodents. The
homopolymer pair, polyriboinosinic-polyribocytidylic acid was the most
effective of the synthetics, with polyriboadenylic-polyribouridylic acid being
significantly less so. As little as 0.5 µg of poly I:poly C given intravenously
to a rabbit induced detectable interferon. In some tissue culture cells,
even less of the compound is effective. In general, single-stranded RNAs
are less active as inducers; although under some conditions, they can cause
the production of significant amounts.

The observations regarding poly I:poly C's capacity to induce interferon
in rodents triggered a search for compounds that would be even more effective. From these studies there has emerged the realization that a number
of structural requirements must be combined in a compound in order for it
to be a good interferon inducer. For a more detailed review of the structural modifications that have been examined, see the review by DeClercq
[16].

(1) There needs to be a secondary structure that is stable at the temperature of the test. The two strands of each double-stranded RNA disassociate
from each other at a specific transition temperature, the melting temperature (T_m), which is a measure of the stability of that double-stranded RNA.
If one attempts to correlate the T_m values of a group of double-stranded
RNAs with their ability to induce interferon, one can discern a trend toward
correlation. However, there are so many exceptions that it is obvious that
other factors in addition to the degree of thermal stability are important.
Single-stranded RNAs that have secondary structure can induce interferon
both in vitro and in tissue cultures although, in general, not nearly so well
as double-stranded RNA [17,18,19,20]. It would appear that secondary
structure, not necessarily double-strandedness, is a requirement for activity.

(2) Another factor that is important, though not dominant, in determining the degree of activity of a double-stranded RNA is its resistance to the
action of ribonucleases. The single-stranded RNA, poly AU, is a poor

inducer of interferon. When thiophosphates are substituted for the phosphate groups, the resultant poly (AsUs) is much more resistant to nuclease action and is a better inducer than poly AU [21]. However, there are exceptions to this generality. The effect of differences in the amount of nuclease action in the sera of different animal species will be mentioned later.

In the one case where it has been possible to study a series of chemically identical double-stranded RNAs with differing molecular weights, it appears that a certain minimum molecular weight is necessary for action [22]. Poly I:poly C with a molecular weight of 1.5×10^5 is inactive, but the compound with a molecular weight of 2.7×10^5 or higher is active.

However, the differences according to others are small [16]. In particular the size of the poly I strand is more important than that of the poly C strand; complexes made with poly I of s values equal to 12.5 S in tissue culture yield slightly more interferon than do complexes made with poly I of s = 2.5 S. Here s is the sedimentation coefficient and S is the svedberg unit (10^{-13} sec).

(3) A ribose backbone is needed. Single- or double-stranded DNAs induce little or no interferon [23] in spite of generally high T_m values. If the 2'-hydroxy groups on the ribose are esterified with a methyl group, the double-stranded RNA loses its interferon-inducing activity.

The list of antiviral drugs of any type that are effective in vivo is small indeed. Poly I:poly C is the most successful. Its effect has been largely limited to rodents and rabbits. This fact will be referred to again later. Two examples of the antiviral action are as follows. When rabbit eyes are abraded and infected with herpes virus, they develop a keratoconjunctivitis resembling the human disease. Figure 1 shows the data obtained by Park and Baron in treating this disease with poly I:poly C in the form of eye drops [24]. The abscissa is the time in days after infection; the ordinate is a number obtained by combining the evaluation of several clinical parameters. The higher the number, the more severe the disease. It can be seen that if treatment is begun on the same day as infection, no disease develops. One can wait as long as three days after infection to begin treatment and still have significant curative effect. However, if treatment begins on day 4, the drug is without therapeutic value.

In other experiments by Worthington and Baron [25], mice were infected with Semliki Forest virus (SFV), a virus that causes fatal encephalitis. Figure 2 plots the percentage of the animals that die as a function of days after infection, with and without treatment by poly I:poly C. It can be seen that untreated animals were dying by day 5. Virus was replicating in the brain by day 4. However, initiation of treatment even after virus was in the brain resulted in a significant decrease in the mortality rate.

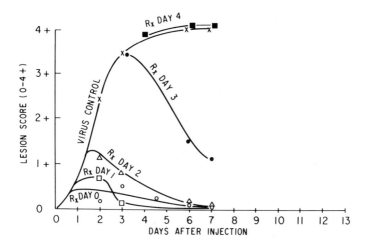

FIGURE 1. Response of herpetic keratoconjunctivitis to topical treatment with poly I: poly C. R_X indicates treatment.

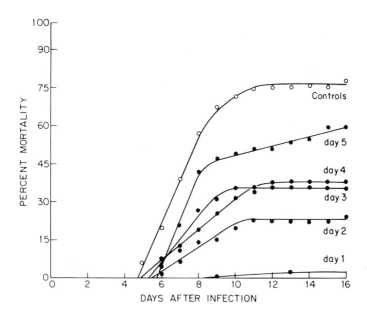

FIGURE 2. Treatment of Semliki Forest virus (SFV) infection in mice with poly I: poly C.

IV. DOUBLE-STRANDED RNA AND TUMORS

Levy et al. studied the effect of poly I: poly C on tumors [26]. Table 2
gives a partial list of the tumors looked at. The sensitivity of different
tumors to the drug is quite variable, with some being quite sensitive, and
some, the fast growing leukemias, being affected just barely significantly
[27,28,29]. With the more sensitive tumors, there were up to one-third
survivors. The mechanism of this antitumor action is complex and will
not be discussed in detail, but there appears to be at least three factors
involved. The first is that poly I: poly C induces the formation of interferon
in mice, and interferon has antitumor action [30]. Second, poly I: poly C
is a potent enhancer of immune reactivity, particularly cell-mediated
immunity, the type that is thought to play an important role in natural host
defense mechanisms against tumors [31,32]. Third, there is a more or
less specific inhibition of tumor macromolecule synthesis in some of the
animal tumor systems [33]. These three elements may interplay in different quantitative degrees in the different tumors.

V. POLY I: POLY C IN PRIMATES

Unfortunately, human response to poly I: poly C is very weak, even with
high doses of the drug [34-36]. Levels of 50 U/ml of serum were found,
but usually not much more, as contrasted with perhaps 50,000 U/ml in
mice. Rhesus monkeys and chimpanzees were totally nonresponsive to
poly I: poly C.
     A possible explanation for poor primate response to poly I: poly C is
that there is present in primate serum a relatively high concentration of
nucleolytic enzymes that hydrolyze and inactivate poly I: poly C, much more
than is present in rodent serum [37]. By and large those species of animals
whose sera showed a large capacity to hydrolyze were poor responders,
and good responders had low hydrolytic capacity. Efforts were made, therefore, to develop a derivative that would be more resistant to hydrolysis.

VI. STABILIZED POLY I: POLY C (POLY ICLC)

Poly I: poly C forms a complex with poly-lysine, but the complex is not
soluble and, therefore, is not useful clinically. However, if a hydrophilic
complex between poly-L-lysine and carboxymethyl cellulose is first formed,
then poly I: poly C will combine with this hydrophilic poly-L-lysine to give
a derivative (poly ICLC) that is soluble in saline and partially resistant to
hydrolysis (Figure 3) [38].
     That poly ICLC is a more stable structure to thermal denaturation
than is poly I: poly C is shown in Figure 4. Poly ICLC in 0.15 M NaCl

TABLE 2.   Effect of Poly I: Poly C on Animal Tumors[a]

Tumor	Percentage of increase in median survival over control
J96132 rcticulum cell sarcoma (subcutaneous)	130[b]
J96132 reticulum cell sarcoma (ascites)	96[b]
Carcinosarcoma Walker 256	100
Reticulum cell sarcoma RCSL	89
Ehrlich ascites tumor	70
S91 Melanoma	55
Fibrosarcoma	52
B1237 lymphoma (ascites)	45
L1210 leukemia	42
Plasma cell YPC-1	39
B1237 lymphoma (subcutaneous)	28
MT-1 tumor (subcutaneous)	26
Reticulum cell sarcoma ovarian	20
Leukemia P388	16
Leukemia K1964	12

[a]Treatment, in most cases, was 150-200 µg/mouse, three times weekly, by intraperitoneal route. With the exception of the J96132 reticulum cell sarcoma, some Ehrlich ascites tumors, and a few Walker carcinosarcoma, all animals ultimately died.

[b]Mean day of death of the animals that died. About 30% of all the animals treated have survived, although treatment had been stopped at about day 50.

does not denature below 100°C, whereas poly I:poly C has a T_m of 62.5°C. It is necessary to dilute the salt to 0.01 5 M to obtain a T_m of 87°C for the complex, while plain poly I:poly C melts at about 49°C.

The compound was slightly more effective in mice as an interferon inducer than poly I:poly C, as shown in Figure 5. Serum interferon was detectable slightly earlier, rose to a somewhat higher titer, and was present longer. Not surprisingly, poly ICLC is a somewhat better antiviral agent in mice than is poly I:poly C (L. Glasgow, unpublished data).

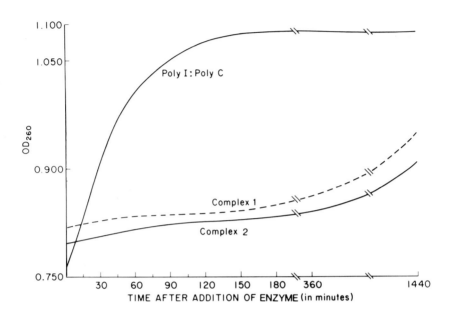

FIGURE 3. Hydrolysis of poly I: poly C and two different lots of the poly-L-lysine complex of poly I: poly C by pancreatic RNase. The complexes, at a concentration of 50 μg poly I: poly C/ml in 0.15 M NaCl and 0.001 M phosphate buffer (pH 7.2), were exposed to 5 μg pancreatic RNase/ml at room temperature (about 24°C). Optical density (OD) readings at 260 nm were taken at 10 min intervals.

Of greater interest was the fact that poly ICLC was an effective inducer in monkeys (Figure 6) and chimpanzees. Interferon levels as high as 15,000 U/ml of serum have been found in cynomolgus monkeys under conditions where no interferon was induced by poly I: poly C. However, levels between 200 and 2000 U are more regularly seen.

The new compound is an effective antiviral agent in monkeys. Monkeys infected with street rabies virus could be effectively protected by poly ICLC together with antirabies vaccine, as shown in Table 3 [39]. Vaccine alone had little or no protective effect in several experiments.

Comparable results were obtained with yellow fever virus, Tacharibe virus, Japanese encephalitis virus, Pichinde virus, and with simian hemorrhagic fever virus, all of which are ordinarily lethal for monkeys [40,41], as well as with Russian spring-summer encephalitis and vaccinial keratitis [42,43].

There is an animal model of chronic hepatitis in young chimpanzees. Figure 7 shows the effect of treatment of such infected chimps with poly

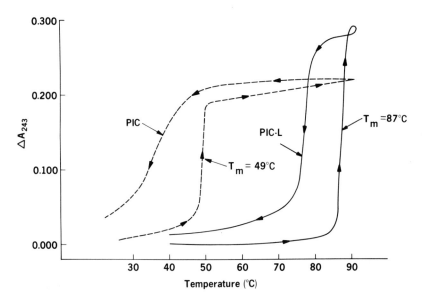

FIGURE 4. Thermal denaturation of poly I:poly C and the poly-L-lysine complex of poly I:poly C (PIC-L). The compounds, at a concentration of 50 μg poly I:poly C/ml in 0.1 standard saline-citrate, were heated to the indicated temperatures in a recording spectrophotometer set at 243 nm. (T_m = melting temperature.)

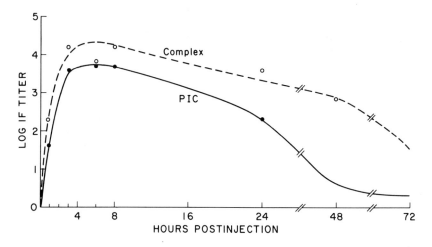

FIGURE 5. Kinetics of induction of serum interferon (IF) in mice after intravenous administration of 5 mg/kg poly I:poly C or poly ICLC.

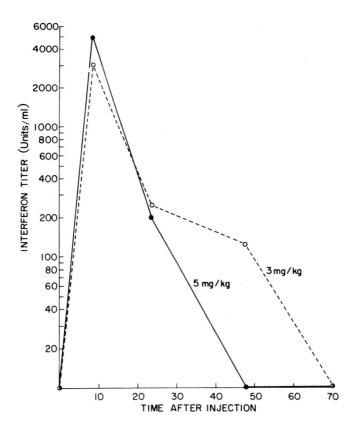

FIGURE 6. Kinetics of induction of serum interferon in rhesus monkeys by administration of 3 or 5 mg/kg poly ICLC.

TABLE 3. Effects of Poly ICLC Treatment in Postexposure Prophylaxis of Rabies in Monkeys

Treatment	No. dead/No. treated
Poly ICLC + vaccine 24 and 72 hr postinfection	1/8
Vaccine 24,48, and 72 hr postinfection	7/8
Controls, untreated	8/8

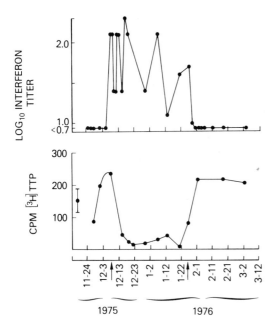

FIGURE 7. The treatment of chronic hepatitis in young chimpanzees with poly I: poly C. The interferon titer is shown above, and the polymerase activity is shown below. The beginning and end of the treatment period are indicated by arrows on the abscissa. The dot and bar on the graph of DNA polymerase response indicate the mean (+1 SD) of polymerase activity detected in six serum samples obtained during the five weeks immediately preceding the experiment.

ICLC [44]. It can be seen that when the animals are injected with poly ICLC, they produce interferon. A marker of the progress of the infection is the level of DNA-dependent polymerase in the blood. During the course of the treatment the polymerase activity fell to background level. When treatment stopped, evidence of the disease returned. Whether really prolonged treatment would have a more permanent effect has yet to be determined.

Vaccinia virus infection in the skin in rabbits can be a severe, sometimes fatal infection. Rabbits were injected intradermally with vaccinia virus. After the lesions became visible, some rabbits were treated daily with an ointment containing the drug. A comparison of the treated and the nontreated rabbits is seen in Figure 8. The infection essentially did not progress after initiation of treatment [45].

One last effect of poly ICLC should be mentioned. It has proven to be a potent booster of antibody response to at least two virus vaccines, Vene-

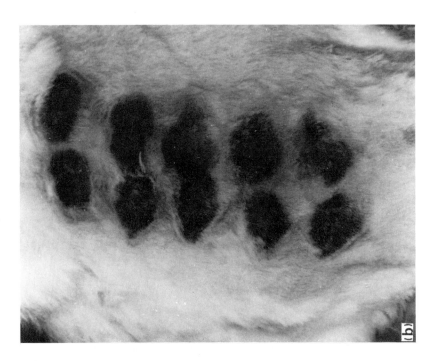

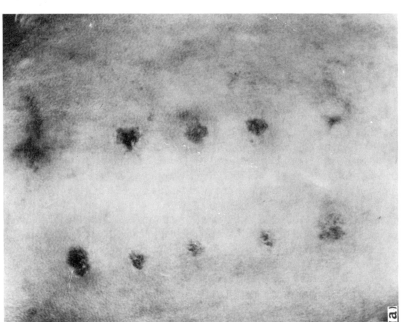

FIGURE 8. Effect of poly ICLC ointment on cutaneous vaccinia infection in rabbits. (A) Poly ICLC treated. (B) Placebo treated.

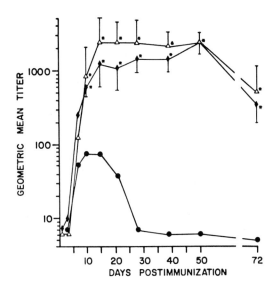

FIGURE 9. Adjuvant effects of poly ICLC on inactivated Venezuelan equine encephalitis virus vaccine in rhesus monkeys. Standard errors are shown where significant differences occur as compared to controls. Key: △, KVEE + 3 mg/kg;◆ , KVEE + 1 mg/kg; ●, KVEE controls; *, P = < 0.01.

zuelan equine encephalitis virus vaccine [46] and swine flu vaccine [47], and to a bacterial vaccine, Hemophilus influenzae (H. Levy, E. Stephen, and A. Anderson, unpublished data). Figure 9 shows some of the results obtained with Venezuelan equine encephalitis virus vaccine. It can be seen that one dose of the drug, together with the vaccine, boosts antibody response by about 80-fold and increases the time during which antibody can be detected.

VII. STUDIES IN HUMANS WITH POLY I: POLY C

Several studies in humans are ongoing. Levine et al. have completed a phase I study of human response and toxicity in terminal cancer patients [48] to determine (1) a dose response curve and (2) the highest tolerated level of drug. In this group of 35 patients, serum interferon levels of about 100 U/ml were seen at a dose of about 100 μg/kg body weight. Peak levels of up to 15,000 U/ml of serum were seen at 510 and 770 μg/kg body weight. These latter levels of drug were associated with unacceptable levels of toxicity; 350 μg/kg was judged to be the highest acceptable dose, with mean peak titers of interferon of about 2000 U/ml of serum being achieved. A relative absence of hyporesponsiveness was seen at higher drug levels in rhesus and cynomolgus monkeys [49].

We (A. M. Lerner, J. Crane, and H. B. Levy) are currently testing the drug as a topically applied ointment in a double-blind study of herpes genitalis. Champney, Lerner, and Levy [50] gave the drug intravenously to a few patients with St. Louis encephalitis (as described later). Levels of serum interferon comparable to those noted by Levine et al. [48] were found. Engel et al. [51] have given poly ICLC to two patients with amyotropic lateral sclerosis (ALS) and to one patient with a chronic relapsing neuropathy, possibly associated with an immunological distrophy. These patients responded with slightly higher levels of serum interferon than did the other groups. There was no clinical improvement in the ALS patients. However, the patient with chronic relapsing neuropathy showed a dramatic clinical improvement. In addition, his cerebrospinal fluid protein fell from 105 to 40 μg/ml. At this writing he is continuing to improve.

VIII. TOXICITY OF POLY I: POLY C

Some problems with poly ICLC should be mentioned. All double-stranded RNAs are pyrogenic, and this one is no exception. In humans, temperatures up to 40.5° C have been seen, although 39.5° C is usual. The fever usually is gone in 5-6 hr. Some differences have been found in other reactivities among the three human studies mentioned above. Levine and Levy found, particularly at the higher levels of drug, that leukopenia (down to 2000 WBC/mm^3) and hypotension (to below 90 mm systolic) occurred in about 30% of the cases. Lerner and Levy found leukopenia and hypotension in most of their cases (patients with high fevers from the disease at the onset of treatment), and Engel et al. [51] found leukopenia but no hypotension. A frequent finding is myalgia and a group of flu-like symptoms. There are suggestions that the use of lower-molecular-weight poly I: poly C in the complex may result in a drug with fewer side effects (A. M. Lerner, B. Gatmaitan, and H. B. Levy, unpublished data). It might be noted that treatment of humans with interferon has itself elicited many of the same undesirable effects as those mentioned above with poly ICLC. In none of the studies has it been necessary to abandon treatment except with the highest levels of drug.

It was mentioned earlier that primates hydrolyze poly I: poly C faster than do rodents, and the suggestion was made that this increased hydrolysis might explain the weak response of primates to poly I: poly C. Consistent with this suggestion are the observations made with poly ICLC preparations which have been made with different molecular weights of poly-L-lysine. With poly-L-lysine of molecular weight 2000, the complex formed is perhaps twice as resistant to hydrolysis as plain poly I: poly C, in contrast to 8-10 times more resistant for the complex made with poly-L-lysine of molecular weight 25,000. The former complex induces perhaps 10-20% as much interferon in monkeys as does the complex made with high-molecular weight poly-lysine.

IX. OTHER MODIFICATIONS OF POLY I: POLY C

In the past the induction of interferon by any means has generally been associated with a certain level of undesirable side effects. In humans and in many animal species, at least some of these symptoms were found when interferon itself was administered. Attempts to dissociate the reactogenicity from the interferon or interferon induction have not been particularly rewarding. Recently a group of workers have reported some success in such dissociation [52-54]. These workers postulate that the several biological effects of the polynucleotide inducers—interferon induction, pyrogenicity, possible effects on blood cell elements, etc.—require different lengths of time of contact with the responsible specific cell population, and that interferon induction requires the shortest length of time of cell contact. They prepared complexes of poly I with other copolymers containing either 13 cytosine to one uracil molecule or 29 cytosine to one guanine, to yield $rI_n \, r(C_{13}, \, U)_n$, or $rI_n \, r(C_{29}, \, G)_n$. These compounds are thermodymically less stable than poly I: poly C and more readily hydrolyzable by RNase. According to the hypothesis of these workers, when these compounds are administered to an animal, they will be hydrolyzed and eliminated rapidly, with an existence only sufficiently long to stimulate the production of interferon and resistance to viral infection. The data presented are indeed consistent with their hypothesis. These authors point out the difficulty in defining toxicity and therefore take as their definition that toxicity is any biological alteration other than the induction of interferon. One of the mismatched analogs of poly I: poly C induced significant interferon and resistance to virus infection, both in tissue culture and in rodents, although perhaps not quite so much interferon as poly I: poly C [53]. The mismatched compounds appeared less pyrogenic in rabbits, caused less stimulation of spleen cells, as measured by thymidine uptake, and required larger amounts for acute toxicity in mice when compared with poly I: poly C. In addition, in rodents there were somewhat less chronic effects, such as lymphopenia and anemia, occasioned by the mismatched analogs than by poly I: poly C. No studies were made in primates. It may indeed be that the ease of hydrolysis of these compounds does reduce their half-life in rodents, and consequently their reactogenicity. However, it may also prove to be that the ease of hydrolysis will render them ineffective in primates.

X. GENERAL CONSIDERATIONS

There are several general considerations that should be mentioned in a discussion of polynucleotide inducers of interferon. In one limited sense, the use of the inducer can be thought of as just an alternative way of administering interferon. As such, the drug has some advantages; it is very much cheaper, it is available on a scale that makes it a practical item in materia medica, and it is able, under certain conditions, to result in the presence of higher serum levels of interferon than can presently be obtained through the use of exogenous interferon.

On the other hand, there are some major differences between the administration of interferon and the administration of the polynucleotide inducers. While interferon does cause the same type of undesirable side effects that poly ICLC does, it may be that the inducers show stronger reactions. It is possible that these quantitative differences are associated with the higher levels of interferon induced, or it may be that the drug per se is more reactogenic. It does seem that the drug induces more fever than interferon. In addition, interferon, at least in tissue culture systems, appears to inhibit most immune reactions tested. Whether this will hold true in the intact host is not known. Poly ICLC, on the other hand, acts as an immune stimulant where it has been tested. Indeed, this may turn out to be a clinically useful feature, because such immune stimulation has been found at levels of drug well below those that induce any adverse reactions.

One potential drawback of the inducers is that they require biological response on the part of the host to produce interferon. There may be some patients who cannot make the response. If the undesirable manifestations of inducers are separable from the interferon induced, then further work might produce more effective, less reactogenic inducers.

REFERENCES

1. A. Isaacs and J. Lindemann, Virus interference. I. The interferon. Proc. Roy. Soc., Ser. B. 147:258 (1957).
2. Y. Nagano and Y. Kojima, Inhibition de l'infection vaccinale par un facteur liquide dans le tissu infecté par le virus homologue. C. R. Soc. Biol. 152:1627 (1958).
3. C. Chany, An inhibiting factor of intracellular multiplication of viruses called interferon originating from cancer cells. C. R. Acad. Sci. 250: 3903 (1960).
4. A. Isaacs, Interferon. Sci. Amer. 204:51 (1961).
5. R. E. Shope, An antiviral substance from Penicillium funiculosum. II. Effect of helenine upon infection in mice with Semliki-Forest virus. J. Exp. Med. 97:627 (1953).

6. K. W. Cochran and T. Francis, Jr., Antiviral action of helenine on experimental poliomyelitis. Proc. Soc. Exp. Biol. Med. 92:230 (1956).

7. U. J. Lewis, E. L. Rickse, L. McCleeland, and N. G. Brink, Purification and characterization of the antiviral agent, helenine. J. Amer. Chem. Soc. 81:4115 (1959).

8. M. W. Rytel, R. E. Shope, and E. D. Kilbourne, An antiviral substance from Penicillium funiculosum. V. Induction of interferon by helenine. J. Exp. Med. 123:577 (1966).

9. G. P. Lampson, A. A. Tytell, A. K. Field, M. M. Nemes, and M. R. Hilleman, Inducers of interferon and host resistance. I. Double-stranded RNA from extracts of Penicillium funiculosum. Proc. Nat. Acad. Sci. U.S. 58:782 (1967).

10. G. T. Banks, K. W. Buck, E. B. Chain, F. Himmelweit, J. E. Marks, J. M. Tyer, M. Hollings, and F. T. Lost, Viruses in fungi and interferon stimulation. Nature 218:542 (1968).

11. A. K. Field, A. A. Tytell, G. P. Lampson, and M. R. Hilleman, Inducers of interferon and host resistance. II. Multistranded synthetic polynucleotide complexes. Proc. Nat. Acad. Sci. U.S. 58:1004 (1967).

12. A. K. Field, G. P. Lampson, A. A. Tytell, M. M. Nemes, and M. R. Hilleman, Inducers of interferon and host resistance. IV. Double-stranded replicative RNA (MS 2-FF-RNA) from E. coli infected with MS2 coliphage. Proc. Nat. Acad. Sci. U.S. 58:2102 (1967).

13. A. K. Field, A. A. Tytell, G. P. Lampson, and M. R. Hilleman, Inducers of interferon and host resistance, V. In vitro studies. Proc. Nat. Acad. Sci. U.S. 61:340 (1968).

14. A. A. Tytell, G. P. Lampson, A. K. Field, and M. R. Hilleman, Inducers of interferon and host resistance. III. Double-stranded RNA from reovirus type 3 virions. Proc. Nat. Acad. Sci. U.S. 58:1719 (1967).

15. A. K. Field, A. T. Tytell, G. P. Lampson, M. M. Nemes, and M. R. Hilleman, Double-stranded polynucleotides as interferon inducers. J. Gen. Physiol. 56:905 (1970).

16. C. DeClercq, Structural variations of polynucleotide inducers. In Symposium on Preparation, Standardization and Clinical Use of Interferon, Zagreb, June 1977, Yugoslav Acad. Sci. and Arts, Zagreb.

17. S. Baron, N. N. Bogomolova, A. Billiau, H. B. Levy, C. E. Buckler, R. Stern, and R. Naylor, Induction of interferon by preparations of synthetic single-stranded RNA. Proc. Nat. Acad. Sci. U.S. 64:67 (1969).

18. A. Billiau, C. E. Buckler, F. Dianzani, C. Uhlendorf, and S. Baron, Induction of interferon mechanism by single-stranded RNA: Potentiation by polybasic substances. Proc. Soc. Exp. Biol. Med. 132:790 (1969).

19. A. Billiau, C. E. Buckler, F. Dianzani, C. Uhlendorf, and S. Baron, Influence of basic substances on the induction of the interferon mechanisms. Proc. Soc. Exp. Biol. Med. 132:790 (1969).

20. A. Billiau and E. Schome, Induction of the interferon mechanism by natural RNA. Life Sci. 9: 69 (1970).
21. E. DeClercq, F. Eckstein, and J. C. Merigan, Interferon induction increased through chemical modification of a synthetic polynucleotide. Science 165: 1137 (1969).
22. P. Jameson and S. E. Grossberg, Interferon induction in mice by complexes of polynucleotides of varying sizes. Bacteriol. Proc., p. L55 (1970).
23. J. Vilček, M. H. Ng, A. E. Friedman-Kein, and T. Krauciu, Induction of interferon synthesis by synthetic double-stranded polynucleotides. J. Virol. 2: 648 (1968).
24. J. H. Park and S. Baron, Herpetic keratoconjunctivitis therapy with synthetic double-stranded RNA. Science 162: 811 (1968).
25. M. Worthington and S. Baron, Late Therapy with an interferon stimulator in an arbovirus encephalitis in mice. Proc. Soc. Exp. Biol. Med. 136: 323 (1971).
26. H. B. Levy, L. W. Law, and A. S. Rabson, Inhibition of tumor growth by polyinosinic-polycytidylic acid. Proc. Nat. Acad. Sci. U.S. 62: 357 (1969).
27. H. V. Gelboin and H. B. Levy, Polyinosinic-polycytidylic acid inhibits chemically induced tumorigenesis in mouse skin. Science 167: 205 (1970).
28. P. S. Sarma, G. Shiv, S. Baron, Inhibitory effect of interferon on murine sarcoma and leukaemia virus infection in vitro. Nature 223: 845-846 (1969).
29. L. D. Zeleznick and B. K. Bhuyan, Treatment of leukemia (L-1210) mice with double-stranded polyribonucleotides. Proc. Soc. Exp. Biol. Med. 130: 126 (1969).
30. I. Gresser, L. Berman, G. De Thé, D. Brouty-Boyé, J. Coppey, and E. Falcoff, Interferon and murine leukemia. V. Effect of interferon preparations on the evolution of Rauscher disease in mice. J. Nat. Cancer Inst. 41: 505 (1968).
31. H. Cantor, R. Asofsky, and H. B. Levy, The effect of polyinosinic-polycytidylic acid upon graft-vs-host activity in BALB/c mice. J. Immunol. 104: 1035-1038 (1970).
32. W. Turner, S. P. Chan, and M. A. Chirigos, Stimulation of humoral and cellular antibody formation in mice by Poly Ir: Cr. Proc. Soc. Exp. Biol. Med. 133: 334-338 (1970).
33. H. B. Levy and F. Riley, The effect of polyinosinic: polycytidylic acid on tumor metabolism. Proc. Soc. Exp. Biol. Med. 135: 141-145 (1970).
34. D. A. Hill, S. Baron, H. B. Levy, J. Bellanti, C. E. Buckler, G. Cannellos, P. Carbone, R. M. Chanock, V. DeVita, M. A. Guggenheim, E. Homan, A. Z. Kapikian, R. L. Kirschstein, J. Mills, J. E. Vankirk, and M. Worthington, Clinical studies of induction of interferon

by polyinosinic-polycytidylic acid. In Perspectives in Virology, Vol. 7: From Molecules to Man (M. Pollard, ed.), Academic Press, New York, 1971, pp. 198-222.

35. R. A. Robinson, V. T. Devita, H. B. Levy, S. Baron, S. P. Hubbard, and A. S. Levine, A phase I-II trial of multiple-dose polyriboinosinic-polyribocytidylic acid in patients with leukemia or solid tumors. J. Nat. Cancer Inst. 57:599 (1976).

36. C. W. Young, Interferon induction in cancer, with some observations on the clinical effects of poly I:C. Med. Clinics N. Amer. 55:721-728 (1971).

37. J. J. Nordlund, S. M. Wolff, and H. B. Levy, Inhibition of biologic activity of poly I:poly C by human plasma. Proc. Soc. Exp. Biol. Med. 133:439-444 (1970).

38. H. B. Levy, G. Baer, S. Baron, C. E. Buckler, C. J. Gibbs, M. J. Iadarola, W. T. London, and J. Rice, A modified polyriboinosinic-polycytidylic acid complex that induces interferon in primates. J. Infec. Dis. 132:434-439 (1975).

39. G. M. Baer, J. H. Shaddock, S. A. Moore, H. B. Levy, and S. Baron, Successful Prophylaxis against rabies in mice and rhesus monkeys: The interferon system and vaccine. J. Infec. Dis. 136:286-271 (1977).

40. H. B. Levy, W. London, D. A. Fuccillo, S. Baron, and J. Rice, Prophylactic control of Simian hemorrhagic fever in monkeys by an interferon inducer, polyriboinosinic-polyribocytidylic acid poly-L-lysine. J. Infec. Dis. 133:A256-A259 (1975).

41. E. L. Stephen, M. L. Sammons, W. L. Pannier, S. Baron, R. O. Spertul, and H. B. Levy, Effect of a nuclease-resistant derivative of poly I:poly C on yellow fever in Rhesus monkeys. J. Infec. Dis. 136:122-126 (1977).

42. M. P. Burgasova, D. G. Andzaparidze, T. A. Bektemirov, N. N. Bogomolova, and Yu. S. Boriskin, Influence of Poly (I)-Poly(C) complex with poly-L-Lysine on the experimental tick-Eorne encephalitis. Vop. Virusologie 4:438-441 (1977).

43. D. G. Andzhaparidze, T. A. Bektemirov, and M. P. Burgasova, The effect of poly (I)-poly(C) complex with poly-L-Lysine on the course of vaccinia infection in monkeys. Vop. Virusologie 3:339-343 (1977).

44. R. H. Purcell, W. T. London, V. J. McAliffe, A. E. Palmer, P. M. Kaplan, H. B. Levy, J. L. Gerin, J. Wagner, H. Popper, E. Lvovsky, and D. O. Wong, Modification of chronic hepatitis-B virus infection in chimpanzees by administration of an interferon inducer. Lancet, p. 757 (Oct. 9, 1976).

45. H. B. Levy and E. Lvovsky, Topical treatment of vaccinia virus infection with an interferon inducer in rabbits. J. Infec. Dis. 137:78-81 (1978).

46. W. E. Houston, C. L. Crabbs, E. L. Stephen, and H. B. Levy, Modified polyinosinic-polycytidylic acid, an immunological adjuvant. Infec. Immun. 14:318-319 (1976).

47. E. L. Stephen, D. E. Hilmas, J. A. Mangeafico, and H. B. Levy, Swine influenza virus vaccine: Potentiation of antibody responses in rhesus monkeys. Science 197:1289-1290 (1977).

48. A. S. Levine, M. Sivilich, P. Wiernick, and H. B. Levy, Phase I-II trial of stabilized polyriboinosinic-polyribocytidylic acid in leukemia and solid tumors. AACR Proc. in press (1978).

49. M. L. Sammons, E. L. Stephen, H. B. Levy, S. Baron, and D. E. Hilmas, Interferon induction in cynomolgus and rhesus monkeys after repeated doses of a modified polyriboinosinic-polyribocytidylic acid complex. Antimicrob. Agents Chemother. 11:80-83 (1977).

50. K. Champney, H. B. Levy, and A. M. Lerner, Sustained interferon in human serum following Poly ICLC. Proc. Amer. Soc. Clin. Invest. Clin. Res. 24:451 (1976).

51. W. K. Engel, R. Cuneo, and H. B. Levy, Treatment of neuropathy with stabilized polyinosinic-polycytidylic acid. Lancet i:503 (1978).

52. W. A. Carter, P. M. Pitha, L. W. Marshall, I. Tazania, and Tazaia, 6-T P.O.P. Synthesis of interferon induction in mismatched analogues of polycytidylic acid. J. Mol. Biol. 70:567-587 (1972).

53. P. O. Ts'o, J. L. Alderfer, J. Levny, L. W. Marshall, J. O'Malley, J. S. Horoszewicz, and W. A. Carter, Antiviral and other biological properties of PolyI.PolyC and its mismatched analogues. Mol. Pharmacol. 122:299-312 (1976).

54. W. A. Carter, J. O'Malley, M. Beesan, P. Cunnington, A. Kelvin, A. Ver-Hodge, J. L. Alderfer, and P. O. Ts'o, Mismatched analogues of PolyI.PolyC. Mol. Pharmacol. 123:440-453 (1976).

8

TILORONE HYDROCHLORIDE
AND RELATED MOLECULES

Gerald D. Mayer and Russell F. Krueger
Merrell-National Laboratories
Division of Richardson-Merrell Inc.
Cincinnati, Ohio

I. INTRODUCTION

Among the large number and variety of agents that induce interferon, tilorone hydrochloride represented a significant advance. The first synthetic compound of low molecular weight recognized to induce interferon in vivo by the oral route [1,2], it was also demonstrated to be an orally and parenterally active broad-spectrum antiviral agent in the laboratory [3,4]. Subsequently, it was found to stimulate the reticuloendothial system [5] and influence the primary immune response to sheep red blood cells in mice [6]. These initial observations were vastly extended by Megel and associates through their studies on the selective effects on humoral and cell-mediated immunity [7].

Although tilorone has been the most prominent member of the low-molecular-weight compounds synthesized at the Merrell Research Center and other laboratories, it was not the first important compound. The initial

TABLE 1. Structures and LD_{50} Values of Tilorone Analogs

Compound[a]	Structure	Mol. wt.[b]	Mouse LD_{50} (mg/kg)[c] Oral	Subcutaneous
Tilorone hydrochloride		411	1520	111
RMI 10,024		439	1560	110
RMI 10,874		370	1780	353
RMI 11,002		392	>4000	353

Table 1 (continued)

Compound[a]	Structure	Mol. wt.[b]	Mouse LD$_{50}$ (mg/kg)[c]	
			Oral	Subcutaneous
RMI 11,513		352	1410	304
RMI 11,567		338	2700	1000
RMI 11,645		373	2590	930

Table 1 (continued)

Compound[a]	Structure	Mol. wt.[b]	Mouse LD$_{50}$ (mg/kg)[c]	
			Oral	Subcutaneous
RMI 11,877		354	2930	820

RMI 12,358		380	>1000	420

[a]All compounds are dihydrochloride salts, as the free bases are insoluble in aqueous solutions at physiologically compatible pH.
[b]Mol. wt. = molecular weight of free bases.
[c]After a 7-day observation period.

compound, designated by Richardson-Merrell Inc. RMI 2557 DA (2·HCl), was a bis-basic ester of fluorenone that had modest antiviral activity but only by the parenteral route [8]. Furthermore, its interferon-inducing capacity was minimal. Following the discovery of RMI 2557, a more extensive chemical synthesis program was undertaken to elucidate the structure activity relationships of bis-basic tricyclic compounds and to develop compounds that were orally active, more potent, and which possessed other pharmacodynamic differences. Over 800 compounds were synthesized, including representatives of many different chemical series of bis-basic substituted polycyclic aromatic compounds. The structure activity relationships of many of the chemical series were first reviewed in presentations at the 1970 meeting of the American Chemical Society [9] and in 1971 at Leuven, Belgium [10].

The structures and LD_{50} values of nine orally active compounds, including tilorone, that were chosen for further evaluations are shown in Table 1. The selections were based on structural differences, relative toxicity, and oral potency against encephalomyocarditis (EMC) virus; all compounds were also active subcutaneously. Several different tricyclic nuclei are represented, namely, fluorenone (tilorone), anthraquinone (RMI 10,024), xanthone (RMI 10,874), fluorene (RMI 11,002), xanthene (RMI 11,513), dibenzofuran (RMI 11,567), fluoranthene (RMI 11,645), dibenzothiophene (RMI 11,877), and acenaphthene (RMI 12,358). Side chain linkages are ethers, represented by tilorone, RMI 10,024, and RMI 10,874, and ketones, represented by the rest of the analogs shown. Tilorone, RMI 11,002, RMI 11,567 and RMI 11,877 appeared to be good representatives with potential for clinical activity and so were evaluated more extensively than the other five. All of the compounds were tested as dihydrochloride salts, which improved their solubility for testing under physiological conditions. Physicochemical properties were reported by Albrecht [11]. The structure activity relationships of each Richardson–Merrell chemical series among these particular antiviral agents are reported elsewhere [9,10,12-16].

The size of the molecule appeared to be important for oral activity. Molecular weights of these orally active interferon inducers ranged from 338 to 439. Many analogs with longer side chains or substituents that added to their molecular weight were active subcutaneously but not orally. The upper limit for a subcutaneously active compound to display oral activity appeared to be about 450. No lower molecular size limit was established except that which was required to maintain the functional integrity of the basic compound structure necessary for interferon induction.

II. INTERFERON INDUCTION

The interferon-inducing capabilities of tilorone-related compounds were compared in mice (Table 2) and rats (Table 3). Sera from treated rodents displayed characteristics associated with interferon, namely, species specificity, a broad antiviral spectrum, nondialyzability, trypsin sensitivity, and resistance to ribonuclease. All of the compounds induced high levels of interferon in mice when given orally or subcutaneously; yet only tilorone, RMI 11,002, and RMI 11,513 were good inducers in rats by either route. Although not shown in Table 1, 6-hr titers after oral or subcutaneous treatment of mice were <25 with all of the compounds. Titers in mice 12 or 24 hr after oral treatment were generally comparable with each other (RMI 11,645was the significant exception). In all cases of subcutaneous administration, 12-hr titers were higher than those at 24 hr. Our experiences

TABLE 2. Serum Interferon Levels of Treated Mice

	Interferon titers					
	Oral (250 mg/kg)			Subcutaneous (100 mg/kg)		
Compound	12 hr	24 hr	48 hr	12 hr	24 hr	48 hr
Ethers						
Tilorone	6,400	6,400	50	12,800	800	< 25
RMI 10,024	3,200	12,800	100	12,800	1,600	< 25
RMI 10,874	6,400	3,200	25	1,600	800	< 25
Ketones						
RMI 11,002	3,200	1,600	< 25	3,200	200	< 25
RMI 11,513	6,400	3,200	< 25	3,200	800	< 25
RMI 11,567	12,800	25,600	50	6,400	3,200	25
RMI 11,645	400	1,600	200	3,200	1,600	< 25
RMI 11,877	6,400	6,400	100	12,800	800	< 25
RMI 12,358	3,200	3,200	< 25	800	400	< 25

with tilorone have shown that interferon titers reached maximum some
16-18 hr after oral treatment and 12 hr after subcutaneous treatment.
Stringfellow and Glasgow, however, reported similar patterns of interferon
induction by tilorone administered orally or subcutaneously [17]. Polymeric
inducers such as poly I:poly C and endotoxin are "early" (within 6 hr) inducers. Tilorone then must be considered a "late" inducer. Declercq and
Merigan suggested that slow absorption of tilorone from the gastrointestinal
tract accounted for the delay in the onset of interferon by tilorone [18].

    We have not been successful in stimulating interferon nor providing
antiviral protection with intravenous administration of tilorone to mice.
Significant protection against Semliki Forest virus (SFV) was obtained by
intravenous administration of tilorone to rats, but no interferon measurements were made.

    Differences in potency of the compounds were evaluated by single oral
treatment of mice with three different dose levels and selecting serum
samples at the predetermined maximal time for interferon to be assayed
(Table 4). In this study all nine compounds induced good interferon levels
at 250 mg/kg, with RMI 11,567 eliciting the highest titer. RMI 11,645
was the most potent inducer at 50 and 10 mg/kg. No interferon was detectable with 50 or 10 mg/kg of RMI 11,877.

TABLE 3. Serum Interferon Kinetics in Rats

	Interferon titers (hour after treatment)								
	Oral (250 mg/kg)				Subcutaneous (100 mg/kg)				
Compound	12 hr	18 hr	24 hr	30 hr	6 hr	12 hr	18 hr	24 hr	30 hr
Ethers									
Tilorone	400	200	200	25	100	400	200	25	25
RMI 10,024	<25	50	50	50	<25	50	50	25	<25
RMI 10,874	<25	50	50	50	<25	50	<25	<25	<25
RMI 11,043	<25	<25	25	<25	<25	<25	50	<25	<25
Ketones									
RMI 11,002	50	≥200	100	25	<25	400	<25	<25	<25
RMI 11,513	50	100	200	50	25	400	100	<25	<25
RMI 11,567	<25	50	25	<25	<25	25	25	<25	<25
RMI 11,645	<25	<25	<25	<25	<25	<25	<25	<25	<25
RMI 11,877	<25	<25	25	<25	<25	<25	<25	<25	<25

TABLE 4. Interferon Dose Response of Mice to Oral Treatment

Compound	Hour after treatment	Dose (mg/kg)		
		250	50	10
Ethers				
Tilorone	24	6,400	400	25
RMI 10,024	24	12,800	200	25
RMI 10,874	12	6,400	400	25
Ketones				
RMI 11,002	12	3,200	100	25
RMI 11,513	12	6,400	100	25
RMI 11,567	24	25,600	50	25
RMI 11,645	24	3,200	1600	25
RMI 11,877	12	6,400	25	25
RMI 12,358	24	3,200	25	25

DeClercq and Merigan found that mouse thymus and lymph nodes contained the highest levels of interferon among organs after oral administration of tilorone [18]. Analysis of the kinetics of interferon induction in mouse and rat organs offered some interesting observations. Figure 1 shows that spleen, kidney, and lung interferon titers in mice were maximum 18 hr after oral tilorone treatment; peak thymus levels occurred 6-12 hr later. The appearance and duration of interferon in organs of orally dosed rats is seen in Figure 2. It is significant that rats, which have been shown to produce much less serum interferon than mice in response to tilorone and analogs, showed no detectable thymic interferon in direct contrast to the high levels found in mice. Again, spleen, kidney, and lung interferons all peaked at 18 hr after oral treatment of both mice and rats with tilorone. We thought perhaps that serum interferon might be due to organ "spillover" (this may yet be the case in mice). Although splenectomy reduced serum interferon levels in mice significantly, splenectomized rats treated with tilorone had as much serum interferon as tilorone-treated, sham-operated controls. No evidence for interferon stimulation in the gastrointestinal tract of mice was found after orally administered tilorone [17, 18].

The interferogenic responses to tilorone of different strains and ages of mice, as well as mice subjected to various types of stress, have been investigated. $C_{57}BL$ mice made less interferon than Swiss outbred albino mice [19]. Nude athymic mice produced respectable levels of interferon

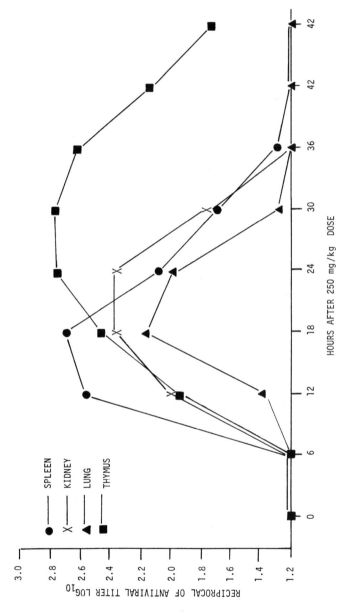

FIGURE 1. Interferon titers of mouse organs after tilorone treatment.

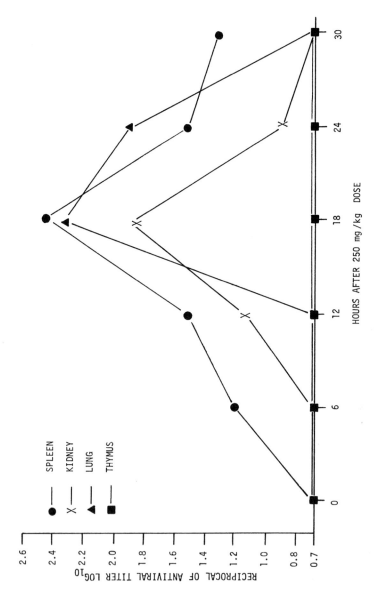

FIGURE 2. Interferon titers of rat organs after tilorone treatment.

but which were consistently less than those found in their phenotypically normal littermates [20,21]. Ten-gram mice made less interferon than 25-g mice given the same amount of tilorone; this age response was also reflected in tilorone's capacity to protect mice from SFV infection [22]. We found that adrenalectomized mice made significantly less interferon in response to orally administered tilorone than did their sham-operated counterparts.

The induction of interferon by tilorone in mice depends on protein synthesis [18,23,24]. Nonlethal doses of cycloheximide, given during the initial and peak phases of interferon induction, reduced the amount of interferon normally induced by tilorone. If cycloheximide treatment was delayed until the declining phase was in progress, however, the protein synthesis inhibitor enhanced the interferon response. Although interferon levels were diminished, cycloheximide given 1 hr prior to tilorone did not delay the onset of interferon induction. The degree of inhibition by cycloheximide was age-dependent; young mice were more adversely affected than older mice. In spite of the apparent requirement for protein synthesis for in vivo interferon induction by tilorone, it is still uncertain whether this reflects a direct consequence of new protein synthesis or if the primary effect is an event preceding actual interferon stimulation.

Table 5 compares the molecular weights of interferons elicited by tilorone and some of its congeners in mice and rats. In mice, tilorone, an ether, induced interferon of a single molecular species. The molecular weight of mouse interferon induced by the ether RMI 10,024 was not determined. Another ether analog, not among the primary nine compounds, induced interferons characteristic of the tilorone type. By contrast, the ketone compounds induced two distinct molecular species of interferons in mice. Rat serum interferons of two molecular species were found regardless of which inducer was used.

TABLE 5. Molecular Weights of Mouse and Rat Serum Interferons

| Inducer | Molecular weights | |
	Mouse	Rat
Ethers		
Tilorone	34,800	27,000 and 80,000
RMI 10,024		27,000 and 81,000
Ketones		
RMI 11,002		33,000 and 85,000
RMI 11,877	32,000 and 69,000	
RMI 11,645	31,000 and 68,000	
RMI 11,513	35,500 and 67,000	32,000 and 77,000
RMI 11,567	35,500 and 62,000	

TABLE 6. In Vitro Interferon Responses to Tilorone[a]

Induction	No induction
Human embryo lung fibroblasts [28]	Mouse L 929 cells [18,27]
Normal human leukocytes [28]	Mouse embryo fibroblasts [18]
Normal human lymphocytes [29]	Mouse spleen lymphocytes and macrophages [18][b]
Leukemic human lymphocytes [29]	Mouse thymus lymphocytes and macrophages [18]
Lymphoblastoid cell lines [28] B_3HRl and EB_4	Mouse peritoneal lymphocytes and macrophages [17,18]
Mouse embryo fibroblasts [30]	Rabbit kidney (RK_{13}) [31]
	Human skin fibroblasts [27]
	Mouse peripheral leukocytes[b]
	Rat peripheral leukocytes[b]
	Monkey peripheral leukocytes[b]

[a]Reference numbers are shown in brackets.
[b]Personal observation of author (GDM).

    No interferon stimulation by orally or parenterally administered tilorone
could be demonstrated in rabbits, hamsters, ferrets, cats, or dogs. Only
one report describes interferon induction by tilorone in monkeys [25]; we
have been unable to confirm or expand upon such data with orally or subcutaneously administered tilorone, RMI 11,002, RMI 11,567, or RMI
11,877. Furthermore, no interferon could be demonstrated in rabbits
treated orally with RMI 11,002 or RMI 11,567. Topical application of
tilorone to human eyes did not stimulate interferon secretion in tears [26].
    The notion that low-molecular-weight synthetic compounds do not
stimulate interferon production in vitro is not valid (Table 6 [17,18,27-31]).
In most cases, however, near cytotoxic concentrations of tilorone were
required to elicit a positive response. Contradictions could be explained
as simply a matter of different tilorone concentrations used. Furthermore,
the cytotoxic concentration of tilorone has varied among different cell types.
Table 6 includes only those cell types from which interferon was directly
sought and does not include observations relating to protection of cells
from virus infection by compound itself.
    Tilorone and poly I: poly C in the presence of diethylaminoethyl (DEAE)-
dextran were synergistic for interferon induction in mouse L929 cells and

mouse embryo cells [27]. However, this only resulted with concentrations of poly I: poly C-DEAE-dextran mixtures that induced low levels of interferon, and the degree of potentiation was directly proportional to the tilorone concentration up to cytotoxic concentrations. No synergism was seen in human foreskin fibroblasts, nor in primary rabbit kidney cells. Although mixtures of the individual ribonucleotides, polyinosinic and polycytidylic acids, were effective, mixtures of polyadenylic and polyuridylic acids were not. Individual ribonucleotide homopolymers, as well as extracted mouse brain RNA and mouse spleen RNA, were also ineffective. DEAE-dextran has been shown to enhance infectivity of viral nucleic acids and increase the activity of synthetic polynucleotides as interferon inducers [30].

Hyporeactivity, a condition whereby an initial dose of a compound interferes with the response of the host to a subsequent dose, is common to all interferon inducers. The overall subject is dealt with in detail by Ho [32], but information on tilorone is lacking.

The extent and length of the hyporeactive period depends at least on the dose level, the host itself, and the inducer. For example, a dose of 50 mg/kg tilorone given orally, although inducing a substantial level of interferon, did not establish hyporeactivity in mice to a subsequent 250 mg/kg dose. Hyporeactive states established in mice by some inducers were not seen in rabbits [32]. We found that prior administration of tilorone failed to establish hyporeactivity to poly I: poly C in rats but did so for another dose of tilorone. It is obvious from the information presented in Table 7 [18,33,37,76-78], which shows hyporeactivity of tilorone with nonviral and viral inducers, that the extent of hyporeactivity varied with the inducer. Stringfellow [33] proposed that the hyporeactive phenomenon was responsible for the lack of therapeutic activity of interferon inducers. Mouse infections caused by EMC virus, SFV, influenza A_2, and murine cytomegalovirus (CMV) all made the host refractory to a subsequent dose of tilorone, poly I: poly C, Newcastle Disease virus (NDV), or Rochester murine virus (RMV). Mice inoculated with herpesvirus hominis (HVH) type 2, either intraperitoneally or intravaginally, were hyporeactive to a subsequent dose of NDV or RMV but not to the nonviral inducers poly I: poly C or tilorone. NDV used as the first inducer did not establish hyporeactivity to tilorone. In mice we found that tilorone used as the first inducer established a severe hyporeactive state to statolon given 72 hr later. Statolon as the first inducer, on the other hand, failed to establish a hyporeactive state to tilorone given 72 hr later.

The time of administration between the first and the second dose of inducer was important. Maximum development of the hyporeactive state in mice occurred with tilorone when the two doses were separated by 72 hr. The normal interferon response of the host returned 144 hr after the first dose. Although all of the active analogs established hyporeactivity to themselves and tilorone in mice, the length of time of the hyporeactive period was variable. Thus, RMI 10,874, RMI 11,002, RMI 11,567, and

TABLE 7. Tilorone Hyporeactive Responses of Mice

First inducer	Second inducer	Response	References
Nonviral inducers			
Tilorone	Poly I: poly C	Moderate	18
Tilorone	Endotoxin	None	18
Tilorone	Tilorone	Severe	18,37
Poly I: poly C	Tilorone	Severe	18
Endotoxin	Tilorone	Moderate	18
Maleic acid divinyl ether	Tilorone	Moderate	18
Mycoplasma arthritidis	Tilorone	Moderate	76
Mycoplasma arthritidis	Tilorone	None	76
Viral inducers			
EMC	Tilorone	Severe	33,77
SFV	Tilorone	Severe	33
Influenza A_2	Tilorone	Severe	33
CMV	Tilorone	Severe	33
HVH, type 2	Tilorone	None	33
NDV	Tilorone	None	33,78

RMI 11,877 all induced their maximum hyporeactive state earlier in mice than did tilorone and the other analogs.

Ho et al. [34] suggested that hyporeactivity resulted from a reduced capacity of the reticuloendothelial system to clear an inducer from the blood. Metabolic studies have suggested that the length of the hyporeactive period may coincide with the disappearance of the compound from the host. The hyporeactive state could not be established in mice with single doses of non-interferon-inducing compounds given 72 hr earlier than their active analogs. Invariably, the inactive congeners were cleared more rapidly than the active analogs. One inactive Merrell analog that, like tilorone, was cleared relatively slowly did establish hyporeactivity to tilorone. Hyporesponsiveness, then, does not appear to depend on the quantity of interferon induced because it can be established with structurally related compounds that are inefficient interferon inducers. Thus, it appears that the faster the clearance, the shorter the hyporeactive period. However, more extensive work is indicated to support this hypothesis. Hyporeactivity is not an absolute condition. Tilorone incorporated into the drinking water of mice provided a continual low level of serum interferon while the mice were supplied with the treated water [35]. We found that incorporation of low levels of tilorone into their drinking water one week before using mice experimentally for other studies protected mice from the lethal effects of an infection of unknown etiology that appeared to be transmissable. Hyporeactivity, as measured by interferon response, correlated directly with activity against EMC virus. We were able to show that incorporation of tilorone into feed protected mice from viral challenge 1 week later.

Several other theories have been advanced to account for hyporeactivity. Stringfellow et al. [33] found evidence of a serum hyporeactive factor (SHF) in EMC virus, SFV, CMV, and influenza A_2 virus-infected mice, all of which caused a severe hyporeactive state to induction by poly I: poly C, NDV, RMV, or tilorone. On the other hand, HVH type 2, which did not cause hyporeactivity to poly I: poly C or tilorone interferon induction, but did to the virus inducers, had the lowest SHF levels. We looked for a similar SHF that might be stimulated by tilorone but found none. Furthermore, we found tilorone not to be antigenic. With serum collected from tilorone-treated mice during the period of maximum hyporeactivity, we could not (1) prevent tilorone from inducing interferon in vivo when such serum was mixed with tilorone and administered orally or subcutaneously to mice; (2) suppress the in vitro activity of serum interferon derived from tilorone-treated mice; (3) suppress stimulation of interferon in mouse L929 cells by poly I: poly C in the presence of DEAE-dextran. Youngner and Stinebring [36] could not transfer the hyporeactive response passively in serum taken from animals treated with endotoxin 48 hr earlier. Cycloheximide given 1 hr before an initial dose of tilorone failed to prevent the induction of the hyporeactive state in mice. It can be inferred, then, that new protein synthesis is not required for the development of hyporeactivity.

III. ANTIVIRAL ACTIVITY

Antiviral activity with tilorone and congeners has been demonstrated in mice, rats, rabbits, and monkeys as judged by an increased number of survivors, increased length of the survival time, prevention of viremia, and prevention of antibody response to live virus or attenuation of eye and skin lesions. Activities were primarily seen with prophylactic regimens and could be obtained with oral, topical, or parenteral treatment, depending on the type of infection. Viruses against which some of these compounds were found to be effective in laboratory animal experimentation include: SFV [4,22,31,38]; encephalymyocarditis viruses, including EMC, MM, and Mengo [4,8,9,10,11,12,13,14,15,16,31,37,38,39,40,41,42]; Venezuelan equine encephalomyelitis (VEE) virus [43,44,45]; influenza viruses [4,37,46,47,48]; herpes viruses [37,49,50,51,52]; vaccinia virus [4,37]; vesicular stomatitis (VS) virus [18,37,52]; tick-borne encephalitis (TBE) virus [53,54]; foot and mouth disease (FMD) virus [55]; Friend leukemia virus [56,57,58,59,60,61,62,63]; rabies virus [64]; scrapie virus [65]; spring-summer meningoencephalitis virus [66]; and flaviviruses [67]. Table 8 summarizes the activities of all nine compounds against key virus types.

TABLE 8. In Vivo Antiviral Spectrum of Tilorone Analogs

Compound	EMC	SFV	VEE	Influenza A_2	Influenza PR_8	TBE	Vaccinia	HVH[a]
Tilorone	+[b]	+	+	+	+	+	+	+
RMI 10,024	+	+	NT	0	0	NT	+	NT
RMI 10,874	+	+	+	0	NT	NT	+	NT
RMI 11,002	+	+	+	0	0	+	0	+
RMI 11,513	+	+	NT	+	NT	NT	0	NT
RMI 11,567	+	+	+	0	0	+	+	+
RMI 11,645	+	+	NT	0	NT	NT	0	+
RMI 11,877	+	+	+	+	0	+	+	+
RMI 12,358	+	+	NT	+	NT	NT	+	NT

[a]Type 1, topical treatment.
[b]+ = active; NT = not tested; 0 = inactive.

Activity was demonstrated in mice with a single oral dose of tilorone as early as 96 hr prior to inoculation with EMC virus. Maximum activity was seen when compound was administered approximately 24 hr before subcutaneous inoculation. When the virus was inoculated intracranially, the best activity was obtained with compound administered 48 hr before challenge. In general, the minimal orally effective dose in fatal EMC virus infections ranged from 10 to 25 mg/kg, and maximal effectiveness occurred with 100-250 mg/kg. Similar data were obtained against SFV, except that activity could be demonstrated when tilorone was given as early as 120 hr before virus and as late as 24 hr after inoculation. Hyporeactivity was not nearly so striking with tilorone when measured against SFV infection as it was against EMC virus challenge. Tilorone and its congeners were usually found to be less active against the influenza viruses than against the EMC virus and SFV. Considerably greater numbers of mice were protected by orally administered tilorone if they were vaccinated with inactivated influenza A_2 (Jap/305) or influenza B/Mass and later challenged with homologous live virus than mice that were (1) not vaccinated; (2) treated with tilorone only; (3) challenged with a heterologous live influenza virus. Although usually less active than amantadine, tilorone was more active than this anti-influenza compound if the virus was given by aerosolization instead of by nasal instillation.

Anti-influenza effects were additive when both tilorone and amantadine were given to the same mice. However, tilorone had to be given in a multiple-dose regimen to supplement amantadine activity.

A comparison of tilorone with RMI 11,002, RMI 11,567, and RMI 11,877 revealed that multiple-dose regimens were required to achieve optimal activity against influenza A_2 (Jap/305) virus. The order of anti-influenza activity of these compounds did not follow the order of potency for interferon induction. Only tilorone was active against influenza $A_0 PR_8$ and only when mice were infected by aerosolization.

Activity with tilorone administered orally to mice was also seen against VEE, TBE, and vaccinia viruses but not HVH type 1. Topical application of tilorone to hairless mice infected percutaneously with HVH type 1 was effective but somewhat irritating to the skin. No activity in mice could be demonstrated with tilorone against fatal infections established by intraperitoneal inoculations of polio, type II, or coxsackie A-21 viruses.

When tested for the ability of the compound to protect cells from viral infection, tilorone was active against vesicular stomatitis virus (VSV) at 1 and 2 μg/ml on L929 or Hep 2 cells. A level of 5 μg/ml was cytotoxic. No interferon was detectable in cells that were treated with tilorone for 24 hr. No antiviral activity was demonstrated in rabbit kidney (RK13) cells. Tilorone had antiviral activity in nonconfluent L929 mouse cell cultures in direct proportion to concentration and duration of exposure of cells to compound. Tilorone was also active in vitro against HVH type 1 [68] and the monkey oncogenic herpes virus saimiri [69].

RMI 11,002 was orally active against EMC and TBE viruses in mice and against SFV in mice and rats. Although oral activity was demonstrated against VEE virus in both mice and rhesus monkeys, interferon was detected only in mice [43]. Even with evidence of interferon in the serum of mice, no activity against influenza viruses or vaccinia virus was seen. Topical application of RMI 11,002 suppressed the development of ulcerated zosteroid lesions in mice caused by HVH types 1 and 2; however, systemic administration was ineffective.

When given systemically, RMI 11,002 did not prevent the development of blister-like lesions caused by HVH type 1 on mouse tails. No activity against HVH type 1 was seen in rabbits when RMI 11,002 was given subcutaneously or applied topically [51].

RMI 11,567 is as potent in mice as tilorone, but the spectrum of activity differs. Like tilorone, it was active against EMC, VEE, TBE, SFV, HVH type 1, and vaccinia viruses but was not active against influenza A_2 (Jap/305) and $A_0 PR_8$ viruses. RMI 11,567 had an oral ED_{50} of 15 mg/kg against SFV in mice. Activity against VEE virus was also demonstrated in both mice and rhesus monkeys; however, as with RMI 11,002, interferon was detected only in mice [43].

Oral doses of RMI 11,567 were ineffective in reproducibly influencing HVH types 1 and 2 cutaneous lesions in mice and rats. An investigation of mice treated with the compound showed high levels of serum interferon. However, in tissue culture, HVH type 1 was not sensitive to mouse interferon induced by RMI 11,567.

RMI 11,567 was found to inactivate HVH type 1 upon direct exposure. This demonstration of activity prompted topical evaluation of the compound against this virus in mice. The compound was formulated in polawax A-31 and propylene glycol at 1, 3, and 5% concentrations. Three applications of 3 or 5% given at 2, 4, and 6 hr after inoculation of the mouse tail with type 1 were as effective as when treatment was continued q.i.d. for 1, 2, 3, or 4 days. Topical application of 3 and 5% concentrations of RMI 11,567 at 2, 4, and 6 hr after inoculation plus q.i.d. for the next 4 days also prevented full skin lesion development and paralysis in hairless mice. In either the tail or skin lesion models of infection, a 1% concentration was not effective.

Antiviral efficacy was obtained with RMI 11,877 in rodents and monkeys. As with the previously described compounds, interferon was detected only in mice and rats. RMI 11,877 was orally, topically, and parenterally active.

Mice were protected by oral and subcutaneous administration of RMI 11,877 against infections caused by EMC virus. It also was active in mice and rats against SFV. Protection was dose- and time-dependent with maximal activity achieved with administration 24 hr before virus inoculation. The minimum effective dose orally in mice was 21 mg/kg, which was comparable to that seen with tilorone. However, when the LD_{50} was considered,

RMI 11,877 had a higher therapeutic index than tilorone. At the minimum effective oral and subcutaneous dosages, no interferon could be detected in the serum of mice or rats. The compound was also shown by serum antibody and virus titers to be orally active in monkeys against VEE virus. Although no interferon was detected in the monkey, it was detected in mice at a dose effective against a fatal infection of VEE virus. Mice were also protected against TBE virus. RMI 11,877 was active orally in mice infected with influenza A_2 (Jap/305) but not against influenza $A_0 PR_8$.

The severity of vaccinia-virus-induced tail lesions of mice was reduced by over 50% with prophylactic and therapeutic regimens using multiple oral doses of RMI 11,877. A single prophylactic dose was ineffective. RMI 11,877 was evaluated against herpes viruses rather extensively. No activity could be demonstrated against the development of lesions on the tails of white mice infected subcutaneously with HVH types 1 or 2. Despite high serum interferon levels induced by oral administration of RMI 11,877, the development of HVH-type-1-induced lesions in hairless mice was not prevented. Topical application, however, was as effective as RMI 11,567. RMI 11,877 also directly inactivated HVH type 1. In rabbits, a 5% aqueous solution of RMI 11,877 applied directly to the eye when HVH-type-1-induced lesions were first detectable effectively prevented progressive lesion development after eight doses were given.

The remaining five compounds are somewhat different chemically and were evaluated against a spectrum of RNA and DNA viruses in vivo and in vitro. All of the compounds showed a dose-dependent antiviral response with maximal activity obtained with prophylactic treatment.

RMI 11,645 was active in mice against EMC virus and SFV. No activity was seen against influenza A_2 (Jap/305) or vaccinia viruses. RMI 11,645 inactivated viruses on exposure to light [70]. RMI 10,024 and RMI 10,874 were similar in their antiviral spectrum, with activity seen against EMC, SFV, and vaccinia viruses but not against influenza A_2 (Jap/305). RMI 10,874 was active in mice against VEE virus; RMI 10,024 was not evaluated in this test. RMI 11,513 and RMI 12,358 were both active against EMC, SFV, and influenza A_2 (Jap/305) viruses, but only RMI 12,358 was active against vaccinia virus.

IV. IMMUNOLOGICAL EFFECTS

Interferon inducers usually impose other effects on the host that involve the immune system and tilorone and analogs are no exception. Megel et al. have recently reviewed many of the immunological responses elicited by tilorone [71,72].

The initial report on immunomodulation by tilorone was by Hoffman and Ritter [6], who showed that a single dose of tilorone to mice enhanced the primary immune response to sheep red blood cells and increased serum

TABLE 9. Summary of Immunological Responses with Tilorone
and Related Compounds

| Compound | Humoral immunity stimulation | | Cell-mediated immunity suppression |
	IgG	IgM	EAE
Tilorone	Yes	Yes	Yes
RMI 10,024	Yes	No	No
RMI 10,874	Yes	Yes	Yes
RMI 11,002	Yes	No	Yes
RMI 11,513	Yes	No	No
RMI 11,567	Yes	Yes	Yes
RMI 11,645	Yes	Yes	Yes
RMI 11,877	Yes	No	Yes
RMI 12,358	Yes	Yes	Yes

hemolysin titers as well. Subsequent reports confirmed these findings
[59, 67, 73-75].

Table 9 summarizes the consistent immunomodulatory effects of
tilorone and some of its analogs in rodents. Many of the compounds were
selective in their effects, stimulating humoral immunity, indicated by
elevated IgG and IgM antibody to sheep red blood cells, and suppressing
cell-mediated immunity, indicated by a reduced incidence of paralysis in
the Lewis rat experimental allergic encephalomyelitis model [7, 71, 74, 79].
RMI 10,874, RMI 11,567, RMI 11,645, and RMI 12,358, like tilorone,
enhanced IgG and IgM antibody response and suppressed cell-mediated
immunity. Tilorone also has been shown to stimulate IgE antibody levels
[71]. RMI 10,024 and RMI 11,513 stimulated IgG antibody levels but had
no effect on IgM levels or on cell-mediated immunity. RMI 11,002 and
RMI 11,877 differed from tilorone only in that they failed to stimulate production of IgM antibody. Interferon inducers of the synthetic polymeric
type enhanced antibody production [80,81] and cell-mediated immunity [82].
Interferon itself has been shown to stimulate antibody production [83].

Administration of tilorone to mice produced anergy to tuberculin-
mediated delayed hypersensitivity [84]. Tilorone and some of its analogs
have been shown to cause a transient lymphopenia in mice and rats with
depletion of lymphocytes in T-cell areas of the spleen, thymus, and lymph

nodes of mice and rats [85-90]. T lymphocytes in blood and reticuloendothelial organs were rapidly repopulated by B-cell lymphocytes [20,86,91].
Athymic nude mice failed to develop a lymphopenia upon tilorone treatment
[21]. Although the majority of the data support a suppressive role on cellular immunity, others have shown cell-mediated immune-stimulatory effects
with tilorone [92-94].

Tilorone extended the survival time of transplants. Mouse tail skin
allografts were prolonged by tilorone given continuously in the drinking
water [95]. NDV and statolon also prolonged survival of such allografts
but not as long as tilorone. Megel et al. [72,96] showed that tilorone given
to donor rats for three consecutive days suppressed a graft-versus-host
(GVH) reaction in recipient rats, but one- or two-day treatments were
ineffective. Prolongation of skin and heart allografts in rats [97-99] and
renal allographs in dogs [99,100] was demonstrated in tilorone-treated
animals. Tilorone administered orally to 6-week-old chickens suppressed
delayed hypersensitivity but not the GVH reaction. Hemagglutination antibody was not stimulated in chickens [101].

Stimulation of humoral immunity by tilorone-like compounds in mice
is cause to consider such compounds as potential adjuvants. Tilorone
administered with, or distal to, A_2 influenza vaccine significantly elevated
hemagglutination-inhibition titers in guinea pigs over those achieved with
aqueous influenza vaccine of comparable antigenic content in guinea pigs
not given tilorone [71]. Concomitant use of tilorone with alum or water
in oil emulsion showed no adjuvant effect. The polymeric interferon inducer
poly I:poly C was used as an adjuvant with VEE virus in mice [102].
Tilorone has been used successfully as an immunoadjuvant against murine
tumors [103,104].

Spleen weights of tilorone-treated mice were increased [5,20,86,91].
Tilorone enhanced chromated sheep red blood cell vascular clearance and
hepatic uptake in mice [5]. Interferon has been shown to enhance phagocytosis by peritoneal macrophages in vitro [105].

Several interferon inducers, including tilorone, enhanced the spreading
of peritoneal macrophages freshly plated on a glass surface, but a significant correlation between interferon titers and percent of spread macrophages
could not be determined [106]. Splenectomy did not influence the spreading
response of macrophages to tilorone. In the presence of tilorone peritoneal
exudates, containing macrophages and lymphocytes from unsensitized C_3H
mice, completely protected C_3H mouse embryo fibroblast cells from destruction by HVH type 2 or vaccinia virus [107]. Macrophages with or
without lymphocytes were protective while lymphocytes in the absence of
macrophages were not. Tilorone inhibited endotoxin-induced production
of leukocyte-inhibiting factors in human lymphocytes [108].

Tilorone has been shown to stimulate complement, presumably by
inhibiting complement consumption, in vivo and in vitro [72]. RMI 11,645
inhibited complement to some extent in vitro. RMI 11,002, RMI 12,358,

RMI 11,567, RMI 10,024, RMI 10,874, RMI 11,513, and RMI 11,877 had
no effect on complement in vitro.

McGuire et al. [109] found that tilorone and other known immunomodulators suppressed the yield of prostacyclin from activated mouse
peritoneal cells. Prostacyclin formation was not blocked by immunomodulators applied directly to cell homogenates, therefore they were not prostacyclin synthetase inhibitors.

Although antibody levels did not seem to be altered in NZB/NZW mice
treated with tilorone, Walker [110] suggested that tilorone-induced suppression of cell-mediated immunity may have caused young NZB/NZW mice to
die prematurely with severe glomerulonephritis and vasculitis. Tilorone
enhancement of tumor growth in mice and rats, which could be accounted
for by stimulation of blocking antibody and/or suppression of cell-mediated
immunity, was seen by Gazdar and co-workers [111-113].

The anti-inflammatory properties of tilorone have been extensively
reviewed by Megel [72]. In summary, tilorone (1) inhibited the primary
inflammatory response and the secondary immunologically-induced inflammatory response in the adjuvant arthritis test in rats; (2) inhibited carrageenan-
induced paw edema and abscess in rats; (3) inhibited the direct passive
Arthus reaction in rats. RMI 11,002 inhibited carrageenan-induced paw
edema but not carrageenan-induced abscesses nor the Arthus reaction.
RMI 12,358 inhibited carrageenan-induced paw edema but not the direct
Arthus reaction. RMI 11,567 modestly inhibited carrageenan-induced paw
edema but not the carrageenan-induced abscess. RMI 11,645 did not inhibit
carrageenan-induced paw edema nor the direct Arthus reaction. RMI 10,024
had no effect on carrageenan-induced abscess nor on the direct Arthus reaction. RMI 10,874 inhibited carrageenan-induced paw edema but not
abscess. RMI 11,513 inhibited neither carrageenan abscess formation nor
the direct Arthus reaction. RMI 11,877 inhibited neither carrageenan-
induced paw edema nor abscess formation.

Subcutaneous administration of tilorone did not increase the susceptibility of mice to infection with Staphylococcus aureus [114]. In contrast,
susceptibility of mice to infection with Listeria monocytogenes was significantly increased [114]. Collins [115] found increased numbers of organisms
in livers and spleens of tilorone-treated mice infected with L. monocytogenes, Mycobacterium tuberculosis, and Salmonella enteritidis. Tilorone
enhanced infection by Salmonella and increased antibiotic dosage requirements for protection [116]. We found that tilorone administration to mice
24 hr prior to challenge with S. aureus ablated the protective response of
chloramphenicol. The effect was not evident when penicillin or sulfonamide
were substituted for chloramphenicol. Neither tilorone itself nor serum
collected from mice 24 hr after tilorone treatment affected the in vitro
action of chloramphicol against S. aureus. Munson et al. [59] found that
although tilorone did not protect against S. aureus challenge 24 hr later,
RMI 11,002 did.

TABLE 10. Rodent Antitumor Responses to Tilorone

Response	Tumor	References
Active	Mammary carcinoma 13762	117
	Reticulum cell sarcoma A-RCS	118
	Walker carcinosarcoma 256	118, 120-123
	Mammary adenocarcinoma R35	117, 123
	Morris hepatoma 3942A	120, 121
	Morris hepatoma 7777	118, 121
	Morris hepatoma 7794	121
	Lewis lung carcinoma (oral treatment)	124
	B_{16} melanoma	125
	Friend leukemia	56-63
	Leukemia K 1964	126
	Leukemia YLL	126
	Leukemia YALL	127
	Spontaneous lymphoma; development in immunosuppressed mice	128
Equivocal	B_{16} melanoma	117, 123, 129
	Murine sarcoma	111
Inactive	Ehrlich adenocarcinoma	59
	Prostatic adenocarcinoma	130
	Ependymoblastoma	123
	Mast cell tumor P815	118
	Plasma cell tumor YPC-1	118
	Lewis lung carcinoma (parenteral treatment)	123, 129
	L1210 leukemia	118, 123, 124
	P388 leukemia	118, 123, 124

V. ANTITUMOR ACTIVITY

Antitumor activity was demonstrated with tilorone in mice and rats. Table 10 provides the references for individual studies with tilorone [56-63, 111, 117, 118, 120-130]. Only an occasional discrepancy was observed, as noted by the B_{16} melanoma studies and subcutaneous vs. oral treatment of Lewis lung carcinoma. Oral administration provided better activity than did parenteral treatment. Generally, a single daily dose of tilorone was active in mice with responsive tumors, and in some cases, even a single weekly dose was active. Activity was reported against four of six leukemic and against eight of 14 solid tumors evaluated, excluding B_{16} melanoma and murine sarcoma, which must be considered equivocal. When used in sequence with 1,3-bis(2-chloroethyl)-1-nitrosourea therapy during remission of murine lymphoid leukemia, long-term survival resulted. Some of the analogs were more effective than tilorone.

The anticancer properties of RMI 11,002 were studied in several research laboratories in various animal models. Activity was demonstrated in mice against Ehrlich adenocarcinoma and Friend leukemia [59], Lewis lung carcinoma and B_{16} melanoma [124], and P388 lymphocytic leukemia [117]. No activity was seen in mice against L1210 leukemia [59,117,124] or in rats against R35 mammary adenocarcinoma [59].

RMI 11,567 was evaluated in vitro and in vivo for anticancer activity. Activity in cell culture at 2.6-3.6 µg/ml was demonstrated against a human epidermoid carcinoma of the nasopharynx [119]. In mice, oral administration inhibited sarcoma 180 [131]. An increase in survival time was obtained when RMI 11,567 was given intraperitoneally to P388 lymphocytic leukemic mice [117,119]. No activity was seen when intraperitoneal therapy was used for L1210 leukemic mice [117]. The compound was not effective in mice when evaluated against a transplantable fibrosarcoma which was induced by methylcholanthrene [131].

RMI 11,877 also was evaluated in vitro and in vivo for anti-cancer activity. It was active in cell cultures against a human epidermoid carcinoma of the nasopharynx [119]. In mouse models of L1210 lymphoid and P388 lymphocytic leukemias, no activity was found with intraperitoneal therapy.

The other four tilorone-related compounds have been tested for antitumor activity in mice. RMI 10,024 was active against Ehrlich adenocarcinoma and lymphocytic P388 leukemias and the solid tumors sarcoma 180, B_{16} melanoma, and a methylcholanthrene-induced fibrosarcoma. RMI 10,874 was active in mice against Friend leukemia, Lewis lung carcinoma, and Ehrlich adenocarcinoma but was inactive against L1210 and P388 leukemias as well as sarcoma 180 and the methylcholanthrene-induced fibrosarcoma. RMI 11,513 and RMI 11,645 were active in mice only against Ehrlich adenocarcinoma and were inactive against L1210 and P388 leukemias and sarcoma 180, B_{16} melanoma, and methylcholanthrene-induced fibrosarcoma. RMI 12,358 was tested only against L1210 leukemia and was inactive.

VI. CLINICAL STUDIES

The laboratory animal studies have suggested that tilorone hydrochloride and its analogs might have clinical utility against viral diseases, cancer, and in various immunologic disorders. Tilorone was the initial as well as most extensively studied representative investigated in humans.

Phase I clinical trials of tilorone were conducted in normal subjects [132] and in stage IV cancer patients who were refractory to all modes of

TABLE 11. Summary of Tilorone-Rubella Study in Humans

Parameter	Placebo	Tilorone
Total symptomatology	19.5 days	16.3 days
Average antibody response	299	68
Average length of time virus shed	8.0 days	5.0 days
Number of virus isolations (first passage)	13	3

therapy previously attempted with them [133]. The tolerated oral daily dose was about 500 mg, and the weekly tolerated single dose was 1500 mg. Side effects included nausea, vomiting, diarrhea, and stimulation of the central nervous system (CNS). After long-term therapy, transient corneal dysplasia developed in three of 120 patients [134]. The only clinical laboratory abnormality observed was the development of leukocyte inclusion bodies. Efforts to detect circulating interferon after a single, oral, 500-, 1000-, or 1500-mg dose of tilorone were unsuccessful.

Tilorone was evaluated against rubella virus in a double-blind challenge study in healthy male volunteers [135]. A single oral 750-mg dose of tilorone was given to four subjects 24 hr before intranasal inoculation with 1000 $TCID_{50}$ of virus. Four placebo subjects were treated similarly. Clinical and laboratory measurements indicated that tilorone did not prevent clinical infection but appeared to shorten illness by 3 days, suppress virus shedding, and prevent full antibody response (Table 11). The number of virus isolations on first passage indicated higher virus titers in controls. No remarkable side effects associated with therapy were observed. No interferon was found in the serum of subjects given tilorone 24 hr earlier. Lymphocyte transformation, dermal hypersensitivity, and peripheral blood T-cell numbers were assessed in these rubella-infected individuals [136]. Tilorone alone, or with rubella, had no effect on any of the parameters studied.

Since tilorone was very active against group A arboviruses causing neurotropic infections, SFV and VEE virus, an attempt to show clinical activity against a similar type virus was conducted [137]. Sandfly fever is a self-limiting febrile illness of viral etiology transmitted by the Phlebotomus fly. The virus is an ungrouped arbovirus. Temperatures of about 102° F are common after infection, with fever lasting from 1 to 3 days. Experience gained by the U.S. military has made it possible to understand and characterize viral pathogenesis so that it can be described with confidence as a well-defined acute viral infection, self-limiting, with no mortality or sequelae and a very predictable clinical course. The infection appears

to be well suited for assessing the antiviral activity of compounds like
tilorone in humans. Tilorone was given orally as a single, low dose of
500 mg to 10 male subjects, six of whom were inoculated intravenously
with plasma containing sandfly fever virus one day later. Four subjects
were infected but not treated. Conclusive evidence of interferon in tilorone-
treated noninfected subjects was not found. The proportion of subjects
with viremia was approximately the same among the tilorone and non-
tilorone-treated individuals. Both groups showed essentially the same
temporal onset and persistence of viremia. It was concluded that tilorone
was inactive against sandfly fever virus infection in humans.

    Five children with subacute sclerosing panencephalitis were treated
with tilorone [138]. Two children who received a single weekly oral dose
of 20 mg/kg for more than a year showed definite improvement. Two others
on the same tilorone regimen have been treated for less than six months
and cannot yet be conclusively evaluated at this stage. The fifth child with-
drew because of nausea and vomiting.

    A renal transplant patient, who had been on immunosuppressive therapy
and developed progressive multifocal leukoencephalopathy (PML), was
placed on a twice-a-week regimen of 750-mg tilorone per dose after cessation of azathioprine but continuance of prednisone [139]. After 16 months
of tilorone treatment, T-cell rosettes increased and phytohemagglutinin
T-cell-stimulated mitogenesis improved. Delayed hypersensitivity to
Candida appeared. B-cell stimulation to S. aureus antigen was greater
than in normals. Serum immunoglobulin normalized and cerebrospinal
fluid (CSF) IgG was increased. Neurological status and renal function remained unchanged in a condition that generally gets progressively worse.
It was felt that continual immunosuppressive therapy prompted the expression of PML. Tilorone was chosen to treat this particular patient because
it suppresses T-cell function, stimulates humoral immunity, and is antiviral. Although the findings were positive and tilorone could have accounted
for the enhanced humoral response and arrest of virus activity, cessation
of azathioprine alone could possibly have accounted for the improvements
measured.

    A therapeutic, double-blind, placebo-controlled trial with 16 amyo-
trophic lateral sclerosis patients showed no evidence of any benefit from
tilorone treatment [140]. Poly I: poly C: poly lysine was also not effective
in patients with this disease [141].

    In stage IV cancer, positive responses were seen in patients with
malignant melanoma [133]. No bone marrow depression was seen, and
there appeared to be a transient stimulation of platelet production. Because
of the encouraging responses seen in this initial and limited investigation,
phase II trials were conducted in 66 patients who were beyond hope of cure.
No significant benefits were observed in 13 melanoma patients. Partial
responses were seen in patients with breast and renal cancer [142]. As
part of the Eastern Oncology Multi-Clinic Cooperative Study Group, 25

advanced breast cancer patients were also studied. No significant responses were seen, and the drug was not considered of value when used as a single agent [143].

Tilorone was also evaluated against cancer in humans in France [144]. It was given orally alone or in combination with other therapy to 48 patients with disseminated or inoperable cancer. The only detectable response was the temporary arrest of tumor growth in six of 11 patients with measurable metastatic lung lesions where tumor doubling time was known.

In an ongoing investigation of tilorone in children with acute leukemia in relapse, changes in leukocytes other than inclusion bodies have been reported. A transient decrease in percent of T cells was found in five of seven patients, in three there were increases in active T cells, and in four a transient increase in B cells [145].

The only other tilorone-related compound where data have been published involves RMI 11,002 [146]. The drug was given orally to advanced cancer patients who were beyond surgical, radiotherapeutic, or chemotherapeutic cure. In 32 patients, given 1.6-25 mg/kg of the compound daily for up to 91 days, no tumor regression nor stabilization was observed. Side effects were similar to those seen with tilorone. In addition, three cases of acute allergic dermatitis were noted that responded promptly to drug withdrawal. Maximum tolerated dose was 22 mg/kg per day, which was greater than that found with tilorone.

VII. CONCLUSION

The antiviral chemotherapist prefers to deal with well-defined chemical entities, and the advent of the low-molecular-weight interferon inducer offers promising possibilities to explore new classes of compounds and new concepts of antiviral chemotherapy. The opportunities for molecular modification to achieve optimal structure activity relationships and minimize toxicity are manifold. Tilorone hydrochloride, the first, and still one of the most potent low-molecular-weight interferon inducers, represents the standard by which other compounds of its kind are measured.

Dosage requirements for expression of full activity by these compounds are generally high. Toxicity in higher animals is increased considerably as one goes up the phylogenetic ladder, so the therapeutic ratio against any infection is likely to be diminished. Just as variation among viruses in interferon sensitivity exists [147], so is there an order of virus sensitivity to inducers in vivo [148]. Add to this the fact that the challenge dose of virus used to assure infection surely is greater than that encountered under natural conditions and the chances for clinical success are reduced substantially. The exclusive requirement for prophylactic treatment, other than shortly after viral exposure, is another handicap to clinical interest and usage.

That interferon induction is a major factor in the antiviral activity of tilorone and related compounds has been proved. Serum interferon levels and the degree of activity against vesicular stomatitis virus, Semliki Forest, and encephalomyocarditis viruses showed close correlation [18,37], although Giron et al. could not establish that point with low doses of tilorone against MM virus [40]. We have shown the interferon-antiviral relationship in several ways with Semliki Forest and encephalomyocarditis viruses, namely, through (1) dose response curves, (2) time response curves, and (3) hyporeactive responses. Furthermore, we have been unable to induce interferon in hamsters with tilorone, and this compound will not protect hamsters against paralysis caused by Semliki Forest virus, in our hands, the most sensitive virus to interferon inducers in vivo. Herpes viruses were insensitive to interferon stimulated in mice by tilorone and related compounds. The same compounds, active when applied topically to hairless mice infected with herpes viruses, failed to prevent lesion development if they were given orally or subcutaneously.

Although interferon induction by these compounds most assuredly plays a protective role in some infections, it obviously does not represent the whole story. Direct inactivation of viruses and topical activity against herpes viruses with some of the compounds in the presence or absence of white light do not involve an interferon function. Tilorone, RMI 11,002, RMI 11,567, and RMI 11,877 all induce substantial amounts of interferon in mice, yet only tilorone was active against influenza PR_8. No interferon was detected in monkeys treated with these four compounds, yet all were active against Venezuelan equine encephalomyelitis virus.

There is ample reason to suspect that the immunoregulatory and even the anti-inflammatory properties of tilorone and related compounds could influence certain other disease states. Also, template binding by tilorone and some of its related compounds affected polymerase action of oncogenic viruses, which might account, in part, for some of the antitumor actions observed [149-155]. The ultimate success of these low-molecular-weight interferon inducers, then, may not be marked by their interferon-inducing potential but by their other actions. Their broad biological profile must be considered. Besides interferon induction and direct virus inactivations, some decrease cell-mediated immunity while others stimulate it (this may be dosage and regimen dependent); many stimulate humoral immunity, phagocytosis, inhibit reverse transcriptases, and influence complement and prostacyclin formation and/or action. Tilorone stimulates complement. The specific clinical indication where compounds with such actions might be useful include, of course, acute viral, bacterial, and fungal infections, slow virus infections, tumors, transplants, arthritis, and possible use as vaccine adjuvants.

Currently a laboratory curiosity, these low-molecular-weight interferon inducers still seek their niche among the drugs of the future.

REFERENCES

1. G. D. Mayer and B. A. Fink, Fed. Proc. 29: 635 (1970).
2. G. D. Mayer and R. F. Krueger, Science 169: 1214 (1970).
3. R. F. Krueger and S. Yoshimura, Fed. Proc. 29: 635 (1970).
4. R. F. Krueger and G. D. Mayer, Science 169: 1213 (1970).
5. W. Regelson, J. A. Munson, R. F. Krueger, A. E. Munson, and
   G. D. Mayer, Presentation at the International Meeting of the Reticuloendothelial Society, Freiburg, Germany, 1970.
6. P. F. Hoffman and H. W. Ritter, J. Ret. Soc. 9: 638 (1971).
7. H. Megel, A. Raychaudhuri, S. Goldstein, C. R. Kinsolving,
   I. Shemano, and J. G. Michael, Proc. Soc. Exp. Biol. Med. 145:
   513 (1974).
8. A. D. Sill, W. L. Albrecht, E. R. Andrews, R. W. Fleming, S. W.
   Horgan, E. M. Roberts, and W. Sweet, J. Med. Chem. 16: 240 (1973).
9. W. L. Albrecht, E. R. Andrews, R. W. Fleming, J. M. Grisar,
   S. W. Horgan, A. D. Sill, F. W. Sweet, and D. L. Wenstrup,
   Presentation at the Meeting of the American Chemical Society, Chicago,
   Ill., 1970.
10. R. W. Fleming, W. L. Albrecht, E. R. Andrews, J. M. Grisar,
    S. W. Horgan, A. D. Sill, F. W. Sweet, and D. L. Wenstrup, Int.
    Colloq. on Interferon and Interferon Inducers, Leuven, Belgium (1971).
11. W. L. Albrecht, in Modulation of Host Immune Resistance in the Pre-
    vention or Treatment of Induced Neoplasias (M. A. Chirigos, ed.),
    U.S. Government Printing Office, Washington, D.C., 1974, p. 83.
12. W. L. Albrecht, R. W. Fleming, S. W. Horgan, J. C. Kihm, and
    G. D. Mayer, J. Med. Chem. 17: 886 (1974).
13. W. L. Albrecht, R. W. Fleming, S. W. Horgan, and G. D. Mayer,
    J. Med. Chem. 20: 364 (1977).
14. E. R. Andrews, R. W. Fleming, J. M. Grisar, J. C. Kihm, D. L.
    Wenstrup, and G. D. Mayer, J. Med. Chem. 17: 882 (1974).
15. A. A. Carr, J. F. Grunwell, A. D. Sill, D. R. Meyer, F. W. Sweet,
    B. J. Scheve, J. M. Grisar, and R. W. Fleming, J. Med. Chem. 19:
    1142 (1976).
16. A. D. Sill, E. R. Andrews, F. W. Sweet, J. W. Hoffman, P. L.
    Tiernan, J. M. Grisar, R. W. Fleming, and G. D. Mayer, J. Med.
    Chem. 17: 965 (1974).
17. D. A. Stringfellow and L. A. Glasgow, Antimicrob. Agents Chemother.
    2: 73 (1972).
18. E. DeClercq and T. C. Merigan, J. Infec. Dis. 123: 190 (1971).
19. M. J. Kanady and W. R. Smith, Proc. Soc. Exp. Biol. Med. 141: 794
    (1972).
20. H. Megel, A. Raychaudhuri, and J. P. Gibson, in Control of Neoplasia
    by Modulation of the Immune System (M. A. Chirigos, ed.), Raven
    Press, New York, 1977, p. 409.

21. J. P. Gibson, H. Megel, K. P. Camyre, and J. G. Michael, Proc. Soc. Exp. Biol. Med. 151:264 (1976).

22. R. F. Krueger, G. D. Mayer, S. Yoshimura, and K. A. Ludwig, in Antimicrob. Agents Chemother. 1970 (G. L. Hobby, ed.), American Society of Microbiology, Bethesda, Md., 1971, p. 486.

23. G. D. Mayer, R. F. Krueger, K. P. Camyre, F. Bray, and C. R. Hull, Bacteriol. Proc. p. 195 (1971).

24. E. DeClercq and T. C. Merigan, Virology 42:799 (1970).

25. Z. V. Ermolieva, L. E. Korneeva, G. I. Balezina, D. V. Nikolaeva, I. S. Gvazava, and L. L. Fadeeva, Antibiotiki 18:517 (1973).

26. H. E. Kaufman, Y. M. Centifanto, E. D. Ellison, and D. C. Brown, Proc. Soc. Exp. Biol. Med. 137:357 (1971).

27. J. W. Groelke, K. P. Camyre, and G. D. Mayer, Proc. Soc. Exp. Biol. Med. 148:1044 (1975).

28. M. Degre and E. T. Glaz, Acta Pathol. Microbiol. Scand. B85:189 (1977).

29. A. J. Dennis, H. E. Wilson, A. D. Barker, and M. S. Rheins, Proc. Soc. Exp. Biol. Med. 141:782 (1972).

30. F. Dianzani, P. Cantagalli, S. Gagnoni, and G. Rita, Proc. Soc. Exp. Biol. Med. 128:708 (1968).

31. R. F. Krueger, G. D. Mayer, K. P. Camyre, and S. Yoshimura, Presentation at 11th Intersci. Conf. Antimicrob. Agents Chemother., Atlantic City, N.J., 1971.

32. M. Ho, in Interferons and Interferon Inducers (N. Finter, ed.), American Elsevier, New York, 1973, p. 100.

33. D. A. Stringfellow, E. R. Kern, D. K. Kelsey, and L. A. Glasgow, J. Infec. Dis. 135:540 (1977).

34. M. Ho, B. Postic, and Y. H. Ke, in Interferon: March 1967 Ciba Foundation Symposium (G. E. W. Wolstenholme and M. O'Connor, eds.), Churchill, London, 1968, p. 19.

35. E. T. Glaz and M. Talas, Acta Virol. 17:168 (1973).

36. J. S. Youngner and W. R. Stinebring, Nature 208:456 (1965).

37. G. D. Mayer and R. F. Krueger, Proc. 5th Int. Congr. Infec. Dis., Vienna p. 245 (1970).

38. W. L. Albrecht, Presentation at Univ. of Illinois Coll. Pharm., Urbana, 1972.

39. W. L. Albrecht, E. R. Andrews, A. A. Carr, R. W. Fleming, J. M. Grisar, S. W. Horgan, A. D. Sill, F. W. Sweet, and D. L. Wenstrup, Med. Chem. Symposium, Iowa City (1972).

40. D. J. Giron, J. P. Schmidt, and F. F. Pindak, Antimicrob. Agents Chemother. 1:78 (1972).

41. D. A. Stringfellow, J. C. Overall, Jr., and L. A. Glasgow, J. Infec. Dis. 130:470 (1974).

42. A. Vickenstedt and M. Horn, Chemotherapy (Basel) 20:235 (1974).

43. G. D. Mayer, A. C. Hagan, and F. Bray, Fed. Proc. 32:704 (1973).

44. R. W. Kuehne, W. L. Pannier, and E. L. Stephen, Antimicrob. Agents Chemother. 11:683 (1977).
45. E. L. Stephen, R. D. Spertzel, W. L. Pannier, and R. L. Mundy, Fed. Proc. 33:555 (1974).
46. G. D. Mayer, R. F. Krueger, and S. Yoshimura, Bacteriol. Proc. p. 188 (1972).
47. J. Portnoy and T. C. Merigan, Clin. Res. 19:139 (1971).
48. J. Portnoy and T. C. Merigan, J. Infec. Dis. 124:545 (1971).
49. J. F. Fitzwilliam and J. F. Griffith, J. Infec. Dis. 133 (Suppl.):A221 (1976).
50. E. Katz, E. Margalith, and B. Winer, Antimicrob. Agents Chemother. 9:189 (1976).
51. G. D. Mayer, F. Bray, and K. P. Camyre, Presentation at 14th Intersci. Conf. Antimicrob. Agents and Chemother., San Francisco, 1974.
52. T. Tokumaru, Res. Commun. Chem. Pathol. Pharmacol. 11:289 (1975).
53. H. Hofmann and C. Kunz, Arch. Ges. Virusforsch. 37:262 (1972).
54. L. M. Vilner, E. V. Finogenova, N. S. Tikhomirova-Sidorova, I. M. Rodin, V. A. Kropachev, E. M. Kogan, and L. B. Trukhmandva, Vop. Virusologie 1:70 (1976).
55. J. Y. Richmond and C. H. Campbell, Arch. Ges. Virusforsch. 42:102 (1973).
56. A. D. Barker, M. S. Rheins, and H. E. Wilson, Bacteriol. Proc. p. 188 (1971).
57. A. D. Barker, M. S. Rheins, and H. E. Wilson, Proc. Soc. Exp. Biol. Med. 137:981 (1971).
58. A. D. Barker, Diss. Abstr. Int. B32:2881 (1971).
59. A. E. Munson, J. A. Munson, W. Regelson, and G. L. Wampler, Cancer Res. 32:1397 (1972).
60. M. S. Rheins, A. D. Barker, and H. E. Wilson, Can. J. Microbiol. 17:1257 (1971).
61. M. W. Rana and H. Pinkerton, Anat. Rec. 178:444 (1974).
62. M. W. Rana, H. Pinkerton, and A. Rankin, Proc. Soc. Exp. Biol. Med. 150:32 (1975).
63. M. S. Rheins, A. D. Barker, and H. E. Wilson, Bacteriol. Proc. p. 188 (1971).
64. F. Fornosi, M. Talas, and G. Weiszfeiler, Acta Microbiol. Acad. Sci. Hung. 18:327 (1971).
65. K. W. Cochran, Abstr. Amer. Soc. Microbiol., 72nd Meeting (1972).
66. H. Hofmann and C. Kunz, Zbl. Bakteriol. (Orig. A) 225:305 (1973).
67. V. V. Vargin, W. Zschiesche, and B. F. Semenov, Acta Virol. 21:114 (1977).
68. E. Katz, B. Winer, and E. Margalith, J. Gen. Virol. 31:125 (1976).
69. R. H. Adamson, D. V. Ablashi, G. R. Armstrong, and V. W. Ellmore, Antimicrob. Agents Chemother. 1:82 (1972).

70. K. P. Camyre, J. W. Groelke, and W. L. Albrecht, Abstr. Amer. Soc. Microbiol., 73rd Meeting (1973).

71. H. Megel, I. Shemano, A. Raychaudhuri, and J. P. Gibson, in Modulation of Host Immune Resistance in the Prevention and Treatment of Induced Neoplasias (M. A. Chirigos, ed.), U.S. Government Printing Office, Washington, D.C., 1974, p. 103.

72. H. Megel, Presentation at the International Symposium on New Anti-inflammatory Drugs, Pisa, Italy, 1976.

73. T. Diamantstein, Immunology 24: 771 (1973).

74. H. Megel, A. Raychaudhuri, S. Goldstein, C. R. Kinsolving, I. Shemano, and J. G. Michael, Fed. Proc. 32: 1021 (1973).

75. A. E. Munson, J. A. Munson, and W. Regelson, Int. Colloq. on Interferon and Interferon Inducers, Leuven, Belgium (1971).

76. B. C. Cole, J. C. Overall, Jr., P. S. Lombardi, and L. A. Glasgow, Infec. Immun. 12: 1349 (1975).

77. D. A. Stringfellow and L. A. Glasgow, Infec. Immun. 6: 743 (1972).

78. C. E. Buckler, H. G. Du Buy, R. R. Rafajko, and S. Baron, Int. Colloq. on Interferon and Interferon Inducers, Leuven, Belgium (1971).

79. S. Levine and R. Sowinski, Amer. J. Pathol. 82: 381 (1976).

80. W. Brown and M. Makano, Science 157: 819 (1967).

81. T. J. Chester, E. DeClercq, and T. C. Merigan, Infec. Immun. 3: 516 (1971).

82. H. Cantor, R. Asofsky, and H. B. Levy, J. Immunol. 104: 1035 (1970).

83. T. J. Chester, K. Paucker, and T. C. Merigan, Nature 246: 92 (1973).

84. R. M. Massanari, Clin. Res. 25: 380A (1977).

85. S. Levine, R. Sowinski, and W. L. Albrecht, Toxicol. Appl. Pharmacol. 40: 137 (1977).

86. H. Megel and A. Raychaudhuri, Presentation at a meeting of the Reticuloendothelial Society, Miami Beach, Fla., 1975.

87. J. P. Gibson and J. W. Newberne, Lab. Invest. 34: 316 (1976).

88. G. Zbinden and E. Emch, Acta Haematol. 47: 49 (1972).

89. S. Levine, J. P. Gibson, and H. Megel, Proc. Soc. Exp. Biol. Med. 146: 245 (1974).

90. S. Levine, in Modulation of Host Immune Resistance in the Prevention or Treatment of Induced Neoplasias (M. A. Chirigos, ed.), U.S. Government Printing Office, Washington, D.C., 1974, p. 89.

91. A. Raychaudhuri and H. Megel, J. Ret. Soc. 20: 127 (1976).

92. K. S. Johansen, T. S. Johansen, and D. W. Talmadge, J. Allergy Clin. Immunol. 54: 86 (1974).

93. G. E. Freidlaender, M. B. Mosher, and M. S. Mitchell, Cancer Res. 34: 304 (1974).

94. R. E. Kavetsky, Vop. Onkol. 23: 88 (1977).

95. L. E. Mobraaten, E. DeMaeyer, and J. DeMaeyer-Guignard, Transplantation 16: 415 (1973).

96. H. Megel, A. Raychaudhuri, and L. L. Thomas, Transplantation 21: 81 (1976).
97. A. Wildstein, L. E. Stevens, and G. Hashim, Clin. Res. 23:299A (1975).
98. A. Wildstein, L. E. Stevens, and G. Hashim, Transplantation 21: 129 (1976).
99. A. Wildstein, L. Stevens, H. Applebaum, R. McCabe, G. Hashim, and H. Fitzpatrick, Proc. Clin. Dial. Transplant Forum 5:47 (1975).
100. A. Wildstein, L. E. Stevens, H. Applebaum, R. E. McCabe, G. A. Hashim, and H. Fitzpatrick, Transplantation 22:205 (1976).
101. J. P. Donahue, J. Giambrone, O. J. Fletcher, and S. H. Kleven, Amer. J. Vet. Res. 38:2013 (1977).
102. W. E. Houston, C. L. Crabbs, E. L. Stephen, and H. B. Levy, Infec. Immun. 14:318 (1976).
103. S. J. Mohr and M. A. Chirigos, in Modulation of Host Immune Resistance in the Prevention or Treatment of Induced Neoplasias (M. A. Chirigos, ed.), U.S. Government Printing Office, Washington, D.C., 1974, p. 131.
104. J. W. Pearson, S. D. Chaparas, M. A. Chirigos, and N. A. Sher, J. Nat. Cancer Inst. 52:463 (1974).
105. K. Huang, R. M. Donahue, F. B. Gordon, and H. R. Dressler, Infec. Immun. 4:581 (1971).
106. M. Rabinovitch, R. E. Manejias, M. Russo, and E. E. Abbey, Cell. Immunol. 29:86 (1977).
107. D. A. Stringfellow, Abstr. Amer. Soc. Microbiol., 77th Meeting (1977).
108. E. Jirillo, D. Fumarola, R. Monno, and I. Munno, Boll. Soc. Ital. Biol. Sper. 53:20 (1977).
109. D. A. Stringfellow, F. A. Fitzpatrick, F. F. Sun, and J. C. McGuire, Prostaglandins 16:901-910 (1978).
110. S. E. Walker, Clin. Immunol. Immunopathol. 8:204 (1977).
111. A. F. Gazdar, A. D. Steinberg, and S. Baron, Int. Colloq. on Interferon and Interferon Inducers, Leuven, Belgium (1971).
112. A. F. Gazdar, A. D. Steinberg, G. F. Spahn, and S. Baron, Proc. Soc. Exp. Biol. Med. 139:1132 (1972).
113. A. F. Gazdar, J. Nat. Cancer Inst. 49:1435 (1972).
114. R. Gruenewald and S. Levine, Infec. Immun. 13:1613 (1976).
115. F. M. Collins, Antimicrob. Agents Chemother. 7:447 (1975).
116. F. E. Durr and N. A. Kuck, Abstr. Amer. Soc. Microbiol., 73rd Meeting p. 251 (1973).
117. NCI: CCNSC Screening Report to Merrell-National Laboratories, Merrell-National Laboratories Project Rept. No. 0-72-32 (1973).
118. R. H. Adamson, J. Nat. Cancer Inst. 46:431 (1971).
119. NCI: CCNSC Screening Report to Merrell-National Laboratories, Merrell-National Laboratories Project Rept. No. 0-73-08.

120. A. Rhoads, D. Roye, W. West, and H. P. Morris, Proc. 162nd
     Meeting Amer. Chem. Soc. (1971).
121. A. R. Rhoads, W. L. West, and H. P. Morris, Res. Commun.
     Chem. Path. Pharmacol. 6: 741 (1973).
122. R. H. Adamson, Arch. Int. Pharmacodyn. 192: 161 (1971).
123. NCI: CCNSC Screening Report to Merrell-National Laboratories,
     Merrell-National Laboratories Project Rept. No. 0-71-46 (1971).
124. G. L. Wampler and W. Regelson, in Modulation of Host Immune
     Resistance in the Prevention or Treatment of Induced Neoplasias
     (M. A. Chirigos, ed.), U.S. Government Printing Office, Washington,
     D.C., 1974, p. 123.
125. E. V. Turner and J. H. Wallace, Abstr. Amer. Soc. Microbiol.,
     77th Meeting (1977).
126. D. G. Johns, S. M. Sieber, and R. H. Adamson, in Modulation of
     Host Immune Resistance in the Prevention or Treatment of Induced
     Neoplasias (M. A. Chirigos, ed.), U.S. Government Printing Office,
     Washington, D.C., 1974, p. 117.
127. S. T. Yancey and W. A. Bleyer, Cancer Res. 34: 1866 (1974).
128. S. E. Walker and M. R. Anver, Clin. Res. 22: 612A (1974).
129. P. S. Morahan, J. A. Munson, L. G. Baird, A. M. Kaplan, and
     W. Regelson, Cancer Res. 34: 506 (1974).
130. G. R. Burleson and M. Pollard, Fed. Proc. 35: 624 (1976).
131. Sloan-Kettering Institute for Cancer Research, Merrell-National
     Laboratories Project Rept. No. 0-73-75 (1973).
132. G. M. Schiff, C. C. Linnemann, T. Rotte, G. Mayer, and S. Trimble,
     Presentation at Symposium on Antivirals with Clinical Potential,
     Stanford Univ., Stanford, Calif., 1975.
133. G. L. Wampler, M. Kuperminc, and W. Regelson, Cancer Chemo-
     ther. Rep. 57: 209 (1973).
134. M. Cawein, B. C. Lampkin, I. Tsukimoto, G. Mayer, W. Regelson,
     and G. Schiff, Presentation at Symposium on Antivirals with Clinical
     Potential, Stanford Univ., Stanford, Calif., 1975.
135. G. M. Schiff, C. C. Linnemann, T. Rotte, G. Mayer, and S. Trimble,
     Clin. Res. 21: 882 (1973).
136. C. A. Kauffman, J. P. Phair, C. C. Linnemann, Jr., and G. M.
     Schiff, Inf. Immun. 10: 212 (1974).
137. J. E. Hill, Ann. Progr. Rept. FY 1973 p. 189 (1973).
138. G. M. Fenichel, G. Saavedra, and H. N. Cooper, Presentation at
     Child Neurology Society Conference, Monterey, Calif., 1976.
139. J. B. Selhorst, K. F. Ducy, J. M. Thomas, and W. Regelson,
     Presentation at American Academy of Neurology, 1978.
140. W. H. Olson, J. A. Simons, and G. W. Halaas, Neurology 28: 1293
     (1978).
141. W. K. Engel, R. A. Cuneo, and H. B. Levy, Lancet i: 503 (1978).
142. P. Richter, G. L. Wampler, M. Kuperminc, and W. Regelson, in
     Modulation of Host Immune Resistance in the Prevention or Treat-

ment of Induced Neoplasias (M. A. Chirigos, ed.), U.S. Government Printing Office, Washington, D.C., 1974, p. 141.

143. M. Kuperminc and R. Gelber, Proc. Am. Assoc. Cancer Res. 17: 260 (1976).

144. L. Israel, P. Miller, and R. Edelstein, in Modulation of Host Immune Resistance in the Prevention or Treatment of Induced Neoplasias (M. A. Chirigos, ed.), U.S. Government Printing Office, Washington, D.C., 1974, p. 145.

145. B. C. Lampkin, D. A. Hake, and S. Granger, Abstr. 16th Int. Congr. Hematol. p. 224 (1976).

146. P. Richter, G. L. Wampler, M. Kuperminc, and W. Regelson, in Modulation of Host Immune Resistance in the Prevention or Treatment of Induced Neoplasias (M. A. Chirigos, ed.), U.S. Government Printing Office, Washington, D.C., 1974, p. 139.

147. W. E. Stewart, W. D. Scott, and S. E. Sulkin, J. Virol. 4: 147 (1969).

148. G. D. Mayer and R. F. Krueger, in Antimicrob. Agents Chemother. 1969 (G. L. Hobby, ed.), American Society of Microbiology, Bethesda, Md., 1970, p. 182.

149. P. Chandra, F. Zunino, and A. Gotz, FEBS Lett. 22: 161 (1972).

150. P. Chandra, F. Zunino, A. Zaccara, and A. Wacker, FEBS Lett. 23: 145 (1972).

151. P. Chandra, F. Zunino, V. P. Gaur, A. Zaccara, and G. Luoni, FEBS Lett. 28: 5 (1972).

152. P. Chandra and M. Woltersdorf, FEBS Lett. 41: 169 (1974).

153. P. Chandra, G. Will, D. Gericke, and A. Gotz, Biochem. Pharmacol. 23: 3259 (1974).

154. M. Green, G. F. Gerard, D. P. Grandgenett, C. Gurgo, A. M. Rankin, M. R. Green, and D. M. Cassell, Cancer 34: 1427 (1974).

155. M. Green and G. F. Gerard, in Progress in Nucleic Acid Research and Molecular Biology, Vol. 14 (W. E. Cohn, ed.), Academic Press, New York, 1974, pp. 255 and 322.

9

INTERFERON INDUCERS: PROPANEDIAMINES AND RELATED MOLECULES

Robert F. Betts and R. Gordon Douglas, Jr.
University of Rochester School of Medicine
Rochester, New York

I. INTRODUCTION

Because of the diversity of viral families and serotypes that produce common colds and related syndromes, control by specific vaccine seems unlikely. Therefore, the use of exogenous interferon or interferon inducers to prevent or treat respiratory viral infections is particularly attractive. Some success already has been achieved with the use of interferon and interferon inducers in this setting. For example, in studies in volunteers, the intranasal application of large quantities of human leukocyte interferon has been shown to reduce the symptoms of rhinovirus illness [1], and topical application of poly I:poly C was shown to have some effect in reducing incidence of rhinovirus infections [2].

This success has stimulated further efforts, since respiratory viral infections constitute our most common afflictions and are the most important cause of days lost from school and industry in this country. Further trials with human leukocyte interferon, as discussed elsewhere in this book, have been limited to a few life-threatening conditions because of the cost and limited supply, and it is generally agreed that poly I:poly C is too toxic for use in acute self-limited infections. Thus, a search for other, cheaper sources of human interferon, or less toxic inducers continues.

A series of low-molecular-weight interferon inducers was developed by Pfizer Research, Groton, Connecticut. Of these, two that appeared most promising—a propanediamine called CP-20,961 [3] and a xylenediamine, CP-28,888 (J. F. Niblack, personal communication)—have been tested clinically.

II. CHEMISTRY

CP-20,961* is a white microcrystalline solid with a melting point between 37° and 39°C (see Figure 1). It is a lipoidal diamine with an aqueous solubility so low that using it requires formulation in an aqueous emulsion using surfactive dispersants. For clinical trials, it has been fused with equal weights of polysorbate 80 and glycerol [3].

---

*N,N-Dioctadecyl-N',N'-bis(2-hydroxyethyl)propanediamine.

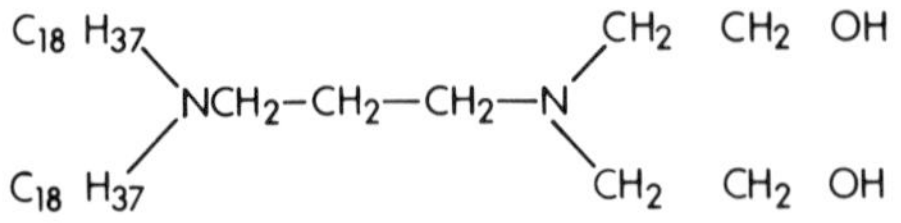

FIGURE 1. Chemical structure of CP-20,961 (N,N-dioctadecyl-N',N'-bis(2-hydroxyethyl)propanediamine).

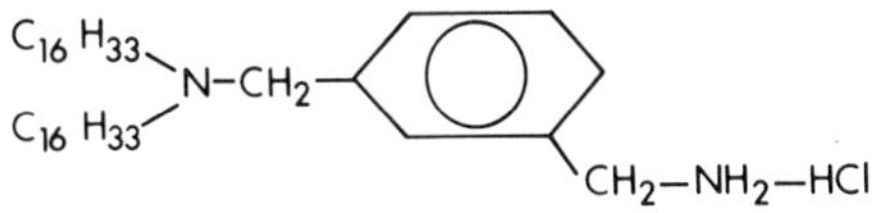

FIGURE 2. Chemical structure of CP-28,888 (N,N-dihexadecyl-m-xylylenediamine).

CP-28,888* is a molecule related to CP-20,961, but it is a substituted xylenediamine rather than a propanediamine, as shown in Figure 2 (J. F. Niblack, personal communication). Like CP-20,961, it possesses low aqueous solubility and also requires emulsification for clinical trials.

III. ACTIVITY IN EXPERIMENTAL ANIMALS

A. CP-20,961

Although oral administration has not been effective, administration of CP-20,961 to mice intraperitoneally markedly reduces mortality of these animals from challenge with encephalomyocarditis virus [3]. Semliki Forest virus infection in mice is even more sensitive to the effects of CP-20,961, and pox resulting from injection of vaccinia virus into the tail of weaning mice are suppressed by intraperitoneal administration of this drug. However, no protective effect was observed in mice when CP-20,961 was tested against two RNA viruses, influenza A/Hong Kong/68 H3N2 virus and pneumonia virus of mice [3]. In the encephalomyocarditis virus model infection, CP-20,961 is more effective with lower multiplicity of infection, and its dose response curve is linear. It is most effective when administered between 24 and 6 hr prior to infection. Administration of drug 3 hr postinfection reduces its effect 10-fold, and no effect is discernible if drug is administered 24 hr postinfection. Toxicity in the mice is not detectable except for a low-grade peritonitis which develops in those animals who receive doses greater than 200 mg/kg intraperitoneally [3].

B. CP-28,888

CP-28,888 appears to be a more potent interferon inducer in mice than CP-20,961 (J. F. Niblack, personal communication). Also, interferon stimulation in plasma of rats was demonstrated with CP-28,888 but not with CP-20,961 (J. F. Niblack, personal communication), when given in

---

*N,N-Dihexadecyl-m-xylylenediamine.

equivalent doses of 25 mg/kg intraperitoneally to mice. Protection against
challenge with vaccinia and encephalomyocarditis virus was superior with
CP-28,888. In hamsters, reduction of symptoms due to influenza A virus
was demonstrated with CP-28,888 but not with CP-20,961.

Several features suggest that the drug's effect is mediated by interferon.
First, interferon-like activity can be demonstrated in the plasma of mice
who are injected with these drugs. This activity appears 12 hr after administration of drug and persists for 20 hr. Second, plasma interferon
levels are about 10-fold higher following CP-28,888 administration than
with CP-20,961, and the higher interferon levels correlate with greater
protection. This interferon-like activity is partially inactivated if held at
pH 2 for 24 hr at 5°C, and treatment of the preparation with 0.25% trypsin
for 1 hr at 37°C completely eliminated its activity. These are properties
consistent with type II or immune interferon. Third, the drug itself has no
direct antiviral effect at a concentration of 40 μg/ml, and finally, it does
not stimulate cell-mediated antiviral activity.

In spite of this in vivo effect, neither CP-20,961 nor CP-28,888 stimulates interferon in cell cultures, nor do they protect cell cultures against
challenge with vesicular stomatitis virus ([3]; J. F. Niblack, personal communication). However, both compounds enhance the protective activity of
poly I:poly C in such cultures, and they are equally potent in this regard
(J. F. Niblack, personal communication).

The lack of toxicity of these compounds and their demonstrated efficacy
as inducers of interferon in animal systems prompted initial toxicity studies
in humans; and when these drugs proved to be safe, subsequent studies in
experimental viral infection in humans were carried out.

IV. COMPARATIVE FEATURES OF EXPERIMENTAL
      VS. NATURAL VIRUS INFECTIONS IN HUMANS

Clinical evaluation of antiviral substances, including interferon and interferon inducers, in respiratory viral infections may be carried out in naturally
occurring or experimentally induced infections. In addition, one has to
make choices about which of the many serologically distinct viruses should
be studied. Most often, experimental rhinovirus and influenza A virus
infection are chosen, rhinovirus infection because of its major role in the
etiology of the most frequent respiratory tract syndrome, the common cold,
and influenza A virus infection because of its unpredictable epidemic nature
and resultant mortality. Very few studies have been performed in respiratory syncytial, parainfluenza, coronavirus, adenovirus, and other types of
respiratory viral infections, despite the importance of these agents.

Experimental infections are desirable for study because a suitable number of subjects can be studied at a single point in time so that a well-designed, double-blind placebo evaluation can be carried out. In addition, the timing of drug administration in relation to virus inoculation can be easily manipulated. Study of natural cases of common colds, or other respiratory syndromes, would take many months to complete because of the diverse etiology of such infections. On the other hand, naturally occurring influenza, because of its epidemic nature and high attack rate, lends itself to study.

Since most studies are performed on experimental infections in volunteers, one must understand the closeness with which experimental infection in volunteers approximates natural infection to interpret the results. Intranasal inoculation of volunteers with a rhinovirus results in an infection which closely mimics natural infection in humans [4]. The infectious dose for humans is very small and has been estimated for several serotypes to be 0.01-1.0 fifty-percent tissue culture infectious dose ($TCID_{50}$). Illness very similar to natural illness consisting of rhinitis, pharyngitis, and, in a low frequency, constitutional symptoms and fever, develops 24-48 hr postchallenge and lasts two to five days. Virus shedding in nasal secretions is detected simultaneously with the development of symptoms, and nasal secretory antibody and interferon-like activity can be recovered from nasal wash material. Artificially induced infection confers immunity against subsequent exposure to natural infection. Much of the available information on natural rhinovirus infection suggests that virus is transmitted by inoculation into the anterior nares and, thus, the experimental infection approximates natural illness both in its mode of acquisition and clinical expression.

Experimental influenza A virus infection in humans, on the other hand, has dissimilarities compared to natural influenza [5]. First, a high inoculum of virus into the nose is required to produce infection. The resulting illness is milder than natural infection in that fever and cough are less frequent and less severe, and pulmonary function abnormalities that occur regularly in natural influenza are not detected in experimental influenza [5]. On the other hand, the titer of virus shed in the nasal wash specimens is higher and persists for a longer period in experimental infection compared to natural infection. In fact, much of the data concerning transmission of natural influenza suggests that natural influenza is transmitted by small particle aerosols, which deposit and initiate infection in the lower respiratory tract [6]. Aerosol inoculation of volunteers, which results in more severe illness and requires a low inoculum to initiate infection, more closely mimics natural infection [7]. However, most investigators feel that the resultant illness is too severe for widespread use of this method of inoculation in volunteer studies.

V. STUDIES OF CP-20,961 IN EXPERIMENTAL
RESPIRATORY VIRAL INFECTIONS IN VOLUNTEERS

A. The Initial Preparation in Rhinovirus Infection

All of these studies used placebo-controlled, double-blind design, and the placebo consisted of the vehicle used to emulsify the drug: equal weights of polysorbate 80 and glycerine homogenized in hot buffered saline solution. The first two studies, which differ only in minor respects, were done using rhinovirus challenge of volunteers who were free of antibody to the adminis-tered virus strain [8,9]. In both, drug was administered by nasal spray in a dose of 50 mg per treatment. In one, the drug was administered four time a day for five days beginning one day prior to virus challenge [8], and in the other it was administered three times the day prior to challenge and two times the day of challenge [9]. In both studies, plaque reduction of vesicular stomatitis virus (VSV) assays were used to detect interferon, and in the study performed by Gaitmaitan et al. [9] the nasal secretions were treated at pH 1.5-2.0 overnight before testing for interferon content. In the former study [8], rhinovirus type 13 was used as a challenge and in the latter [9], type 21 was used.

In both studies, nasal interferon was stimulated by the drug. In the study by Douglas and Betts [8], interferon production was significantly

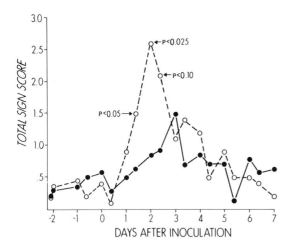

FIGURE 3. Comparison of mean total sign scores of CP-20,961-treated (●—●, 14 patients) and placebo-treated (o--o, 10 patients) subjects. P value calculated from paired sample t tests. (Reprinted from Ref. 8, with per-mission of the American Society for Microbiology.)

greater in recipients of drug compared to placebo recipients, and there was no evidence that the placebo stimulated interferon. In the study by Gaitmaitan et al. [9], among individuals who were challenged with virus, there was no significant difference in the frequency of interferon production by those who received vehicle versus those who received vehicle with drug. However, a buffer-challenged, drug-treated group developed interferon responses, whereas a buffer-challenged, untreated group did not. Both studies showed that interferon was detected earlier after infection in the drug group than in the placebo group, and that interferon titers in nasal washes were higher in the subjects who received drug. There appeared to be a mild therapeutic effect of CP-20,961 in both studies, manifested by decreased symptoms in the first study [8] (see Figure 3) and more rapid recovery from illness in the latter study [9]. However, in the latter study, clearing of the symptoms occurred equally rapidly in drug-treated individuals who were interferon-negative as those who were interferon-positive, suggesting that the drug might produce its effect by a mode of activity other than interferon production.

B. A Microdispersed Preparation in Rhinovirus and Influenza A Virus Infection

As a result of these encouraging findings, and because of concerns about bioavailability of the highly insoluble drug, a new preparation was prepared by altering the formation of the drug so that it was presented in a micro-dispersed form (<2 μm diameter/droplet). Three studies were performed with the microdispersed preparation in volunteers with experimental rhino-virus infections and one in volunteers with experimental influenza.

In the rhinovirus studies carried out by Panusarn and colleagues [10] and by Waldman and Ganguly [11], there were some similarities in mode of administration of drug and in results, but there were important differences as well. In both studies, the drug was administered the day before and the day of virus challenge. In the study carried out by Panusarn and co-workers [10], the method for measuring interferon was altered slightly from their previous work. Instead of the plaque reduction of a low inoculum of VSV, prevention of cytopathic effect caused by 500 fifty-percent tissue culture infectious doses ($TCID_{50}$) of VSV was used to assay interferon activity. In their studies, drug-treated individuals produced significantly higher interferon levels and significantly more prolonged interferon in secretions compared to placebo. Virus titers in nasal washes were not significantly lower in the treated group, but the number of virus-positive days was significantly less. In both studies the most striking effect was an amelioration of symptoms (see Figure 4). Infected individuals who received drug had symptoms identical to the uninfected group who were challenged with buffer. Analysis of virus shedding, clinical symptoms,

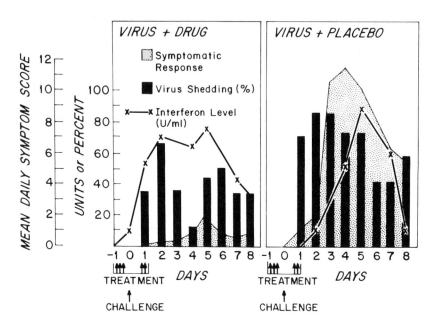

FIGURE 4. Time relations of symptoms, viral shedding, and nasal inter-feron titer in groups of volunteers without specific prechallenge serum antibody. Shown is the effect of drug or placebo treatment for one day before and after nasal instilation (day 0) of approximately 1 TCD$_{50}$ (WI-38 cells) of rhinovirus type 21. (Reprinted from Ref. 10 with permission of the New England Journal of Medicine 291:57 (1974).)

and interferon production suggested that amelioration of symptoms resulted from presence of interferon. In addition to prophylactic administration of drug, both groups carried out additional studies in which drug was adminis-tered to subjects following challenge [11,12]. In such studies, the time of administration was important. If drug was administered 8 hr after challenge, then the rate of infection, the rate of illness, and the severity of symptoms were all diminished without any effect on the frequency of positive speci-mens, but none of these differences were significant [12]. If, as shown by Waldman and Ganguly [11], drug was begun 24 and 48 hr after challenge, there was no effect on the development of symptoms or virus shedding. In fact, these individuals had somewhat greater symptoms than placebo recipi-ents.

Other minor variations of drug administration and virus challenge have been carried out in humans [12].

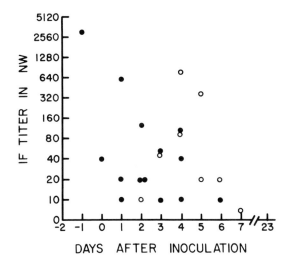

DAYS AFTER INOCULATION

FIGURE 5. Interferon titers, international units per milliliter of nasal wash (NW), detected in relation to days after virus inoculation. Symbols: ● = CP-20,961, o = placebo. (Reprinted from Ref. 13 with permission of the American Society for Microbiology.)

    The microdispersed form of the CP-20,961 was also tested in experimental influenza A/England/42/72 H3N2 virus infection in 20 volunteers. In that study by Douglas and co-workers [13], the drug was administered for five days beginning one day before virus challenge. No appreciable effect on symptoms or on virus shedding was detected. In fact, virus titers and mean total symptom scores were somewhat higher in the CP-20,961 group as compared to the placebo group, but these differences were not significant. Interferon levels were high for the first day after inducer was begun and then the levels diminished, suggesting that with more than two days of treatment, hyporesponsiveness to the inducer developed (see Figure 5). The apparent hyporesponsive state did not explain the failure of the drug, since virus shedding and clinical symptoms were prominent on the first and second day after initiation of inducer, days on which interferon titers were at their peak. The failure of CP-20,961 in influenza infection in volunteers is in keeping with results obtained in experimental influenza infection in mice. However, the difficulty of demonstrating efficacy in acute, mild, self-limited illness and the small numbers of volunteers should be kept in mind in interpreting these results.

VI. STUDIES OF CP-28,888 IN EXPERIMENTAL
     RHINOVIRUS INFECTIONS IN VOLUNTEERS

Because of the apparent superiority in interferon induction of CP-28,888
compared to CP-20,961 in animals, two studies of the clinical effectiveness
of CP-28,888 in experimental rhinovirus infection in volunteers were undertaken. Since the design of the two studies was identical and the results
indistinguishable, the studies were combined for purposes of publication
[14]. Drug or placebo were administered intranasally by spray to 60 volunteers, three times a day on the day prior to challenge and two times on the
day of virus challenge. The total dose was 50 mg.
     Evaluation of total signs and symptoms, frequency of virus shedding,
and serum antibody revealed no differences between the two groups. Interferon content of nasal washes was determined for 30 volunteers: five of 15
in the CP-28,888 and two of 15 in the placebo group had interferon detected
in their nasal washes. The distribution of interferon-positive nasal wash
specimens according to day after inoculation is shown in Table 1. Titers
were low and ranged between 5 and 10 U. Most volunteers had single specimens containing interferon except for two patients in the CP-28,888 group,
each of whom had two positive specimens. Thus, the frequency and quantity
of interferon in nasal secretions was much lower than after CP-20,961
administration, findings in contrast to studies in the mouse and the rat.
It is clear that the failure to ameliorate illness was associated with a failure
to induce interferon. These studies emphasize the significance of species
variation in response to interferon inducers and the lack of predictability
of response in humans from animal data. Furthermore, it is apparent that
such compounds must be tested in humans to determine potential usefulness.

VII. SYNOPSIS OF STUDIES TO DATE

CP-20,961, when applied intranasally, appeared to be nontoxic and induced
interferon in 50-70% of uninfected recipients and in 80-100% of infected
recipients. It is most effective when administered as droplets less than
2 μm in diameter. This microdispersed form of the drug dramatically
reduces symptoms of rhinovirus but not influenza A infection when administered prior to challenge. Its effect is less when administered 8 hr after
challenge, and it has no effect when administered 24 or 48 hr postchallenge.

VIII. DIFFERENCES IN INTERFERON INDUCTION
       IN MICE AND HUMANS

As noted, mice responded to a single dose of drug with production of interferon that developed 9 hr after drug and persisted for about 24 hr. In
humans, a single intranasal dose did not result in interferon production [12],

TABLE 1. Interferon Response to CP-28,888 and
Rhinovirus Infection

	No. of subjects tested	No. with interferon in nasal wash	Distribution of Interferon-positive nasal wash specimens according to day after inoculation						
			1	2	3	4	5	6	7
CP-28,888	15	5	—	—	1	1	3	—	2
Placebo	15	2	—	1	—	—	1	—	—

Source: Adapted from Ref. 14.

but five doses over two days resulted in sustained interferon production
after 24 hr persisting for 96 hr. This lag period and prolonged production
of interferon from a brief exposure to inducer would not have been anticipated from animal data. It is also uncertain whether the physical characteristics of the interferon produced in mice and in humans are the same.
In mice, interferon produced is atypical compared to that stimulated by
other inducers in that it is partially inactivated at pH 2. In humans, no
detailed analysis of properties of the interferon induced by CP-20,961 have
been carried out. However, in the study by Gaitmaitan et al. [9], nasal
secretions were treated at pH 2 prior to assay for interferon, and levels
measured were nearly identical to those in studies where pH treatment was
not used [8]. Results in experimental infections appear to be similar in
mice and in humans. CP-20,961 had its greatest effect when given prior
to infection, and it had a diminished effect when given 3 hr (in the mice)
and 8 hr (in humans) following infection. It was ineffective when given 24
hr (both mice and humans) or later after infection. The most striking difference between the response of mice and humans was the discrepancy of
results obtained in experimental infection with CP-28,888.

IX. ALTERED RESPONSIVE STATE
     PRODUCED BY INTERFERON INDUCERS

From the available studies there has been some evidence that administration
of interferon inducers may render the host more susceptible to viral infection or may result in more severe symptoms. In the studies of Douglas
and Betts [8], three of 15 recipients of drug who did not shed virus initially
became infected after day 4, whereas none of 14 placebo subjects did. In
the study of Gaitmaitan et al. [9], eight subjects were treated with drug
and challenged with buffer. Four of these eight developed a virus infection
by natural mechanisms (two of these apparently acquired challenge virus by

person-to-person transmission). Of the five who received placebo and buffer challenge, none shed virus.

When a single dose of drug was administered 24 hr prechallenge, an apparently paradoxical result occurred. Subjects who received a single dose of drug or of vehicle alone did not secrete interferon after virus challenge, and individuals who received the single dose of drug were more symptomatic following virus challenge than individuals who had received saline or vehicle only [12]. In Waldman's study, individuals who received inducer beginning 24 and 48 hr after challenge seemed to have slightly greater symptoms than placebo recipients [11].

On the other hand, subsequent experiments showed that treatment with four days of drug or vehicle, both of which induced interferon, produced a state of hyporesponsiveness when these subjects were challenged with virus [12]. In spite of this, these subjects were less symptomatic following challenge than were untreated subjects.

When microdispersed CP-20,961 was tested in experimental influenza infection in normal volunteers, high-titered interferon was induced and it appeared before viral infection. However, by day 3 of treatment, interferon levels had decreased at the time when subjects remained symptomatic. In fact, although the differences were not significant, on day 3 of treatment, drug recipients had both lower interferon levels and higher symptom scores than placebo recipients. Taken together, these data suggest that there is a complex interaction between the production of interferon and susceptibility to infection which requires further understanding. Thus, although it is attractive to presume that either a better formulated or a more active interferon inducer would have greater efficacy, it may be that these molecules will have the undesirable feature just alluded to. Perhaps, at least, the hyporesponsive state should have been anticipated since others have observed this finding in animals [15].

X. POTENTIAL USEFULNESS OF INTERFERON INDUCERS

In the case of respiratory viral illnesses, prophylaxis is impractical except for diseases with epidemic behavior because drug would have to be administered year round. Thus, therapeutic effectiveness is essential for most of these infections. However, in the case of influenza, respiratory syncytial virus, parainfluenza types 1 or 2, prophylaxis is possible because of the characteristic epidemiological behavior of the viruses. Thus, prophylaxis would not be administered year round, but only for a few weeks. However, the problems of hyporesponsiveness and potential heightened susceptibilities must be overcome. It should be noted that an agent capable of rendering a therapeutic effect would also be highly desirable in these infections. In either case, topical administration would be desirable to minimize toxicity and maximize efficacy. Although studies to date have shown that these inducers are ineffective when given therapeutically, that is, after onset of sumptoms, it should be noted that therapeutic effects are difficult to demonstrate in acute self-limited illness, and that volunteer studies done to date are limited in scope and numbers of subjects. To prove efficacy, it might be necessary to study larger numbers of subjects with natural rhinovirus infections before it can be concluded that these agents are ineffective therapeutically. In a small, double-blind, placebo-controlled study, 43 of 171 placebo-treated subjects developed "colds" as opposed to a similar number and severity in 171 who prophylactically received CP-20,961 once daily for 30 days [16]. Virological studies were not done, and no measures of interferon production and/or hyporesponsive states were carried out.

The viral diseases in which interferon has been shown to be therapeutically effective may not lend themselves to the use of interferon inducers. For these compounds to be effective in chronic viral infections such as hepatitis, the hyporesponsive state that has been noted with prolonged administration would need to be overcome. In addition, because the infection is disseminated to several organ systems, such inducers should be capable of being administered parenterally.

The studies to date, although not dramatic, do demonstrate some encouraging findings. Symptoms in subjects receiving drug for intermediate periods of time were less than placebo-treated subjects. Usually, although not always, amelioration of symptoms was associated with presence of interferon in nasal secretions. In the instances where there is a lack of a correlation, the explanation might be the method of treatment of specimens before testing, the presence of a substance that does not inhibit VSV but does inhibit rhinovirus, or the fact that another mechanism other than interferon production may account, in part, for the drug effect.

XI. SUMMARY

Two low-molecular-weight interferon inducers, CP-20,961 and CP-28,888, have been tested in experimental respiratory viral infections in humans. Both are insoluble, required emulsification for delivery as nasal sprays, and a microdispersed form appears to have optimal effect. CP-20,961 was shown to induce nasal wash interferon and to decrease symptoms of rhinovirus, but not influenza A virus, infection in volunteers when given prior to or up to 8 hr after virus challenge. When administered for more than 24 hr prior to challenge, the interferon response postchallenge was decreased, but drug efficacy persisted. CP-28,888, although a more potent inducer in mice and rats, failed to induce significant amounts of interferon in humans, and prophylactic efficacy in experimental rhinovirus infection in volunteers was lacking.

REFERENCES

1. T. C. Merigan, S. E. Reed, T. S. Hall, and D. A. Tyrell, Inhibition of respiratory virus infection by locally applied interferon. Lancet i: 563-567 (1973).

2. D. A. Hill, S. Baron, J. C. Perkins, M. Worthington, J. E. VanKirk, J. Mills, A. Z. Kapikan, and R. M. Chanock, Evaluation of an interferon inducer in viral respiratory disease. J. Amer. Med. Assoc. 219:1179-1184 (1972).

3. W. W. Hoffman, J. J. Korst, J. F. Niblack, and T. H. Cronin, N,N-Dioctadecyl N,'N'-bis(2-hydroxyethyl)propanediamine: Antiviral activity and interferon stimulation in mice. Antimicrob. Agents Chemother. 3:498-502 (1973).

4. R. G. Douglas, Jr., Pathogenesis of rhinovirus common colds in human volunteers. Ann. Otol. Rhenol. Laryngol. 79:563-571 (1970).

5. J. W. Little, R. G. Douglas, Jr., W. J. Hall, and F. K. Roth, Attenuated influenza produced by experimental intranasal inoculation. J. Med. Virol. 3:167-176 (1979).

6. R. G. Douglas, Jr., Influenza in Man, in The Influenza Viruses and Influenza (E. D. Kilbourne, ed.), Academic Press, New York, 1975, pp. 395-447.

7. R. H. Alford, J. A. Kasel, P. J. Gerone, and V. Knight, Human influenza resulting from aerosol inhalation. Proc. Soc. Exp. Biol. Med. 122:800-804 (1966).

8. R. G. Douglas and R. F. Betts, Effect of induced interferon in experimental rhinovirus infection in volunteers. Infec. Immun. 9:506-510 (1974).

9. B. G. Gaitmaitan, E. D. Stanley, and G. G. Jackson, The limited effect of nasal interferon induced by rhinovirus and a topical chemical inducer on the course of infection. J. Infec. Dis. 127:401-407 (1973).

10. C. Panusarn, E. D. Stanley, V. Dirda, M. Rubenis, and G. G. Jackson, Prevention of illness from rhinovirus infection by a topical interferon inducer. New Engl. J. Med. 291:57-61 (1974).

11. R. H. Waldman and R. Ganguly, Effect of CP-20,961, an interferon inducer, on upper respiratory tract infection due to rhinovirus type 21 in volunteers. J. Infect. Dis. 138:531-535 (1978).

12. E. D. Stanley, G. G. Jackson, V. A. Dirda, and M. Rubenis, Effect of a topical interferon inducer on rhinovirus infections in volunteers. J. Infec. Dis. 133S:A121-A127 (1976).

13. R. G. Douglas, Jr., R. F. Betts, R. L. Simons, P. W. Hogan, and F. K. Roth, Evaluation of a topical interferon inducer in experimental influenza virus infection in volunteers. Antimicrob. Agents Chemother. 8:684-687 (1975).

14. R. G. Douglas, Jr., R. H. Waldman, R. F. Betts, and R. Ganguly, Effect of an interferon inducer, a substituted xylenediamine, on rhino-

virus challenge in humans. Antimicrob. Agents Chemother. 15:269–279 (1979).

15. J. S. Youngner and W. R. Stineburg, Interferon appearance stimulated by endotoxin bacteria or viruses in mice pretreated with Escherichia coli endotoxin or infected with Mycobacterium tuberculosis. Nature 208:456–458 (1965).

16. J. F. Niblack, Studies with low molecular weight inducers of interferon in man. Texas Repts. Biol. Med. 35:528–534 (1977).

10

INTERFERON INDUCERS: POLYANIONS AND OTHERS

Mary C. Breinig* and Page S. Morahan

Medical College of Virginia
Virginia Commonwealth University
Richmond, Virginia

I. INTRODUCTION

Since the discovery 16 years ago that substances other than viruses could stimulate the production of interferon, the number of nonviral inducers has increased greatly. The list now includes microorganisms such as

*Present affiliation: Graduate School of Public Health, University of Pittsburgh, Pittsburgh, Pennsylvania.

bacteria, chlamydia, mycoplasmas, protozoa and rickettsiae, bacterial
and fungal extracts, endotoxins, mitogens, antibiotics, polysaccharides,
natural and synthetic acids, and synthetic polymers. Many of these nonviral
inducers are, or contain, polyanions, and these inducers are the subject
of this chapter. Polyanions of both natural and synthetic origin have been
reported. The first part of the chapter includes a brief description and
characterization of polyanions in general and their ability to induce interferon. In the latter part of the chapter, synthetic carboxylic polyanions
are discussed with respect to antiviral activity and properties other than
interferon induction. Using pyran copolymer as a model, the role of the
macrophage is outlined as a possible common denominator for the antiviral,
immunomodulator, and antitumor activities of these polyanions.

II. DESCRIPTION AND CHARACTERIZATION
OF POLYANIONS

Polyanions have a wide range of biological activity. Besides inducing the
production of interferon, various polyanions exhibit antiviral [1-21], antitumor [22-40], antibacterial [35,41-43], antifungal [35], and antiprotozoal
[35,41,44] activities. Polyanions also are able to stimulate the reticuloendothelial system (RES) and modulate humoral- and/or cell-mediated
immune responses [45,46]. Many of these host-resistance-enhancing
properties, as well as the toxicities of the synthetic polymers, resemble
bacterial endotoxin, which was the first interferon inducer of nonviral
origin to be described [47,48].

TABLE 1. Examples of Polyanions with Interferon-Inducing Ability
and/or Antiviral Activity

Synthetic	Natural
Polycarboxylates	Endotoxin (LPS)
Pyran (maleic anhydride-divinyl ether)	Lipid A
Polyacrylic acid	Bacterial products
COAM (chlorite-oxidized oxyamylose)	Heparin
Polymethacrylic acid	Fungal polysaccharide
Polysulfates	
Polyvinyl sulfate	
Polyphosphates	
Dextran phosphate	
Polynucleotides	

A variety of polyanionic polymers, natural and synthetic, have been reported to induce interferon and/or antiviral effects (Table 1). The major emphasis in this chapter will be on the synthetic polyanions; discussion of the natural polyanions will be limited to bacterial endotoxin/lipopolysaccharide (LPS), for which considerable biological data are available. Of the synthetic polyanions, the carboxylic acid polyanions have been studied in most detail. The more important features of the carboxylic polymers for interferon induction and antiviral activity are a high density of carboxylate groups pendent from a long-chain polymeric backbone. Polyanionic polymers, in general, have been found to be fairly stable and are not readily biodegradable, which may account for their prolonged activity [49]. One such polyanion which has been studied in considerable detail is pyran, a random copolymer of maleic anhydride and divinyl ether. Figure 1 relates the common struc- tural features between pyran copolymer and several other polyanions. Poly- acrylic acid-maleic anhydride copolymer has biological activities similar to pyran but is not as biologically effective [50]. Maleic anhydride homo- polymer is much less toxic than pyran copolymer but also much less effective against tumor growth and viruses [51]. Polyacrylic acid, polymethacrylic acid, acrylic acid-maleic anhydride copolymer, and maleic anhydride-furan copolymer are among the other purely synthetic polyanionic polymers which have been evaluated [50]. Several polysaccharide derivatives have been studied, and the most active biologically was chlorite-oxidized oxyamylose (COAM) [4]. COAM is a polymer chain with a fairly high carboxylic group density and a possibly more biodegradable polyacetyl backbone, which may account for its rather limited antiviral activity. COAM appears to be rela- tively nontoxic and also inhibits tumor growth [28,29].

Several similarities in structure are apparent in the polymers just described. Among these are a fairly flexible polymer chain and a high density of carboxyl groups situated along the backbone of the polymer. In general, the toxicity of polyanions increases with molecular weight, particu- larly greater than 50,000 [49]. Fortunately, substantial antitumor activity is retained in lower-molecular-weight fractions, less than 10,000 [49]. These fractions are relatively less toxic and are associated with macrophage activation; however, they usually also exhibit less antiviral activity than higher-molecular-weight fractions.

III. INTERFERON INDUCTION WITH POLYANIONS

A. Interferon Induction in Vivo

The ability of synthetic polyanions to induce circulating interferon has been shown most frequently in the mouse, although pyran copolymer has also been reported to induce interferon in humans [52]. Pyran copolymer [53, 54], polyacrylic acid [55], polyvinyl sulfate [12], and COAM [7] have been

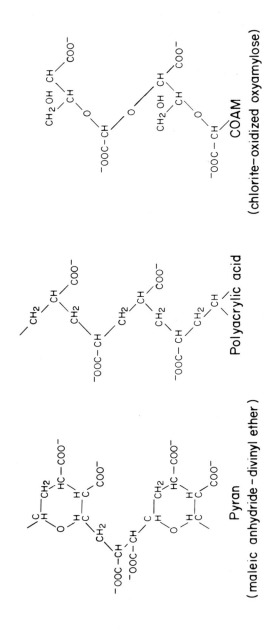

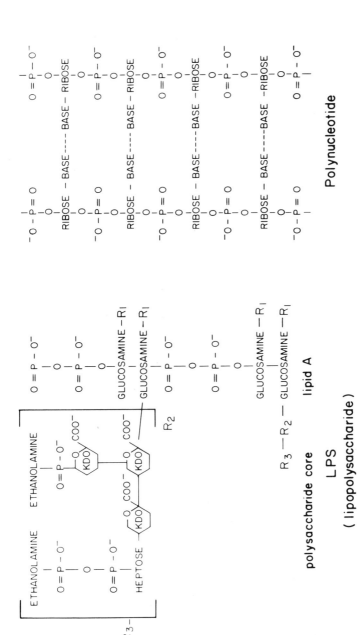

FIGURE 1. Structures of three synthetic polycarboxylates are compared with schematic representations of a polynucleotide and of part of the lipid A and polysaccharide core of LPS. Figures are drawn to illustrate the high density of anionic groups pendent from the various long-chain polymeric backbones. In LPS, R_1 = long-chain fatty acids, R_2 = the KDO (2-keto-3-deoxyoctulonic acid) containing part of the polysaccharide core, and R_3 = rest of core and terminal sugar residues.

shown to induce interferon in the mouse following intraperitoneal injection, and the largest amounts of interferon were usually found within 15-24 hr. Intravenous inoculation of mice with pyran also resulted in the production of interferon [54], with a peak response at 24-48 hr. The natural polyanion, endotoxin, also induces interferon in the mouse [48], rat [56], and rabbit [47] when injected parenterally. In contrast to synthetic-polyanion-induced interferon, however, maximum serum interferon production is attained much earlier, usually within 2 hr.

Polyanions are frequently antiviral out of proportion to the amount of interferon induced and, in fact, may induce antiviral activity in the absence of detectable interferon. Polyacrylic acid protected rabbits against vaccinia virus infection [21] and COAM protected swine against hog cholera virus infection [8], although neither of these polyanions induced detectable interferon in the respective host.

There have been few attempts to characterize the interferons induced by polyanions. This may be due in part to the low levels (< 100 units) usually found in vivo. Endotoxin is also a poor interferon inducer. Paradoxically, although LPS induces low levels of interferon itself, it has the capacity of inducing hyporeactivity (a state of tolerance, during which the interferon response is markedly reduced) to a variety of strong interferon inducers. In general, the injection of a particular interferon inducer renders the animal hyporeactive to interferon production to a second injection with the same inducer. Endotoxin, however, confers broad hyporeactivity. Following the injection of endotoxin, there is a period of a week or more of marked hyporeactivity not only to endotoxin, but to other interferon inducers as well, including viruses and polynucleotides [57-59]. Whether or not synthetic polyanions are able to confer similar broad hyporeactivity has not been examined. Polycarboxylates, however, do follow the general pattern of interferon inducers in which repeated injections of the same inducer results in hyporeactivity [5,55]. With pyran, the hyporeactive period lasted three weeks [5].

It would be interesting to determine the relationship of synthetic-polyanion-induced interferon to endotoxin-induced interferon, both of which are produced in low levels. It is unclear whether polyanion-induced interferon is more typical of the "classical-virus-induced interferon" (type I) or "immune interferon" (type II), pH stable or unstable, temperature stable or unstable, etc. For example, mouse serum interferon induced by pyran copolymer was found to be inactivated by pH 2 treatment [54], whereas mouse serum interferon induced by polyacrylic acid or polyvinyl sulfate was resistant to pH 2 treatment [12,60]. The cellular origin of the circulating interferon has also not yet been determined. Interestingly, however, splenectomy only partially reduced the amount of interferon produced in mice after injection of pyran copolymer [5], whereas splenectomy greatly reduced the amount of interferon after injection of endotoxin [61]. In vivo, the predominant sites of endotoxin-induced interferon synthesis include the spleen, lymph nodes, liver, thymus, and lung [62-64].

B. Interferon Induction in Vitro

While polycarboxylates and endotoxin induce interferon in animals, they are, in general, not very effective as inducers in cultures of many cell lines, primary fibroblasts, or epithelial cells [4,7,12]. Endotoxin is able to induce interferon in cultures of peritoneal cells [65-67] or spleen cells [64,67,68], and the adherent cells produced more interferon than the non-adherent cells. The predominant cells producing interferon on incubation with endotoxin in vitro appear to be the macrophage and B lymphocyte. Interestingly, the interferons produced by these two cells have different stability and biological properties [67]. Peritoneal macrophages produced small amounts of interferon in response to pyran copolymer, but only if the pyran was complexed with arginine [5]. The interferon-producing ability of lymphocytes cultured with pyran or other polyanions has not been well studied.

Synthetic polyanions and endotoxin are therefore, in general, poor inducers of interferon and are usually effective only in the animal, resulting in low yields of interferon. The antiviral protection seen after prophylactic administration of synthetic polyanions has been observed to persist much longer than the interferon response [4,5,20], which suggests that the antiviral protection is probably mediated by factors other than the production of interferon.

IV. OTHER PROPERTIES OF CARBOXYLIC
POLYANIONS

A. Effect of Molecular Weight on Biological
Activity and Toxicity

Activities of anionic polymers vary according to the average molecular weight of the molecular weight distribution of particular samples [49]. The effect of molecular weight on biological activity has been most extensively studied with pyran, where a variety of fractionation, degradation, and synthesizing techniques have been used to produce different molecular weight fractions. These procedures were used in attempts to remove the toxicity inherent in the high-molecular-weight, especially >50,000, compounds. Toxicities associated with high-molecular-weight polyanions have included elevation of liver transaminases, hepatosplenomegaly, thymic involution, anemia, leukocytosis, and decrease in bone marrow cells [49, 69-71,103].

Low-molecular-weight (< 10,000) samples of pyran copolymer with narrow-molecular-weight distribution exhibit less toxicity while retaining the antitumor activity exhibited by higher-molecular-weight samples [49, 70]. Low-molecular-weight fractions, as well as high-molecular-weight

fractions, activate peritoneal macrophages [38]. Activated macrophages
destroy tumor cells nonimmunospecifically while not affecting normal cells
[72]. Phagocytosis is stimulated by low-molecular-weight polymers and
depressed by high-molecular-weight polymers [49, 70]. This finding probably accounts for the biphasic (initial depression followed by elevation)
effects on the reticuloendothelial system of the parent polydisperse pyran
preparation [73]. These data also emphasize the difficulty in determining
the precise mechanisms of action of the polyanions unless they are well
purified and characterized. In regard to toxicity, fractions with low molecular weight and narrow polydispersity isolated from the polydisperse parent
compound showed greater 50% lethal doses than the parent compound, caused
no hepatosplenomegaly, and did not sensitize mice to bacterial endotoxin.
While these fractions retained antitumor activity, they had very limited
antiviral activity [49]. Similar observations have been made with compounds synthesized with varying molecular weights [70]. These data suggest
that different structural features may be required for the antiviral and antitumor activities of polyanions. Unfortunately, the antiviral activity of pyran
and polyribonucleotides has not yet been able to be consistently dissociated
from the toxicity of the compound [49, 70, 74].

B. Immunomodulator Activity

Pyran copolymer, as well as polyacrylic acid, have been shown to have
immunoadjuvant activity in several model systems. Both of these synthetic
polyanions enhanced the primary antibody-plaque-forming response of mice
to sheep erythrocytes in vivo. Polyacrylic acid also increased the background plaques in unimmunized animals, similar to observations reported
for endotoxin [75]. In vivo administration of pyran, on the other hand, did
not stimulate the production of background antibody plaques in unimmunized
mice [1, 46].

The mechanisms of adjuvant activity of polycarboxylic polyanions for
humoral immune responses have been partially defined by using thymec-
tomized, irradiated, and bone-marrow-reconstituted (TxBM) mice that
are deficient in T cells. The splenic-specific, plaque-forming response
of polyacrylic-acid-treated TxBM mice that were immunized with sheep
erythrocytes was significantly less than that observed in normal mice that
were immunized [76]. However, the antibody response in the polyacrylic-
acid-treated TxBM mice was enhanced as measured by plaque-forming
cells and hemolysin titers, as compared with TxBM mice which had received
the antigen without adjuvant. These results suggested that this polycarboxylic
immunomodulator, similar to polynucleotides [76, 77], was able to partially
replace T-cell function or enhance residual T-cell function in T-depleted
mice.

In contrast to the results obtained with polyacrylic acid, pyran was
unable to enhance specific antibody-forming activity to sheep erythrocytes

(plaques per 10^6 spleen cells) in TxBM mice [46]. The substantial immuno-enhancing effect of pyran in normal mice thus appeared to be dependent upon T-cell function. Pyran did cause a slight increase in total plaques per spleen in the immunized TxBM mice. This minimal increase in total antibody plaques in the TxBM mouse treated with pyran was consistent with other data showing that the polyanion caused a modest, nonspecific blastogenesis of the entire spleen cell population in TxBM and normal mice [46].

Data in other systems provide additional evidence that the humoral immunoenhancing effect of pyran is primarily mediated through T lympho-cytes. Pyran was capable of increasing the secondary response of mice to sheep erythrocytes in normal mice, suggesting that the immunomodulator expanded the number of antibody-producing B cells or memory T cells in this T-dependent humoral immune response [46]. The adjuvant effect of pyran in T-dependent humoral immune responses to two different allogeneic cells was variable. Treatment of mice with pyran after immunization with the allogeneic MBL-2 tumor cells caused an enhanced production of comple-ment dependent cytotoxic antibody [46]. However, when pyran was adminis-tered prior to immunization with allogeneic P815 mastocytoma cells, there was no difference in the cytotoxic antibody response between untreated and pyran-treated animals [46]. Immunomodulator treatment at a different time during immunization may be necessary for immunoenhancement. A probable effect of pyran on T cells is supported by other data showing that pyran did not enhance the antibody response to LPS, a T-independent antigen [46].

The effects of polycarboxylate polyanions on cell-mediated immune responses have been investigated primarily with pyran. Although the effects are complex, the general pattern is immunomodulator-induced inhibition of various aspects of cell-mediated immunity. Intravenous treatment of mice with pyran prior to immunization with the allogeneic P815 mastocytoma cells caused a decrease in spleen cell cytolytic activity, in addition to delay-ing the time of the peak response [46]. Unfortunately, experiments were not performed to determine whether the inhibition seen in this in vitro test of cell-mediated immune activity was correlated with enhanced tumor growth in vivo. In the MBL-2 allogeneic tumor system, intraperitoneal treatment of mice with pyran prior to immunization did not alter the initial growth and subsequent cell-mediated immune regression of the tumor [78]. If, however, mice were treated with the immunomodulator 6 days after immu-nization, there was inhibition of the cell-mediated immunological regression of the allograft tumor and the tumor grew progressively. Paradoxically, this inhibition of the in vivo cell-mediated immune response was not due to inhibition of splenic lymphocyte-mediated cytolytic activity, which was similar in untreated or pyran-treated animals. Moreover, pyran treatment caused an increase in specific macrophage-mediated tumoricidal activity. The only index that correlated with the decreased in vivo cell-mediated immune response was a decrease in the number of macrophages that nor-

mally infiltrated the regressing subcutaneous tumor. One can speculate
that the reduced macrophage infiltration into the tumor may be related to
the increased macrophage activity observed in the peritoneal cavity where
the immunomodulator was administered, i.e., that there is a change in the
normal macrophage migration patterns.

Pyran administration has also been reported to cause a delay in skin
graft or tumor allograft rejection [79], although the mechanism of the
inhibition of this cell-mediated immune response has not been established.
The administration of pyran has, in a few instances, caused enhanced growth
of chemical-induced [80] or virus-induced [24,25,81] tumors in mice.
Whether the mechanisms underlying these adverse immunomodulatory
events involve immunologic effects on T cells or macrophages or other
physiological processes is not yet clear.

In an effort to define some of the immunological bases responsible for
the observed effects, the effect of pyran on mitogenic responses has been
measured. As mentioned earlier, in vivo administration of pyran does
cause a modest mitogenic effect on both T and B cells [46]. A similar
slight mitogenic activity (stimulation ratio of 8) is observed in vitro when
normal spleen cells are incubated with pyran. However, a single intravenous
injection of pyran depressed significantly the in vitro blastogenic response
of spleen cells to phytohemagglutinin (PHA) and LPS from 2-14 days after
in vivo administration of pyran. This is similar to data presented for the
biological immunomodulator Corynebacterium parvum. However 5 days
after pyran administration, thymidine incorporation in mitogen-treated
cultures of cells from pyran-treated mice was significantly higher than
that of normal cells incubated with mitogen. As this corresponded to the
time of peak increase in pyran-induced background incorporation of
[^{3}H]thymidine, it was possible that pyran-primed spleen cells were more
susceptible to the action of PHA or LPS and/or were more resistant to the
inhibitory effect of activated macrophages.

Pyran-induced inhibition of blastogenesis is macrophage-dependent.
Peritoneal exudate cells from pyran-treated animals were more effective
than were normal macrophages in abrogating the PHA or LPS response of
normal spleen cells. Removal of glass adherent cells from the spleens of
pyran-treated mice restored the response to PHA and LPS [82].

In summary, these results are consistent with a dual action of pyran
on T lymphocytes and macrophages in the modulation of the immune response.
The enhancement of the humoral immune responses is compatible with a
direct action on T lymphocytes [46]. The inhibitory effect of pyran on cell-
mediated immunity could be due to a direct action on T cells or, most likely,
an indirect effect mediated by macrophages [78,82]. Further experiments
are needed to clarify these hypotheses. It is likely that some of the carboxylic polyanionic immunomodulators act on more than one cell type. Moreover, the target cell(s) for a specific polyanion is (are) probably to a certain
extent dependent on the model system used to determine immune reactivity.

As the present review indicates, polycarboxylate polyanions are capable of producing a wide spectrum of effects on immune reactivity, and the effect of a given immunomodulator on the response to a given antigen may be even more complex than anticipated. Polyanions represent a class of compounds with potent immunoadjuvant activity. These agents have potential as adjuvants with bacterial, viral, and tumor vaccines and as general stimulators of the immune response in clinical situations where immunological inhibition is present.

C. Antimicrobial Activity

Polyanions are able to confer resistance to bacterial, fungal, and protozoal infections. Following treatment with pyran copolymer or polyacrylic acid, mice exhibited enhanced resistance to both gram-positive and gram-negative bacteria, including Listeria monocytogenes [41], Diplococcus pneumonia [35,43], Klebsiella pneumonia [42], and Pasteurella tularensis [43]. The antifungal activity of pyran was demonstrated in mice using Cryptococcus neoformans [35]. Enhanced survival of mice challenged with Toxoplasma gondii [41], Trypanosoma duttoni [35], or the sporozoite stage of Plasmodium berghei [44] was seen following treatment with pyran copolymer or polyacrylic acid.

Certain features of the antimicrobial activity of polyanions are similar to those observed concerning the antiviral activity. For example, greatest protection is observed when the polyanion is administered prophylactically and polyanion treatment can provide prolonged protection (pyran conferred resistance to L. monocytogenes for as long as two months) [41].

D. Antitumor Activity

Synthetic carboxylic polyanions such as pyran, ethylene-maleic anhydride, and polyacrylic acid polymers with molecular weight ranges of 1000 to 100,000 or greater have been tested against a variety of subcutaneous rodent tumors [31-34]. In each case, systemic drug administration was associated with significant tumor regression without excessive weight loss. The higher the molecular weight, the more toxic was the ethylene-maleic anhydride polymer for both the mouse and the dog. Optimum activity was obtained with compounds where carboxamide and ionizable carboxyl groups were interdispersed along the polymer backbone. Monomers were inactive, and when all carboxyl groups were converted to carboxamides, significant tumor inhibitory activity was lost. This is similar to observations on the antiviral action of these compounds.

Of all the carboxylic polyanions, pyran has received the greatest attention with respect to its antitumor activity. Treatment with pyran prior to inoculation of mice with the solid Ehrlich adenocarcinoma inhibited subse-

quent tumor growth [35]. Pyran inhibited tumors induced by Friend leukemia virus [23], Moloney sarcoma virus [28], Rauscher leukemia virus
[23,26], polyoma virus, and Gross leukemia virus in normal or immunosuppressed mice [26,27]. Systemic administration of this polyanion also
inhibited the growth of several syngeneic solid metastasizing tumors,
including the first generation transplant of the mammary carcinoma [32],
Lewis lung carcinoma [36], B16 melanoma [36], and Madison lung carcinoma M109 [37], as well as methylcholanthrene-induced fibrosarcomas
[38]. It should be noted that several of these transplantable tumors, such
as the Lewis lung and Madison lung carcinomas, are quite resistant to
conventional cancer chemotherapy, emphasizing the potential in the antitumor effects of pyran. Pyran was effective against some of these tumors
even when its administration was delayed until 8 days after tumor implantation, a time when the tumors have already metastasized in many animals
[36].

   While administration of pyran alone has produced a significant tumor
growth inhibition and prolonged survival, the combination of pyran treatment with other cancer treatment modalities has provided long-term
survivors. Mohr et al. [39] were the first to demonstrate that pyran could
produce complete cures of mice bearing the LSTRA leukemia, when the
primary tumor burden was reduced with chemotherapy. We have demonstrated that pyran can increase survival in mice bearing the Lewis lung
carcinoma, when the primary tumor is removed by surgery after it has
metastasized [70]. The combination of pyran with other treatments, such
as radiation, to reduce the tumor burden has also proved effective [83].
Moreover, pyran can potentiate the specific immune protective effects
produced by vaccination with killed tumor cell vaccines [84].

   The mechanism of antitumor activity of pyran has received considerable
attention from various laboratories. Possible alternative or cooperating
concepts of antitumor action include immunoenhancing coupling of the polyanion to tumor antigen, direct effect on tumor cells, action of polyanions
on a wide variety of enzymes, alteration of the isoelectric point of proteins,
displacement of nucleohistones, antiviral activities, interferon induction,
enhancement of specific tumor immunity, and macrophage activation. The
antitumor activity does not appear to be due to direct tumor cytotoxicity;
studies of cytotoxicity in vitro have shown that levels greater than 1 mg/ml
of drug are required to destroy 50% of either the tumor or normal cell
targets [36]. These observations of lack of cytotoxicity, together with
the known reticuloendothelial-stimulating activity of pyran, have suggested
that the antitumor activity may be mediated by macrophages. This concept
received additional support by the finding that only those polyanionic preparations which activated macrophages for tumoricidal activity exhibited
antitumor activity in vivo [38].

   The experimental lines of evidence that implicate pyran-activated
macrophages in resistance to the Lewis lung carcinoma and other solid

tumors include: (1) increased infiltration of tumors with histiocytes following systemic immunomodulator treatment [37,85]; (2) recovery of activated
peritoneal macrophages with tumoricidal activity from tumor bearing and
pyran-treated mice [37,85]; (3) inhibition of tumor growth when activated
peritoneal macrophages were mixed with tumor cells in vitro and trans-
planted into syngeneic recipients [38,40]; (4) isolation of macrophages with
antitumor activity from tumors of immunomodulator-treated animals [86],
providing functional significance to the morphological demonstration of
macrophages [37,85]; (5) cytotoxicity and inhibition of tumor growth in
vitro by activated macrophages [38,40]; and (6) lack of a role for specific
transplantation immunity in pyran-induced resistance to tumors [87].
Many of these and other experimental approaches have demonstrated that
other immunomodulators, such as C. parvum, also exert their antitumor
effects via activated macrophages [88]. In fact, the activated macrophage,
rather than lymphocytes, may provide the common denominator in the antitumor mechanism of polyanionic polymers.

In a few instances, pyran treatment has been associated with enhancement of tumor growth. This has been observed with benzo(α)-pyrene-induced
skin tumors [80], the Moloney sarcoma virus in certain strains of mice
[28], and with intravenous pyran treatment against Friend leukemia virus
[24]. The mechanism of these adverse effects is largely unknown. In the
latter situation, we have demonstrated that intraperitoneal administration
of pyran, which is protective against Friend leukemia virus [89], is associated with the increased macrophage activity in the peritoneal cavity and
the spleen. In contrast, the adverse intravenous pyran regimen is associated
with increased erythrocytic stem cell proliferation in the spleen, which provides an increased number of target cells for growth of the virus [25].
These seemingly paradoxical effects exhibited by pyran emphasize the importance of delineating the pharmacology and mechanism of action before
a clinical rationale for immunomodulators can be developed.

V. ANTIVIRAL ACTIVITY OF CARBOXYLIC
POLYANIONS

Many diverse, naturally occurring, and synthetic polyanions exert marked
activity against animal virus replication in vitro [90], against plant viruses
[91,92], and are now being developed for purification of water from contaminating viruses. The mechanism of antiviral activity in these systems
has not been completely defined, but it may involve direct inactivation of
viruses in some situations.

In regard to various animal virus infections in mammals, pyran and
other polycarboxylic polyanions exhibit a broad spectrum of antiviral activity
(Table 2). Polyanion treatment protects mice from mortality following
lethal infection with both RNA and DNA cytopathic viruses and inhibits tumor

TABLE 2.   Antiviral Activity in Vivo of Pyran and Other
Similar Polyanions[a]

Virus	Host	Route of virus administration	Selected references
Cytopathic viruses			
Encephalomyocarditis	Mouse	i.v.[b]	1
MM	Mouse	i.p.	2,3
Mengo	Mouse	i.p.	4,5,6,7
Foot and mouth	Mouse	i.p.	8,9
disease	Guinea pig	Footpad	8,10
Vesicular stomatitis	Mouse	i.n.	11
Influenza	Mouse	i.n., aerosol	4,12,13
Semliki Forest	Mouse	i.p.	4
Hog cholera	Pig	i.m.	8
Herpes simplex	Mouse	i.v., i.p., i. vag.	14,15,16,17
	Rabbit	Corneal	4
Vaccinia	Mouse	i.p., i.v.	4,7,12,18,19,20
	Rabbit	i.d.	21
Tumor viruses			
Friend leukemia	Mouse	i.p.	22,23,24,25
Rauscher leukemia	Mouse	i.p.	23,26
Gross leukemia	Mouse	Spontaneous	27
Moloney sarcoma	Mouse	i.m.	28
Mammary tumor	Mouse	Spontaneous	29
Polyoma	Mouse	i.p.	26
Adenovirus 12	Hamster	s.c.	30

[a]In most cases the polyanion was administered by the systemic route (i.p. or
i.v.).
[b]Abbreviations: i.d., intradermally; i.m., intramuscularly; i.n., intranasally; i.p., intraperitoneally; i.v., intravenously; i. vag., intravaginally;
s.c., subcutaneously.

formation and delays mortality after infection with DNA or RNA tumor
viruses.   This is in contrast to the narrow antiviral spectrum of most conventional chemotherapeutic drugs.
        Our investigations [70,74] have substantiated the importance of molecu-
lar weight and specific polyanionic configuration in the antiviral activity
[5,49].   However, a complete structure activity relationship in regard to
antiviral activity still needs to be performed.   Greatest protection is observed with prophylactic treatment.   Therapeutic treatment often does not
alter the course of disease, particularly with rapidly fatal infections [15].

These results suggest that polyanions may act very early during the viral infection, the drugs may need to be activated by the animal, or the drugs may act through modulation of host responses. Greatest protection is observed when the drug is administered at the same site where virus is subsequently injected [5,11,20]. There is often, however, significant protection, especially with pyran, when the polyanion and virus are injected at different sites. For example, intravenous or intraperitoneal administration of pyran protects mice against lethal vaginal infection with herpes simplex virus [16,17].

In contrast to standard antiviral chemotherapeutic agents, polyanions, especially when the polyanion and virus are both inoculated intraperitoneally, can provide prolonged protection [5,20]. Mice treated with pyran were protected against subsequent picornavirus infection for two months [2] and were resistant to Friend leukemia virus infection for 3 weeks [24]. In contrast to the intraperitoneal route, animals inoculated intravenously with pyran lost protection against picornavirus infection within a week [1].

Considerable emphasis has been directed toward defining the mechanism of antiviral action of polyanions, particularly for pyran and COAM. The major modes of antiviral action that have been considered are listed in Table 3. Polyanions can directly inactivate viruses [5,15]. However, the levels required are greater than those required for antiviral activity in vivo. Inhibition of virus replication by mechanisms similar to conventional chemotherapeutic drugs also does not appear to play an important part in resistance induced by polyanions in vivo. Pyran does inhibit the RNA-dependent DNA polymerase of avian myeloblastosis virus in vitro [93], but the enzyme is present only in oncornaviruses. Moreover, the drug does not have a morphologically toxic effect on normal or transformed mammalian cells at doses far above the effective antiviral dose [36,37].

Considerable effort has been directed toward determining whether induction of the antiviral protein, interferon, accounts for the antiviral action of polyanions [1,2,5,6,11,20,23]. There is no clear evidence that

TABLE 3. Possible Modes of Antiviral Action of Polyanions

---

1. Direct inactivation of virus

2. Inhibition of virus adsorption and/or replication

3. Induction of interferon

4. Stimulation of phagocytosis and inflammation

5. Enhancement of virus-specific, humoral- and/or cell-mediated immune responses

6. Enhancement of macrophage antiviral functions

---

systemic induction of interferon plays any role in the antiviral activity of
pyran or COAM [1,2,5,6,15,20,24]. Although pyran stimulates phagocytosis by the reticuloendothelial system, there is no correlation with antiviral activity. The lower-molecular-weight compounds, which exert potent
RES-stimulating activity, exhibit much less or no antiviral activity [49,70].
Moreover, the kinetics of antiviral activity do not correlate with increased
global phagocytic activity [1,5,73].

Because polyanions are immunomodulators for various humoral and
cell-mediated immune responses, attention has been directed toward specific
immunoenhancement as the mode of antiviral action. The protective effect
of COAM-statolon on Friend leukemia virus has been associated with increased antibody production directed to the p-12 virion antigen [94].
Specific immunostimulation, however, at least in the case of pyran, does
not appear to play a prominent role in the antiviral activity. Pyran is an
effective antiviral agent in animals depleted of T lymphocytes [14,26],
indicating that the drug probably acts independently of these immune cells.
Pyran is also effective against picornavirus infection in splenectomized
animals (authors' unpublished observations). Animals protected by treatment with pyran possess none or low levels of protective antibody against
herpes simplex virus, are not resistant to subsequent rechallenge with the
same virus, and have a decreased virus-specific cellular immune response
[17]. The polyanion appears to inhibit virus replication very early and
efficiently [15,17], so that there is probably little virus antigen to stimulate
a virus-specific immune response.

The major features of pyran-induced protection against herpes simplex
virus type 2 and/or encephalomyocarditis virus are shown in Table 4. Our
recent data substantiates the hypothesis that activated macrophages are
involved in the antiviral action of polyanions [17]. Pyran-activated peritoneal cells can transfer resistance to susceptible recipient mice to infection
with herpes simplex virus or Friend leukemia virus [17,89]. Moreover,
pyran-activated peritoneal macrophages exhibit potent antiviral activity in
vitro [95]. Thus, we have demonstrated that activated macrophages have
the capacity for antiviral activity; however, proof is still needed that these
cells are the major mode of action in vivo in animals treated with polyanions.
This concept is supported by morphological identification of increased numbers of macrophages in the spleen, target organ for Friend leukemia virus,
in animals that were protected by treatment with pyran [24,25]. Moreover,
peritoneal macrophages from these pyran-treated mice exhibited antiviral
activity against Friend leukemia virus, indicating that the virus injected
into the peritoneal cavity might be rapidly inhibited by either peritoneal
or splenic-activated macrophages [89]. Preliminary observations indicate
the presence of macrophages in the vaginal area in pyran-treated mice
protected against vaginal herpes simplex virus (authors' unpublished observations).

Prophylactic treatment with polyanions may be particularly applicable
in special situations with immunosuppressed patients at risk to various viral

TABLE 4. Features of the Antiviral Resistance Induced by Pyran
Against Herpes Simplex Virus Type 2 and/or Encephalomyocarditis Virus

1. Induction of none or minimal levels of interferon
2. No direct antiviral action
3. Early inhibition of virus pathogenesis
4. Lack of virus-specific resistance in survivors
5. Less neutralizing antibody response than in untreated mice
6. Antiviral effect in animals depleted of T lymphocytes
7. Antiviral effect in splenectomized animals
8. Antiviral effect in animals treated with silica
9. Antiviral effect in neonatal animals
10. Systemic as well as local protection
11. Ability of pyran-activated peritoneal cells to transfer resistance in vivo
12. Nonspecific antiviral activity of pyran-activated adherent peritoneal cells in vitro

infections (e.g., cancer patients, renal transplant patients, other immunodeficient patients). Pyran treatment has proven effective in naturally
immunodeficient neonatal animals [16,96], in animals rendered deficient
in cell-mediated immune responses [14,26,27], in animals suppressed by
treatment with silica [16], and in animals treated with steroids [3]. It is
interesting that the polyanion was active against herpes simplex virus [16]
or Friend leukemia virus [89] in animals treated with silica, an agent toxic
for macrophages. The data suggest that the immunomodulator caused an
influx of macrophages into the peritoneal cavity and an hepatosplenomegaly
associated with increased reticuloendothelial capacity, which could decrease
the effectiveness of silica. Moreover, pyran may, as has been reported
for immunomodulators such as C. parvum, amplify the residual reserves
of macrophage stem cells, so that it may be impossible to deplete mice
sufficiently of macrophages in the presence of the immunomodulator [97].

VI. FUTURE PERSPECTIVES

As previously discussed, the polycarboxylic immunomodulators may be
effective in immunodeficient patients. Prophylactic treatment has clearly
been demonstrated in T-depleted and in macrophage-deficient animals [14,
16,26,27,89]. Moreover, several immunomodulators, including pyran

copolymer, can increase the resistance of immature animals to various viral infections. Examples include pyran and Mycobacterium bovis strain BCG against herpes simplex virus [16,98] and picornaviruses ([96]; also authors' unpublished observations) in neonatal mice and levamisole against herpes simplex virus in neonatal rats [99]. Not all immunomodulators have such activity. C. parvum, typhoid vaccine, brucella vaccine, staphage lysate, and levamisole, for example, were without effect in neonatal mice [98]. The mechanisms of the protection in neonatal animals are not known, but they may involve maturation of immature macrophages, as has been demonstrated for several of these immunomodulators in regard to various immune responses [100].

The clinical future of polyanions lies with the separation of the toxicity from the antiviral, antitumor, and immunological effects [49]. Previous clinical studies with pyran used the drug in a direct cancer chemotherapeutic regimen in advanced cancer patients and were limited by drug side effects [49,69,103]. In contrast, proposed trials with less toxic fractions are aimed at adjuvant therapy with the polyanion combined with standard cyto-reductive therapy, i.e., surgery, chemotherapy, or radiation. Such protocols, by using less drug over longer periods, should have much less associated toxicity. Moreover, although polyanions usually exert beneficial effects, treatment with polyanions has also exacerbated tumor formation in a few instances [24,80,81]. As mentioned earlier, protection against, or exacerbation of, Friend-leukemia-virus-induced leukemogenesis depends upon the route of administration of pyran. In the protective (intraperitoneal) regimen, the drug appears to activate the macrophage in the peritoneal cavity and the spleen, while in the adverse (intravenous) regimen, the drug appears to stimulate cells in which the virus replicates. These results may also be related to the presence of both low- and high-molecular-weight species in the polymer preparation, which are known to have different pharmacological effects [49,70]. This illustrates the "yin-yang" aspect of treatment with polyanions, and the absolute necessity of developing well-defined molecular-weight species and of elucidating the parameters affecting the pharmacology and mechanism of action of polyanions before a rationale for clinical treatment can be established.

Perhaps the greatest potential use for polyanions is in combination with virus vaccines. In this situation, the polyanions could act both in an antiviral capacity and as an immunoadjuvant. Campbell and Richmond [101], in a series of studies, have documented that polyanions increase the effec-tiveness of various foot and mouth disease virus vaccines. Moreover, coadministration of pyran with tumor cell vaccines enhanced the specific vaccine-induced protection of the weakly immunogenic L1210 tumor [84]. The tumor cell vaccine and immunomodulator had to be administered by the same route and at the same time, preferably being mixed together. This was not necessary with the virus vaccine; while simultaneous adminis-tration was most effective, administration of the immunomodulator prior to the vaccine or by another route was also effective [101]. The immuno-logical mechanisms underlying these positive immunomodulatory activities, and the possible involvement of macrophages, have not been established.

The new virus vaccines that are currently being advocated are those made of virus protein subunits, without the possible cancer causing or otherwise deleterious nucleic acid [102]. Unfortunately, these vaccines are not as effective as live attenuated virus or whole inactivated virus vaccines. However, in conjunction with polyanions, such vaccines might be prepared that possess adequate effectiveness.

ACKNOWLEDGMENTS

This work was supported by Public Health Service Research Grant CA 16193 from the National Cancer Institute, Training Grant AI 00382 from the National Institute of Allergy and Infectious Diseases, Grant IN-105A from the American Cancer Society, and the Grants-in-Aid Program for Faculty of Virginia Commonwealth University.

MCB was a recipient of National Research Service Award AI 05431 and PSM a recipient of Public Health Service Research Career Development Award AI 70863 from the National Institute of Allergy and Infectious Diseases.

REFERENCES

1. P. S. Morahan, W. Regelson, and A. E. Munson, Antimicrob. Agents Chemother. 2:16 (1972).
2. F. F. Pindak, J. P. Schmidt, D. J. Giron, and P. T. Allen, Proc. Soc. Exp. Biol. Med. 138:317 (1971).
3. D. J. Giron, P. T. Allen, F. F. Pindak, and J. P. Schmidt, Infec. Immun. 3:318 (1971).
4. A. Billiau, J. Desmyter, and P. DeSomer, J. Virol. 5:321 (1970).
5. T. C. Merigan and M. S. Finkelstein, Virology 35:363 (1968).
6. A. Billiau, J. J. Muyembe, and P. DeSomer, Nature 232:183 (1971).
7. P. Claes, A. Billiau, E. DeClercq, J. Desmyter, E. Schonne, H. Vanderhaeghe, and P. DeSomer, J. Virol. 5:313 (1970).
8. J. Leunen, J. Desmyter, and P. DeSomer, Appl. Microbiol. 21:203 (1971).
9. J. Y. Richmond, Infec. Immun. 3:249 (1971).
10. R. F. Sellers, K. A. J. Herniman, and C. W. Hawkins, Res. Vet. Sci. 13:339 (1972).
11. E. DeClercq and T. C. Merigan, J. Gen. Virol. 5:359 (1969).
12. P. E. Came, M. Lieberman, A. Pascale, and G. Shimonaski, Proc. Soc. Exp. Biol. Med. 131:443 (1969).

13. A. Billiau, J. J. Muyembe, and P. DeSomer, Appl. Microbiol. 21: 580 (1971).
14. P. S. Morahan and R. S. McCord, J. Immunol. 115: 311 (1975).
15. R. S. McCord, M. K. Breinig, and P. S. Morahan, Antimicrob. Agents Chemother. 10: 28 (1976).
16. P. S. Morahan, E. R. Kern, and L. A. Glasgow, Proc. Soc. Exp. Biol. Med. 154: 615 (1977).
17. M. C. Breinig, L. L. Wright, M. B. McGeorge, and P. S. Morahan, Arch. Virol. 57: 25 (1978).
18. E. DeClercq and P. DeSomer, Appl. Microbiol. 16: 1314 (1968).
19. A. Billiau, J. J. Muyembe, and P. DeSomer, Infec. Immun. 5: 854 (1972).
20. E. DeClercq and P. DeSomer, Proc. Soc. Exp. Biol. Med. 132: 699 (1969).
21. E. DeClercq and P. DeSomer, Infec. Immun. 8: 669 (1973).
22. W. Regelson, Advan. Exp. Med. Biol. 1: 315 (1967).
23. M. A. Chirigos, W. Turner, J. Pearson, and W. Griffin, Int. J. Cancer 4: 267 (1969).
24. G. B. Schuller, P. S. Morahan, and M. Snodgrass, Cancer Res. 35: 1915 (1975).
25. P. S. Morahan, G. B. Schuller, M. J. Snodgrass, and A. M. Kaplan, J. Infec. Dis. 133: A249 (1976).
26. M. S. Hirsch, P. H. Black, M. L. Wood, and A. P. Monaco, J. Immunol. 108: 1312 (1972).
27. M. S. Hirsch, P. H. Black, M. L. Wood, and A. P. Monaco, J. Immunol. 111: 91 (1973).
28. E. DeClercq and P. DeSomer, Eur. J. Cancer 8: 535 (1972).
29. A. Billiau, R. Leyten, M. Vandeputte, and P. DeSomer, Life Sci. 10: 643 (1971).
30. V. M. Larson, W. R. Clark, and M. R. Hilleman, Proc. Soc. Exp. Biol. Med. 131: 1002 (1969).
31. G. Franchi, S. Garattini, L. K. J. Kram, and L. M. VanPutten, Eur. J. Cancer 9: 383 (1973).
32. J. Sandberg and A. Goldin, Cancer Chemother. Rep. 55: 233 (1971).
33. P. Ferruti and F. Danusso, J. Medicinal Chem. 16: 496 (1973).
34. K. Kapila, C. Smith, and A. A. Rubin, J. Reticuloendothelial Soc. 9: 447 (1971).
35. A. E. Munson, W. Regelson, and W. R. Wooles, J. Reticuloendothelial Soc. 6: 623 (1969).
36. P. S. Morahan, J. A. Munson, L. G. Baird, A. M. Kaplan, and W. Regelson, Cancer Res. 34: 506 (1974).
37. R. M. Schultz, J. D. Papamatheakis, J. Luetzeler, P. Ruiz, and M. A. Chirigos, Cancer Res. 37: 358 (1977).
38. P. S. Morahan and A. M. Kaplan, Int. J. Cancer 17: 82 (1976).
39. S. J. Mohr, M. A. Chirigos, F. S. Fuhrman, and J. W. Pryor, Cancer Res. 35: 3750 (1975).

40. R. P. Harmel, Jr. and B. Zbar, J. Nat. Cancer Inst. 54:989 (1975).
41. J. S. Remington and T. C. Merigan, Nature 226:361 (1970).
42. F. F. Pindak, Infec. Immun. 1:271 (1970).
43. D. J. Giron, J. P. Schmidt, R. J. Ball, and F. F. Pindak, Antimicrob. Agents Chemother. 1:80 (1972).
44. P. J. Van Dijck, M. Claesen, and P. DeSomer, Ann. Trop. Med. Parasitol. 64:5 (1970).
45. W. Braun, W. Regelson, Y. Yajima, and M. Ishizuka, Proc. Soc. Exp. Biol. Med. 133:171 (1970).
46. L. G. Baird and A. M. Kaplan, Cell. Immunol. 20:167 (1975).
47. M. Ho, Science 146:1472 (1964).
48. W. R. Stinebring and J. S. Youngner, Nature 204:712 (1964).
49. D. S. Breslow, E. I. Edwards, and N. R. Newberg, Nature 246:160 (1973).
50. R. Ottenbrite, E. M. Goodell, and A. E. Munson, Polymer 18:461 (1977).
51. E. M. Goodell, R. M. Ottenbrite, and A. E. Munson, J. Reticuloendothelial Soc. 23:183 (1978).
52. T. C. Merigan and W. Regelson, New Engl. J. Med. 277:1283 (1967).
53. W. Regelson, Proc. Int. Symp. Atheroscler. Reticuloendothelial Syst., Lake Como, Italy (1966).
54. T. C. Merigan, Nature 214:416 (1967).
55. P. DeSomer, E. DeClercq, A. Billiau, E. Schonne, and M. Claesen, J. Virol. 2:886 (1968).
56. P. DeSomer and A. Billiau, Arch. Ges. Virusforsch. 19:143 (1966).
57. M. Ho, Y. Kono, and M. K. Breinig, Proc. Soc. Exp. Biol. Med. 119:1227 (1965).
58. J. S. Youngner and W. R. Stinebring, Nature 208:456 (1965).
59. M. Ho, M. K. Breinig, B. Postic, and J. A. Armstrong, Ann. N.Y. Acad. Sci. 173:680 (1970).
60. P. DeSomer, E. DeClercq, A. Billiau, E. Schonne, and M. Claesen, J. Virol. 2:878 (1968).
61. Y. Ito, A. Kunii, N. Mori, and I. Nagata, Virology 44:638 (1971).
62. Y. Kojima, Kitasato Arch. Exp. Med. 43:35 (1970).
63. M. Ho, Y. H. Ke, and J. A. Armstrong, J. Infec. Dis. 128:212 (1973).
64. M. Ho, M. C. Breinig, and N. Maehara, J. Infec. Dis. 133:A30 (1976).
65. T. J. Smith and R. R. Wagner, J. Exp. Med. 125:559 (1967).
66. M. S. Finkelstein, G. H. Bausek, and T. C. Merigan, Science 161:465 (1968).
67. N. Maehara and M. Ho, Infec. Immun. 15:78 (1977).
68. S. Kobayashi, O. Yasui, and M. Masuzumi, Proc. Soc. Exp. Biol. Med. 131:487 (1969).
69. T. J. Leavitt, T. C. Merigan, and J. M. Freeman, Amer. J. Dis. Child. 121:43 (1971).

70. P. S. Morahan, D. W. Barnes, and A. E. Munson, Cancer Chemother. Repts. 62: 1797 (1978).

71. A. E. Munson, W. Regelson, and J. A. Munson, J. Toxicol. Appl. Pharmacol. 22: 299 (1972).

72. A. M. Kaplan, P. S. Morahan, and W. Regelson, J. Nat. Cancer Inst. 52: 1919 (1974).

73. A. E. Munson, W. Regelson, W. Lawrence, Jr., and W. R. Wooles, J. Reticuloendothelial Soc. 7: 375 (1970).

74. P. S. Morahan, A. E. Munson, W. Regelson, S. L. Commerford, and L. D. Hamilton, Proc. Nat. Acad. Sci. U.S. 69: 842 (1972).

75. T. Diamantstein, B. Wagner, I. Beyse, M. V. Odenwald, and G. Schulz, Eur. J. Immunol. 1: 335 (1971).

76. T. Diamantstein, B. Wagner, M. V. Odenwald, and G. Schulz, Eur. J. Immunol. 1: 426 (1971).

77. R. E. Cone and A. G. Johnson, Cell. Immunol. 3: 283 (1972).

78. R. M. Schultz, W. A. Woods, S. J. Mohr, and M. A. Chirigos, Cancer Res. 36: 1641 (1976).

79. S. J. Mohr, M. A. Chirigos, F. Fuhrman, and G. Smith, Cancer Res. 36: 1315 (1976).

80. M. L. Kripke and T. Borsos, J. Nat. Cancer Inst. 53: 1409 (1974).

81. A. F. Gazdar, A. D. Steinberg, G. F. Spahn, and S. Baron, Proc. Soc. Exp. Biol. Med. 139: 1132 (1972).

82. L. G. Baird and A. M. Kaplan, Cell. Immunol. 28: 36 (1977).

83. A. L. Collins and C. W. Song, Radiat. Res. 70: 688 (1977).

84. S. J. Mohr, M. A. Chirigos, G. T. Smith, and F. S. Fuhrman, Cancer Res. 36: 2035 (1976).

85. M. J. Snodgrass, P. S. Morahan, and A. M. Kaplan, J. Nat. Cancer Inst. 55: 455 (1975).

86. P. S. Morahan and A. M. Kaplan, J. Reticuloendothelial Soc. 20: 36a (1976).

87. P. S. Morahan and A. M. Kaplan, in Progress in Cancer Research and Therapy (M. A. Chirigos, ed.), Vol. 2, Raven Press, New York, 1977, p. 499.

88. M. Scott, J. Nat. Cancer Inst. 53: 861 (1974).

89. G. B. Schuller and P. S. Morahan, Cancer Res. 37: 4064 (1977).

90. W. Regelson, Advan. Chemother. 3: 303 (1968).

91. S. Gianinazzi and B. Kassanis, J. Gen. Virol. 23: 1 (1974).

92. D. S. Breslow and A. A. Chadwick, U.S. Patent 3,996,347 (1976).

93. T. S. Papas, T. W. Pry, and M. A. Chirigos, Proc. Nat. Acad. Sci. U.S. 71: 367 (1974).

94. P. A. Marx, Jr. and E. F. Wheelock, Abstr. Ann. Meeting, Amer. Soc. Microbiol. p. 240 (1976).

95. P. S. Morahan, L. A. Glasgow, J. L. Crane, Jr., and E. R. Kern, Cell Immunol. 28: 404 (1977).

96. J. Y. Richmond and C. H. Campbell, Arch. Ges. Virusforsch. 36: 232 (1972).
97. N. Wolmark and B. Fisher, Cancer Res. 34:2869 (1974).
98. S. E. Starr, A. M. Visintine, M. O. Tomeh, and A. J. Nahmias, Proc. Soc. Exp. Biol. Med. 152:57 (1976).
99. G. W. Fischer, J. K. Podgore, J. W. Bass, J. L. Kelley, and G. Y. Kobayashi, J. Infec. Dis. 132:578 (1975).
100. R. M. Blaese, in The Phagocytic Cell and Host Resistance (J. A. Bellanti and D. H. Dayton, eds.), Raven Press, New York, 1975, p. 309.
101. C. H. Campbell and J. Y. Richmond, Infec. Immun. 7:199 (1973).
102. M. R. Hilleman, Cancer Res. 36:857 (1976).
103. W. Regelson, B. I. Shnider, J. Colsky, K. B. Olson, J. F. Holland, C. L. Johnston, and L. H. Dennis, in Progress in Cancer Research and Therapy (M. A. Chirigos, ed.), Vol. 7, Raven Press, New York, 1978, p. 469.

11

INTERFERON AND INTERFERON INDUCERS: IMMUNE MODULATION

Howard M. Johnson

University of Texas Medical Branch
Galveston, Texas

I. INTRODUCTION

A. The Interferon System

Interferon was first recognized as an antiviral system some two decades ago when Alick Isaacs and Jean Lindenmann observed that a virus-infected animal cell produced a protein substance capable of rendering surrounding

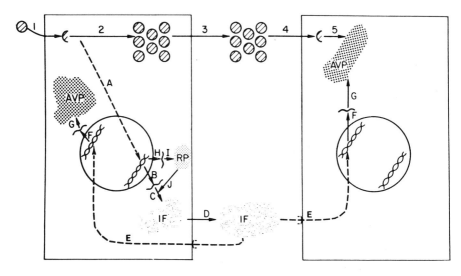

FIGURE 1. Cellular events of the induction and action of interferon (IF).
Virus comes in contact with the cell (1) and penetrates the cell membrane.
The virus then releases its genetic material, and replication of the virus
occurs (2). The new virus leaves the cell (3), enters the fluid around the
first cell, and some of the replicated virus infects a second cell (4), where
the release of the genetic material again takes place (5). During the early
stages of infection of the first cell, some event (viral nucleic acid?) stimulates a gene in the DNA which contains the stored genetic information for
interferon (A). This leads to the production of a messenger RNA (mRNA)
for interferon, which leaves (B) the nucleus and is translated by the cell's
ribosomes (C) into the interferon protein. Several events now occur more
or less simultaneously. Interferon is secreted by the first infected cell
(D), enters the surrounding fluid, where it comes into contact with and
stimulates the second cell (E) by interacting with a membrane receptor for
interferon. The second cell is thereby induced to produce a new RNA (F),
which is translated to a new protein(s) (G), the antiviral protein (AVP).
This in turn modifies the cell's protein-synthesizing machinery such that
cell mRNA is translated into protein, but viral RNA is poorly bound or
translated, or both. In the first cell processes E, F, and G may, in some
instances, also operate to form AVP and thereby reduce the virus yield in
the first cell. Shortly after interferon is synthesized into the first cell,
another mRNA (H) is believed to be synthesized from the cell's DNA which
is translated (I) into a regulatory protein (RP) (hypothesized). This regulatory protein combines with the mRNA for interferon, thereby preventing
the further synthesis of more interferon (J). It has not been determined
whether regulation of the AVP involves mechanisms in addition to the extracellular concentration of interferon. From Ref. 1a. [Reprinted with
permission from H. M. Johnson and S. Baron, Pharmacol. Ther. 1 (1977),
Pergamon Press, Ltd.]

cells resistant to viral infection. Since 1957, many factors governing this antiviral interferon system have been unveiled in laboratories around the world [1]. Evidence indicates that interferon produced during virus infection is one of the more important body defenses against these infections. Figure 1 depicts the function of interferon [1a]. Fundamentally, the interferon system consists of two parts: (1) production of the interferon by the virus-infected cell, and (2) reaction of the secreted interferon with surrounding cells to induce intracellular antiviral protein(s) that inhibit virus multiplication within the cell. This mechanism of controlling viral infections suggests that interferon may have other natural cell-regulatory functions. We will present data that indicate that interferon can play an important role in regulating the immune response in doses that occur naturally.

Based on recent findings, the human and mouse interferon systems could provisionally be classified into two groups. These are virus-type interferons [2-4] and immune interferons [5-10] (Table 1). Virus-type interferons are classically induced by viruses or synthetic polyribonucleotides, while immune interferons are induced in primed lymphocytes by specific antigen or in unprimed lymphocytes by T-cell mitogens (usually). Virus-type interferons are heterogenous, and at least two antigenically distinct types exist [11,12]. They are called fibroblast interferon and leukocyte interferon, indicating their cellular source. Immune interferon is antigenically distinct from the virus-type interferons [13,14]. Antibodies to mitogen-induced immune interferon neutralized both mitogen-induced and antigen-induced interferons to the same extent [14a], so immune interferons induced under various conditions appear to be antigenically the same or similar.

TABLE 1. Provisional Classification of Interferon

A. Virus-type (type I)
    1. Antigenic types
        a. Fibroblast cell origin
        b. Leukocyte cell origin
    2. Inducers
        a. Virus
        b. Polyribonucleotide
        c. Chemicals (tilorone, etc.)

B. Immune-type (type II)
    1. Antigenic types—only one type known to date
    2. Inducers
        a. Antigen
        b. Mitogens (primarily T-cell mitogens)

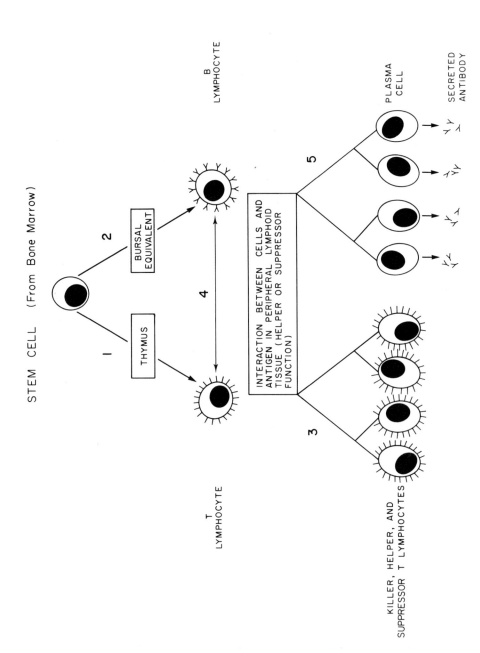

FIGURE 2. Simplified scheme for the origin and function of the cells involved in the immune response. The bone marrow contains stem cells that are destined to become B and T lymphocytes. When the stem cell migrates (1) to an organ under the breast bone called the thymus, it undergoes differentiation to a T lymphocyte and becomes the effector cell for the various aspects of cellular immunity. The T lymphocyte leaves the thymus and migrates to the lymph nodes and spleen, where it is capable of responding to antigen. Another stem cell from the bone marrow migrates (2), to an organ in the lower gut of the chicken called the bursa and in humans probably to the bone narrow, liver, and spleen, where it undergoes differentiation and becomes the effector cell for the production of antibody. The differentiated B lymphocyte migrates from the bursa or its equivalent to the lymph nodes and spleen, where, like the T lymphocyte, it is capable of responding to antigen recognition. Both B and T lymphocytes have specific receptors on their surfaces for antigen recognition and subsequent response. Upon exposure to antigen, the T lymphocyte(s) is capable, with the aid of a phagocytic cell called the macrophage, of being activated (3) to differentiate and to expand in number. The T lymphocyte can interact with the antigen directly and inactivate or kill the antigen. It is also capable, along with the macrophage, of interacting (4) with the B lymphocyte through its helper and suppressor function, either enhancing the differentiation of the B lymphocyte to become a plasma cell (5), which is responsible for antibody production, or suppressing the B lymphocyte from differentiating into a plasma cell. Soluble mediators have been obtained from T lymphocytes, some of which are capable of mediating the helper and suppressor activities. There is evidence that interferon is capable of mediating the suppressor activity of T lymphocytes.

B. The Immune System

Functionally, two major types of lymphocytes are involved in the immune response, one as the humoral and one as the cellular mode of response to antigenic stimulation (Figure 2). Both types of lymphocytes originate as stem cells in the bone marrow, but they take different paths to maturity. From both the historical and anatomical points of view, the paths of differentiation are most clearly seen in the chicken.

One group of cells migrates to an organ known as the bursa of Fabricius in chickens. The counterpart of this organ in mammals is not known, but bursal functions seem to reside in the fetal liver, spleen, and bone marrow. After arriving in the bursa of chickens, or its equivalent in mammals, stem cells differentiate into bursal (B) lymphocytes. The differentiated B lymphocytes leave the bursa, or its equivalent in mammals, and seed regional lymph nodes and the spleen. As a result of genetic coding, these cells have certain immunoglobulins on their surfaces. This surface antibody serves as the cell receptor for antigen, and after reaction with its specific antigen the B cell undergoes clonal expansion and differentiation into antibody-secreting cells known as plasma cells.

The lymphocyte that is responsible for cellular immunity (delayed-type hypersensitivity) is called the thymic (T) lymphocyte, which develops and differentiates in the thymus from a bone marrow precursor cell. The differentiated lymphocytes leave the thymus and, like B lymphocytes, seed regional lymph nodes and the spleen. T lymphocytes are the most numerous lymphocytes in the circulating lymphocyte pool. The T-lymphocyte receptor for antigen does not appear to be an immunoglobulin like that of the B-cell receptor, but its nature is unknown. When the T cell is stimulated by interaction of its receptors with antigen, it reacts in several ways. It performs a "helper" function in that it—or some substance or substances that it releases—interacts with B cells, helping B cells to transform into antibody-secreting plasma cells. Also, stimulation of T cells by antigens results in the development of cytotoxic or "killer" cells, which can carry out the cellular immune responses. (A well-known example is the delayed hypersensitivity to mycobacteria). The T cell also appears to have the additional property of "suppressor" activity, which is the opposite of the helper function and is due primarily to antigen stimulation. It has the effect of inhibiting both antibody response (B-cell activity) and some forms of cellular immunity (some T-cell functions). Together, the helper and suppressor functions of T cells are thought to play a major role in regulating the immune response. These regulatory T-cell activities are thought, in some cases, to be mediated by soluble factors called lymphokines [15]. Evidence will be presented indicating that interferons are candidates for mediation of some forms of suppressor cell activities.

II. ANTIBODY STUDIES WITH INTERFERON

A. In Vivo Systems

Moderate and high doses of virus-type interferon have been reported to
suppress the plaque-forming cell (PFC) response to sheep red-blood cells
(SRBC) in mice [16-18]. Plaque-forming cells are cells that produce antibody against red cells or against an antigen coated to red cells. The reaction of antibody with red cells in the presence of complement results in
a plaque or hole in the lawn of red cells. When mice were injected with
1.5×10^5 U or more of interferon 2 days prior to antigen injection, the
PFC response was suppressed by >80% when assayed 6 days after SRBC
injection [17]. The immunosuppressive effect of virus-type interferon
was more effective against low doses of antigen, and both IgM and IgG
antibody synthesis were affected [18].

The antibody response of mice to Salmonella typhimurium lipopoly-
saccharide (LPS), a thymus-independent antigen, was also significantly
inhibited by virus-type interferon preparations [19]. By removing the
adherent cells from spleen cells of mice treated with interferon and stimulation of the nonadherent cells by LPS in vitro, data were obtained that
suggested that interferon can act directly on B lymphocytes. The immunosuppression effects of the interferon preparations used for the above studies
were shown by several criteria to be due to interferon.

Recently, virus-type interferon at 200 U/ml was shown to significantly
inhibit so-called heterologous adoptive cutaneous anaphylaxis [20]. Briefly,
mice were injected with antigen in a manner that elicited antibody of the
IgE class. Seven to ten days prior to removal of the responding lymphoid
cells, the mice were boosted with the priming antigen. After removal
from the mice, the antigen-sensitized lymphoid cells were treated with
interferon and injected intradermally into Wistar rats. Twenty-four hours
later the site of injection was challenged with the specific antigen for cutaneous anaphylaxis. The findings would suggest that virus-induced interferon
was capable of suppressing IgE antibody production by plasma cells. The
stage of differentiation of the treated cells, however, is unknown. They
could be memory cells from the mice that have subsequently undergone
"activation" by the xenogeneic conditions after injection in the rat.

Related to the above studies on IgE antibody production is the recent
finding that interferon and viral and nonviral inducers of interferon are
capable of enhancing antigen or anti-IgE antibody release of histamine
from human leukocytes [21]. Thus, a new biological role for interferon
that is related to immune function has been discovered. This finding has
clinical potential in virus-induced upper-respiratory allergic reactions.

Very little information is available on the effect of immune interferon
on the in vivo antibody response. One study employed mice sensitized with

the attenuated Calmette-Guérin vaccine (BCG) and challenged with old tuberculin (OT) [22]. This results in high serum levels of immune interferon.
When these mice were immunized with SRBC at the time of high serum levels
of immune interferon, a significant suppression of the splenic PFC response
was observed. Further, the suppression of the anti-SRBC response was
related to the serum concentration of immune interferon. Although sugges-
tive of a suppressive role of immune interferon in the in vivo antibody
response, studies of this type need to carefully monitor the presence and
function of other mediators released into the serum by the challenge with
OT.

B. In Vitro Systems

Most of the information on the role of interferon in antibody formation has
been obtained from in vitro systems. The in vivo studies require large
amounts of interferon, and the concentration and kinetics of administered
interferon in the microenvironment of the immunocompetent cell are unknown. In one series of in vitro studies approximately 3000 U of virus-
type L-cell interferon/ml were required to significantly suppress the in
vitro PFC response of BALB/c mouse spleen cells to SRBC [23]. The
effect was seen when the cultures were pretreated with interferon for 6 hr,
or when interferon was added up to 40 hr after addition of SRBC. The
factor responsible for the inhibition could not be quantitatively dissociated
from the antiviral activity of interferon either in terms of the specific
activity of the interferon or by standard physiocochemical means, such as
treatment of interferon with trypsin, periodate, RNase, and DNase. Trypsin
and periodate treatment, which destroyed the interferon, also destroyed
the PFC inhibitory effect of the interferon preparations. By the use of
separated cell populations, it was claimed that interferon acted directly
on B lymphocytes and had no effect on macrophages or T-lymphocyte helper
effect. This latter observation regarding T-cell helper effect is significant,
since it is the only T-cell function reported not to be affected by interferon
and therefore needs to be investigated further. The aforementioned in vitro
study required lesser amounts of interferon for PFC inhibition than did the
in vivo studies, but the inhibitory concentrations were considerably higher
than the physiological concentrations normally obtained by stimulation of
cultures with interferon inducers [1].

Others [24,25] have demonstrated with C57B1/6 mouse spleen cells
that 20-60 U of virus-type interferon from various sources and specific
activities inhibited the in vitro PFC response to SRBC by 90% or more.
An example of one such inhibition is shown in the PFC inhibition data with
purified mouse virus-type ascites tumor interferon presented in Figure 3.
Interferon, 20 U/culture, inhibited the PFC response by 92%. These inhibitory concentrations of purified interferon did not affect viable cell

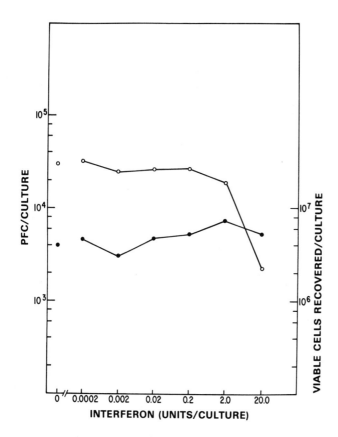

FIGURE 3. The effect of highly purified mouse ascites tumor virus–type interferon (3.2×10^8 NIH reference units/mg protein; P. Lengyel, Yale) on the primary in vitro PFC response. Direct anti–SRBC PFC/culture (o—o) and viable cells recovered per culture (●—●) were determined on day 5. From Ref. 25. [Reprinted with permission from H. M. Johnson, B. G. Smith, and S. Baron, J. Immunol. 114:403 (1975), The Williams & Wilkins Co., Baltimore.]

recovery. Although the above studies involved interferon preparations of different potencies and specific activities, the interferons inhibited the PFC response in proportion to their antiviral activities. In addition, both the antiviral activity and the PFC inhibitory activity of the interferons were neutralized by antibody specific for mouse interferon. Both activities were partially or completely inactivated by heating at 60°C for 1 hr. Human interferons at the concentrations used had neither antiviral activity nor

PFC-inhibitory activity in mouse cells. Limited exposure (4 hr) of cells to interferons significantly inhibits both viral infection and the PFC response. Both the antiviral activity and the PFC inhibitory activity of the interferon preparations are acid stable. It was concluded, therefore, that the inhibition of the primary in vitro PFC response was due to interferon in the preparations [25].

Kinetic data showed that the greater the concentration of interferon added to the cultures, the earlier the effect on the PFC response [25]. Also, the presence of interferon in the culture for the first 4 hr was sufficient to inhibit the PFC response. Interferon, then, appeared to affect some early events which lead to inhibition of the PFC response. These events do not appear necessarily to involve antigen "processing" by macrophages or induction of lymphocytes by "processed" antigen, since kinetic data showed that the B cells could be induced by SRBC to produce PFC on days 3 and 4 in studies involving low dosages of interferon (50 U/culture).

The effect of virus-type interferon on the in vitro PFC response to a thymus- and macrophage-independent antigen has been studied [26]. It required about twice as much interferon (100-200 U) to inhibit the PFC response to Escherichia coli 0127 LPS (thymus-independent) as it did to inhibit the anti-SRBC response. By the use of spleen cells from nude (athymic) mice and spleen cells depleted of macrophages, it was shown that T lymphocytes and macrophages were not required for interferon to exert its inhibitory effect on B lymphocytes. Since it is impossible to remove macrophages completely from the cultures, a possible role for residual macrophages must be considered.

The nature of the cellular events in virus-type interferon inhibition of the in vitro PFC response has recently been further clarified [27]. The findings suggest that interferon appears to affect only "nonactivated" (uncommitted) B-cell precursors by preventing them from becoming activated. Early responding precursor cells, which are already committed to the cell cycle, are refractory to interferon-induced suppression of the in vitro response. Thus, clonal expansion of these refractory B-cell precursors is not affected until late in the immune response and not at the peak of the response. These findings are in agreement with preliminary observations on the effect of virus-type interferon on immunoglobulin production by mouse MOPC-104E plasmacytomas, where the early production (first 4 or 5 days in culture) of immunoglobulin was not suppressed by interferon (H. M. Johnson, E. Blalock, and S. Baron, unpublished data).

From the foregoing studies the general picture emerges of a population of precursor B lymphocytes that are capable of responding to a given antigen (SRBC). The cells are at various stages of differentiation, which in turn determines their relative abilities to differentiate into antibody-producing plasma cells in the presence of various concentrations of virus-type (and perhaps immune) interferon. The lesser differentiated precursor cells are more susceptible than are the highly differentiated precursor cells to inhibition by interferon. Precursor B cells that are sufficiently differentiated undergo normal clonal expansion for a limited time in the presence of interferon.

Virus-type interferon inhibition of the primary in vitro PFC response in C57B1/6 mice involves a dynamic relationship between the nature of the antigen, the concentration of interferon added to antigen-stimulated cultures, and the time of addition of interferon relative to antigen addition [14]. The PFC response to a thymus-dependent antigen, SRBC, was more easily suppressed by interferon than was that to a thymus-independent antigen, E. coli 0127 LPS, both in terms of inhibitory concentrations of interferon and the time at which the interferon could be added to cultures after antigen and still inhibit the PFC response. The anti-SRBC response was effectively inhibited by 150 U of interferon when the interferon was added to mouse spleen cultures up to 16 hr (87% inhibition) after SRBC. At 500 U of interferon, effective inhibition (76%) was obtained when the interferon was added up to 24 hr after SRBC. In the anti-E. coli 0127 response, 150 U of interferon effectively inhibited the PFC response only when added at the time of antigen, and not 8 hr later. With 500 U of interferon, effective inhibition (70%) was obtained when interferon was added to cultures up to 16 hr after E. coli 0127. The anti-SRBC, PFC response was inhibited more extensively by both 150 and 500 U of interferon than was the anti-E. coli 0127 response when interferon was added to cultures at either 8, 16, or 24 hr after antigen.

Evidence has been presented that suggests that splenic memory lymphocytes represent a cell population that differs qualitatively from that of unstimulated spleen cells [28]. Virus-type interferon has been shown to be effective in inhibiting (91% with 120 U of interferon) the generation of PFC from this memory cell pool. The data do suggest that the memory cells are slightly more resistant to interferon inhibition than are virgin lymphocytes. Both virgin and memory lymphocyte populations, then, are inhibited by virus-type interferon in the in vitro PFC response. This is in agreement with the inhibitory effects of interferon on the secondary antibody response in in vivo studies [18]. It is of interest that the in vitro PFC inhibition of memory lymphocytes was obtained with physiological concentrations of interferon.

Both the in vivo and in vitro studies cited above present data that suggest that under certain conditions interferon may also exert a small enhancing effect on the antibody response in addition to its suppressive effects. Injections of interferon into mice or additions to mouse spleen cultures 2 to 3 days after antigen have been shown to slightly enhance the antibody response [19,25]. Similarly, suboptimal immune responses in vitro have been elevated to optimal levels by interferon [23]. Some enhancement has also been noted with low concentrations of interferon [16]. The enhancement data are not as impressive as the data showing the immunosuppressive effects of interferon. Some of the in vitro studies [25] reported above have recently been confirmed [29].

In a related in vitro study a recent report [30] suggested that both virus-type and immune crude interferon preparations possess macrophage migration inhibitory properties. Although interesting, this study must be repeated with more purified interferon preparations in order to be more meaningful. Highly purified virus-type interferon is currently available for such studies. The study does point up the need for purification of immune interferon.

Very little information is available on the immunosuppressive property of immune interferon. This is primarily due to the lack of purified immune interferon for study. One study used sera that were obtained from BCG-sensitized mice that were challenged with OT as the source of immune interferon [22]. The immune-interferon-containing sera suppressed the in vitro PFC response to SRBC when compared to corresponding concentrations of mouse sera that did not contain interferon. The immunosuppressive factor(s) was found primarily in the lower-molecular-weight fraction (40,000) from a Sephadex G-100 column, with minor suppressive activity in the 90,000 fraction. This corresponded to the distribution of the antiviral activity from the column. Other biological activities, such as macrophage migration inhibitory factor and lymphotoxin, have been found at these same or similar molecular weights [31,32]. Since no data were provided on these other biological activities, it is not possible to unequivocally attribute the immunosuppressive property of the sera to immune interferon. It has been suggested that immune interferon may possess several biological activities in addition to its antiviral property, such as macrophage migration inhibitory and soluble immune response suppressor properties [10]. The recent separation of mouse immune interferon and macrophage migration inhibitory activities, however, would suggest that some lymphocyte mediator activities are due to distinct molecules [33].

It is possible to differentiate the immunosuppressive and antiviral effects of virus-type interferon. Suppression of the in vitro antibody response of mouse (C57B1/6) spleen cells to SRBC was blocked by 5×10^{-5} M 2-mercaptoethanol (2-ME) [34]. The blockade was not due to a direct effect on interferon, since 2-ME was capable of blocking the suppression when added to cultures after interferon had established the immunosuppressive state (48 hr after interferon). Similar protective effects of 2-ME were observed during immunosuppression by virus-type interferon inducers, but not T-cell mitogen inducers of interferon (immune interferon). Virus-type interferon inhibited DNA synthesis in unstimulated spleen cell cultures and in 2-ME stimulated cultures, and the degree of inhibition of DNA synthesis appeared to be related to the immunosuppressive property of interferon in the absence or presence of 2-ME. 2-ME did not affect the antiviral properties of either virus-type or immune interferon in nonlymphoid cells. Further, the induction of virus-type interferon in spleen cells was neither inhibited nor enhanced by 2-ME, while the induction of immune interferon was enhanced. This enhancement was consistent with 2-ME enhancement of the immunosuppressive effects of immune interferon inducers.

There are two possibilities for 2-ME blockade of the immunosuppressive effect of virus-type interferon, while not affecting the antiviral property. First, the immunosuppressive and antiviral properties of virus-type interferon may involve different mechanisms at the subcellular level. Second, the selectivity of the blockade by 2-ME could be due to the fact that spleen cells are the target cells in immunosuppression, while L cells are the target cells in inhibition of virus replication. Thus, virus-type interferon may suppress the immune response at the level of the macrophage, and 2-ME may reverse this effect by replacing a blocked macrophage function.

Related to this is the finding that virus-type interferon preparations are capable of activating macrophages as determined by their increased antitumor effects [35,36]. Activated macrophages, as a result of appropriate signals, have very motile cytoplasmic processes and show well-developed intracellular granules. They are capable of more active phagocytosis and killing. In the activated state the macrophage may have a suppressive effect on the immune response and may thus be considered a suppressor cell [37]. Thus virus-type interferon may affect several cell types involved in the immune response.

III. ANTIBODY STUDIES WITH INTERFERON INDUCERS

A. In Vivo Systems

Inducers of interferon, as illustrated in Table 1, can be classified on the basis of whether they induce cells to produce virus-type or immune interferon. Inducers of both types of interferons have been studied in in vivo systems. Virus-type interferon inducers have been reported to have both enhancing and suppressive effects on the antibody response in vivo. Synthetic, double-stranded polyribonucleotides, virus-type interferon inducers, are well known as enhancers or adjuvants of the in vivo antibody response [38-40]. This enhancement has been ascribed to the effect of these polyribonucleotides on the T lymphocytes [41]. Less recognized is the fact that synthetic polyribonucleotides can also inhibit the in vivo antibody response under certain conditions [40,41]. There is a temporal relationship between enhancement and suppression of the immune response when mice are injected intravenously with polyriboadenylate: polyribouridylate (poly rA: poly rU) at various times in relation to intravenous injections of bovine gamma globulin [40]. Poly rA: poly rU, given one day to 12 hr before antigen, profoundly suppressed the antibody response. When given 2 hr before, or at the same time as antigen, a significant enhancement of the antibody response was observed.

The T-lymphocyte mitogens, phytohemagglutinin (PHA) and Con A, which were shown earlier to be inducers of immune interferon in lymphoid cell cultures, are also suppressors of the antibody response in mice [42,43] and rabbits [44] if the mitogens are injected one to two days before antigen. It was found in the rabbit that injection of Con A or PHA at the time of antigen had an enhancing effect on the antibody response [44].

B. In Vitro Systems

In vitro antibody induction studies have shown that poly rA: poly rU can have both a modest enhancing or inhibiting effect on the immune response, depend- ing on the polyribonucleotide concentration and the length of the culture period [45-47]. We have obtained consistent suppression of the in vitro antibody PFC response with polyribonucleotides. Poly rA: poly rU and polyriboinosinate: polyribocytidylate (poly rI: poly rC), at 0.1-1.0 μg/ml, inhibited the anti-SRBC PFC response (Figure 4) in spleen cell cultures by >90% when the polyribonucleotides were added to cultures along with antigen [48]. Functional T lymphocytes were required in the cultures for the poly- ribonucleotides to be effective as inhibitors, thus demonstrating the thymus

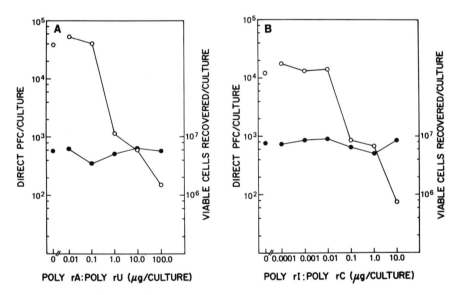

FIGURE 4. The effect of poly rA: poly rU (A) and poly rI: poly rC (B) on the primary in vitro PFC response to SRBC in C57B1/6 mouse spleen cultures. Polyribonucleotides were added at the time of SRBC addition, and direct anti-SRBC PFC/culture (o—o) and viable cells recovered/culture (●—●) were determined on day 5. From Ref. 48. [Reprinted with permis- sion from H. M. Johnson, J. A. Bukovic, and B. G. Smith, Proc. Soc. Exp. Biol. Med. 149:599 (1975).]

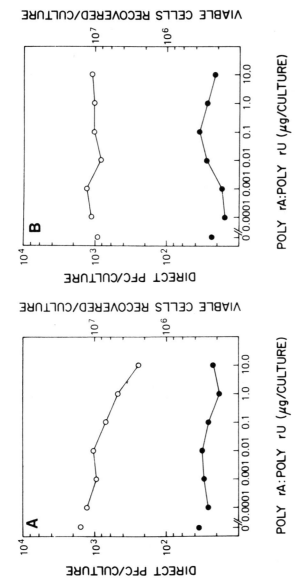

POLY rA:POLY rU (µg/CULTURE)

FIGURE 5. The effect of poly rA:poly rU on the primary in vitro PFC response to E. coli 0127 LPS in C57B1/6 (A) and nude (athymic) (B) mouse spleen cultures. The polyribonucleotide was added at the same time as antigen, and direct anti-E. coli 0127 LPS PFC/culture (o—o) and viable cells recovered/culture (●—●) were determined on day 5. From Ref. 48. [Reprinted with permission from H. M. Johnson, J. A. Bukovic, and B. G. Smith, Proc. Soc. Exp. Biol. Med. 149:599 (1975).]

TABLE 2. Neutralization by Anti-Mouse Interferon Antibody of
Inhibitory Effect of Poly rA: Poly rU on in vitro PFC Response of
C57B1/6 Spleen Cells to SRBC

Antiserum, dilution[a]	Poly rA:poly rU[a] (2 µg/culture)	Anti-SRBC, PFC/culture (mean ± SD for duplicates)	Percentage of inhibition relative to control
None	−	26,750 ± 1,061	
None	+	1,075 ± 742	96
Anti-interferon, 1:100	−	12,025 ± 177	
Anti-interferon, 1:100	+	16,650 ± 530	−29
Anti-interferon, 1:1000	−	21,550 ± 636	
Anti-interferon, 1:1000	+	18,325 ± 2,298	15
NRS,[b] 1:100	−	12,925 ± 1,237	
NRS, 1:100	+	2,400 ± 283	81

[a]Antisera and poly rA: poly rU were added to cultures at the same time.
  Antisera dilutions represent final concentrations after addition to cultures.
[b]Normal rabbit serum (NRS) is a pool of four normal rabbit sera.
Source: Reprinted with permission from Ref. 14.

dependence of the inhibitions. This is illustrated in Figure 5, where
poly rA:poly rU was used to inhibit the PFC response to the T-independent
antigen E. coli 0127 LPS in C57B1/6 mouse spleen cultures and in nude
(athymic) mouse spleen cultures. At 10 µg per culture, poly rA:poly rU
inhibited the response in C57B1/6 cultures by 84%, while having no effect
in the nude spleen cultures. The C57B1/6 cultures contained functional B
cells but lacked functional T cells. Ten to 100 times more polyribonucleotide was required in order to inhibit the in vitro PFC response to the T-
independent antigen E. coli 0127 LPS than was required for the T-dependent
SRBC antigen. This latter observation is further evidence of a differential
effect of interferon and interferon inducers on the in vitro PFC response
to a T-dependent and T-independent antigen. The in vitro PFC response
to SRBC is macrophage-dependent, while the response to E. coli 0127 LPS
is less dependent on macrophages [49]. The above findings, thus, are
consistent with the earlier 2-ME data, which suggested that interferon
suppressed the PFC response by blockade of a macrophage function.

Data in Table 2 show that the inhibitory effect of poly rA: poly rU on the in vitro PFC response to SRBC was neutralized by antibody to virus-type interferon [14]. The same effect was observed with E. coli 0127 LPS antigen. The antiviral property of interferon stimulated in spleen cultures by polyribonucleotide is also neutralized by the same antibody to interferon. The above findings suggest that the in vitro immunosuppressive effect of double-stranded polyribonucleotides is due to their early stimulation of virus-type interferon production by T lymphocytes.

T-cell mitogens are potent inhibitors of the in vitro PFC response [50-53]. They also induce lymphocytes to produce immune interferon [5,8-10]. These T lymphocytes have been shown to possess histamine receptors [54]. In an attempt to obtain some insight into the possible role of immune interferon in the mediation of suppressor T-cell effects, the T-cell mitogens Con A, PHA-P, and SEA were compared for their ability to inhibit the in vitro antibody response and to stimulate the production of immune interferon in mouse spleen cell cultures (Figures 6 and 7) [10].

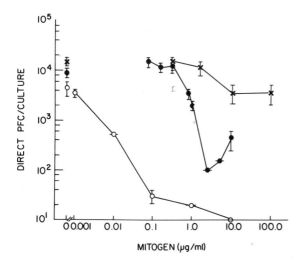

FIGURE 6. The suppressive effect of various T-lymphocyte mitogens on the primary in vitro PFC response to SRBC. Mitogens were added at the time of SRBC addition, and direct anti-SRBC PFC/culture were determined on day 5. PFC responses are representative of three experiments. From Ref. 10. Key: SEA, o—o; Con A, ●—●; PHA-P, ×—×. [Reprinted with permission from H. M. Johnson, G. J. Stanton, and S. Baron, Proc. Soc. Exp. Biol. Med. 154: 138 (1977).]

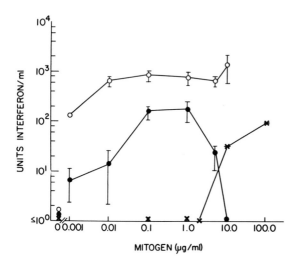

FIGURE 7. Stimulation of the production of mitogen-type interferon in C57B1/6 mouse spleen cell cultures by various T-lymphocyte mitogens. Spleen cells and mitogens were incubated for 48 hr under conditions as described for the PFC response. Interferon concentrations are expressed as the mean of duplicate determinations $\pm$ SD. The SD (not plotted) for 0.001 μg SEA is 146. The responses are representative of three experiments. From Ref. 10. Key: SEA, o—o; Con A, ●—●; PHA-P, ×—×. [Reprinted with permission from H. M. Johnson, G. J. Stanton, and S. Baron, Proc. Soc. Exp. Biol. Med. 154:138 (1977).]

It was found that the ability to inhibit the PFC response to SRBC was proportional to the ability of these mitogens to induce interferon in the cultures. Staphylococcal enterotoxin A (SEA), a simple protein toxin of molecular weight approximately 28,500 that is produced by Staphylococcus aureus, was the most effective inhibitor of the PFC response (Figure 6) and the best inducer of immune interferon (Figure 7), followed by Con A, with PHA-P being the least effective. The data are supportive of previous studies suggesting a role for immune interferon in regulation of the immune response via suppressor T cells [14]. The data also suggest that SEA would be the most suitable inducer of immune interferon in quantity as a prerequisite to purification and characterization of the molecule. Studies in humans, using peripheral blood lymphocytes, also suggest that SEA is more suitable than Con A and PHA-P for induction of immune interferon [54a].

IV. INTERFERON AND CELL-MEDIATED
     IMMUNITY

Along with its inhibitory effects on antibody production, virus-type interferon has also been shown to inhibit cellular immune responses or delayed-
type hypersensitivities. Interferon (2500 U/ml) was shown to inhibit DNA
synthesis of PHA-stimulated and mixed lymphocyte-stimulated mouse spleen
cell suspensions [55]. It is well known that these effects involve the T or
thymus-derived lymphocytes. A similar inhibitory effect has been noted
on Con A-stimulated lymphocytes [56]. Interferon also inhibited the cellular
immune response of mice to allografts [57-59]. Mice with contact sensitivity
to picryl chloride and delayed-type hypersensitivity to SRBC were suppressed
by 3.6×10^5 and 2.1×10^6 U/ml of interferon, respectively, when the interferon was given just prior to challenge with the specific antigens [60].
Sensitization with SRBC was also blocked by virus-type interferon and inducers of virus-type interferon [61]. T-cell function, both afferent and
efferent, then, is also affected by interferon.

Recently, partially purified human interferon was found to inhibit the
response of human lymphocytes in the mixed lymphocyte reaction, while at
the same time enhancing the killer activity of these cells [62]. The mechanisms involved are not known, but the findings are consistent with data that
indicate that interferon increases the surface density of some membrane
antigens [63].

Both human leukocyte and fibroblast interferons were found to suppress
mitogen stimulation of DNA synthesis in peripheral lymphocytes [64]. Interferon had to be continuously present in order to suppress DNA synthesis.
The induction of the antiviral state and the immunosuppressive state in the
in vitro PFC response do not require the continuous presence of virus-type
interferon once these states have been induced [25]. This may be due to
the fact that interferon is much more effective in inducing the antiviral and
immunosuppressive states than in blocking DNA synthesis.

V. INTERFERON AND GRAFT-VS.-HOST
    (GVH) REACTION

Poly rI:poly rC was employed in studies with mice to determine its effect
on the graft-vs.-host (GVH) reaction [65]. This is the reaction of injected
immunocompetent cells against the cells and tissues of a genetically non-
identical recipient. The recipient is unable to reject the graft because of
its immunoincompetence as a result of immaturity or immunosuppression.
When effector spleen cells were removed from mice three days after injection with poly rI:poly rC, the GVH reaction was enhanced in allogenic newborn mouse recipients of these cells. On the other hand, if the effector

spleen cells were removed 7 or 13 days after the injection of poly rI:poly rC, the GVH reaction was suppressed. Thus, poly rI:poly rC either enhanced or suppressed the GVH reaction, depending on the time of removal of the effector spleen cells after injection of the donor mice with poly rI:poly rC.

In a related study, Con A treatment of mouse spleen cells prior to their administration to lethally irradiated allogenic recipients resulted in 80% or greater protection of the animals against development of overt wasting disease (GVH reaction) over a 100-day period [66]. Interferon, based on its suppressor properties, is a good candidate as a possible mediator of the Con A-induced suppression of the GVH reaction. In another study [67], the intensity of the GVH reaction was significantly reduced when the donor mice were injected with large amounts of interferon prior to removal of cells for grafting.

Virus-type interferons from several sources and of different specific activities inhibit the in vitro PFC response in the mouse system in proportion to the antiviral activity [25]. In a system where parent donor spleen cells were treated with various interferons prior to injection into F_1 hybrid newborn mice, it was observed that some virus-type interferon preparations blocked the GVH reaction while others were without effect (H. M. Johnson and J. Georgiades, unpublished data). Blockade was related to the source of interferon and not the specific activity. Thus virus-type interferons may affect the in vitro PFC response and the GVH reaction differently.

VI. RELATIONSHIP OF CYCLIC AMP, IMMUNE INTERFERON, AND THE IMMUNE RESPONSE

It has been proposed that adenosine $3':5'$-cyclic monophosphate (cyclic AMP) has an inhibitory effect on the immunological and inflammatory functions of lymphocytes [68]. Evidence has been obtained that suggests that cyclic AMP may play a role in regulation of interferon production by lymphocytes and suppression of the in vitro PFC response [69]. Figure 8 presents data showing dibutyryl cyclic AMP inhibition of the production of immune interferon in C57B1/6 mouse spleen cell cultures that were stimulated by the two T-cell mitogens Con A and SEA. Dibutyryl cyclic AMP, 2×10^{-5} M, inhibited Con A stimulation of interferon production by 96%, while 1×10^{-4} M inhibited SEA stimulation of interferon production by 85%. When the same concentrations of dibutyryl cyclic AMP were added to the supernatant fluids of mouse spleen cell cultures after complete interferon production, no inhibition of antiviral activity of the interferon was observed, so it is concluded that dibutyryl cyclic AMP blocked the production of immune interferon, and not the established activity of produced interferon.

Table 3 presents data on dibutyryl cyclic AMP blockade of mitogen-induced suppression of the in vitro PFC response to SRBC. SEA inhibited the PFC response by >90% when compared to controls. Protection of the

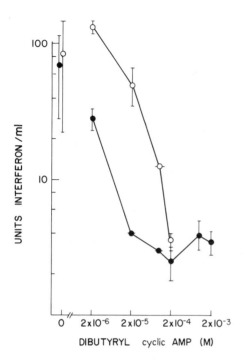

FIGURE 8. Dibutyryl cyclic AMP inhibition of the production of interferon in concanavalin A (Con A, ●—●) and staphylococcal enterotoxin A (SEA, o—o) stimulated C57B1/6 female (8-weeks-old) mouse spleen cell cultures. Cultures consisted of 1.5×10^7 spleen cells/ml and 2 μg and 1 μg Con A and SEA, respectively. Dibutyryl cyclic AMP and mitogens were added to cultures at the same time, and the cells were incubated for 48 hr. Supernatant fluids were obtained by centrifugation of the harvested cultures at 1000 rpm in a RC-3 Sorval centrifuge at 7°C. Data are plotted as units of interferon per milliliter ± SD for duplicated samples. From Ref. 69. [Reprinted with permission from H. M. Johnson, Nature 265:154 (1977).]

PFC responses was essentially complete when dibutyryl cyclic AMP (1.4×10^{-4} M) was added to cultures along with SEA. Dibutyryl cyclic AMP protection of the PFC responses from Con A suppression was also observed. Con A, at 1.0 and 2.0 μg/ml, inhibited the PFC response by >90% when compared to the controls. Dose response studies with various concentrations of dibutyryl cyclic AMP showed that the concentrations (1×10^{-4} to 2×10^{-4} M) of the cyclic ribonucleotide that blocked the development of suppressor activity correlated with those concentrations that blocked the production of interferon in spleen cultures stimulated by the T-cell

TABLE 3. Effect of Dibutyryl Cyclic AMP on Mitogen-Induced
Suppression of the in vitro PFC Response to SRBC

Mitogen	Mitogen concentration (µg/ml)	Dibutyryl cyclic AMP $(1.4 \times 10^{-4}$ M)	PFC/10^6 viable cells $\pm$ SD
SEA	0.25	-	64 $\pm$ 8
SEA	0.50	-	101 $\pm$ 11
SEA	0.25	+	5080 $\pm$ 820
SEA	0.50	+	5508 $\pm$ 1406
—	—	+	4148 $\pm$ 296
—	—	-	5206 $\pm$ 3626
Con A	1.0	-	7 $\pm$ 9
Con A	2.0	-	16 $\pm$ 11
Con A	1.0	+	1577 $\pm$ 505
Con A	2.0	+	1456 $\pm$ 307
—	—	+	3146 $\pm$ 537
—	—	-	2571 $\pm$ 691

Source: Reprinted with permission from Ref. 69.

mitogens (Figure 9) [70]. Dibutyryl guanosine 3':5'-cyclic monophosphate
(cyclic GMP), at the same concentrations, had no effect on either mitogen
stimulation of interferon production or mitogen-induced suppression of the
in vitro PFC response.

The effect of dibutyryl cyclic AMP on SEA-induced immunosuppression
and interferon production was further explored by adding dibutyryl cyclic
AMP $(1.4 \times 10^{-4}$ M) to cultures at various times relative to SEA (0.5 µg/ml)
addition and determining the PFC response (Figure 10) [70]. In a parallel
study, SEA induction of interferon under the same conditions was determined
(Figure 10). When dibutyryl cyclic AMP was added to the cultures at either
-1 or 0 hr, complete blockade of the SEA-induced immunosuppression was
observed. An enhancement of the PFC response was obtained when dibutyryl
cyclic AMP was added to the cultures at 0 hr; however, subsequent experiments did not always show this enhancement. With increasing time between
mitogen addition and dibutyryl cyclic AMP addition to cultures, there was
an increasing amount of interferon produced and a corresponding increase

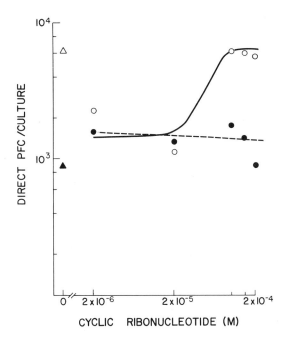

FIGURE 9. Dibutyryl cyclic AMP blockade of SEA (0.5 μg/ml) suppression
of the in vitro anti-SRBC, PFC response in C57B1/6 female (8-weeks-old)
mouse spleen cell cultures. SEA, SRBC, and cyclic ribonucleotides were
added to cultures at the same time, and direct anti-SRBC, PFC/culture
were determined on day 5. The data are expressed as the mean of duplicate
determinations. Mean coefficient of variation for all determinations was
27%. Key: △, SRBC; ▲, SEA + SRBC; o—o, dibutyryl cyclic AMP +
SEA + SRBC; ●---●, dibutyryl cyclic GMP + SEA + SRBC. From Ref. 70.
[Reprinted with permission from H. M. Johnson, J. E. Blalock, and
S. Baron, Cell. Immunol. 33: 170 (1977).

in the suppression of the anti-SRBC, PFC response. The data suggest a
direct relationship, then, between the effect of dibutyryl cyclic AMP on
SEA-induced immunosuppression and on production of interferon by SEA-
stimulated cultures. This is further evidence that mitogen-induced suppression of the in vitro response is related to mitogen induction of interferon
in the cultures.

Cholera toxin (an enterotoxin produced by Vibrio cholerae) raises the
endogenous level of cyclic AMP by stimulating adenylate cyclase activity.
Adenylate cyclase converts ATP to cyclic AMP. The methyl xanthine
3-isobutyl-1-methyl xanthine (IMX) raises the endogenous cyclic AMP level

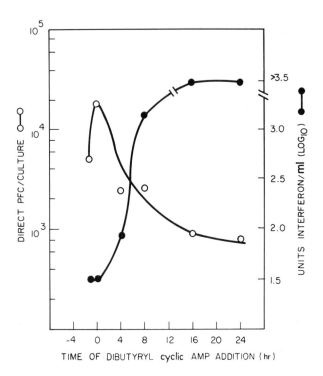

FIGURE 10. Determination of the PFC response and interferon production
after addition of dibutyryl cyclic AMP to spleen cell cultures at various
times relative to SEA addition. SEA (0.5 µg/ml) and SRBC were added at
0 hr to the spleen cells for the PFC response, and dibutyryl cyclic AMP
(1.4×10^{-4} M) was added at the indicated times relative to time 0.
Direct anti-SRBC responses were determined on day 5. Mean PFC
responses/culture $\pm$ SD for the SRBC control and the SEA-suppressed
control were 4610 ± 834 and 350 ± 353, respectively. Parallel studies
were carried out on interferon production under the same culture conditions,
except that SRBC were absent from the cultures and the cultures were
incubated 48 hr after SEA addition at time 0. From Ref. 70. [Reprinted
with permission from H. M. Johnson, J. E. Blalock, and S. Baron, Cell.
Immunol. 33: 170 (1977).]

TABLE 4. Effect of Agents that Increase Endogenous Cyclic AMP
Levels on SEA-Induced Suppression of the in vitro PFC
Response to SRBC

Agent (μg/ml)	SEA (0.5 μg/ml)	PFC/10^6 viable cells $\pm$ SD
—	+	431 $\pm$ 135
Cholera toxin (0.1)	+	2984 $\pm$ 596
Cholera toxin (0.1)	−	4791 $\pm$ 165
—	−	4326
—	+	91 $\pm$ 42
IMX (12.5)	+	3973 $\pm$ 477
IMX (12.5)	−	1366 $\pm$ 571
—	−	2294 $\pm$ 1238

Source: Reprinted with permission from Ref. 69.

by inhibiting phosphodiesterase activity. Both agents blocked SEA suppression of the in vitro anti-SRBC, PFC response in a manner similar to that observed for dibutyryl cyclic AMP (Table 4) [69]. Further, they blocked SEA stimulation of interferon production in mouse spleen cell cultures at concentrations that blocked SEA suppressor activity.

Dibutyryl cyclic GMP (10^{-3} to 10^{-7} M) did not affect the ability of dibutyryl cyclic AMP (1.4×10^{-4} M) to block the suppression of the PFC response by SEA; nor was the effect of dibutyryl cyclic AMP on mitogen stimulation of interferon affected by dibutyryl cyclic GMP [70]. This is further evidence that the phenomena reported here are due to cyclic AMP and are not influenced by cyclic GMP in this system.

The data suggest that immune-induced interferon is associated with mitogen-induced suppressor cell activity, and that the interferon may possibly be a mediator of such activity. In related studies, it has been shown that high concentrations (10^{-3} M) of dibutyryl cyclic AMP can inhibit the yield of interferon from phytohemagglutinin-stimulated human peripheral leukocytes [71] and from virus- or polyribonucleotide-stimulated mouse L-cell cultures [72]. The data presented here show a logical relationship between cyclic AMP, immune interferon activity, suppressor cell activity, and regulation of the immune response. Preliminary studies on the effect of cyclic AMP on induction of virus-type interferon in mouse spleen cultures suggest that this interferon system may be slightly more resistant to blockade of induction.

VII. RELATIONSHIP OF INTERFERONS TO
      OTHER MEDIATORS OF IMMUNE FUNCTION

Immune interferon, induced in leukocyte cultures by PHA, is among the
earliest described lymphokines [5]. A plethora of lymphocyte-regulating,
soluble factors have subsequently been described [15]. Several of these
factors may ultimately be shown to represent additional biological properties
of immune interferon. Mitogen-stimulated T lymphocytes, for example,
produce a soluble immune response suppressor(s) (SIRS), which inhibits
the in vitro PFC responses [73]. Sensitized T lymphocytes that are stimulated by specific antigen also produce an inhibitor of the in vitro antibody
response, which may be the same as SIRS [74]. Contained within the SIRS
supernatant fluid are immune interferon and macrophage migration inhibitory
factor [10,31]. To date the three activities have not been separated, and
thus they may represent different biological activities of the same molecule.
     Recently, mouse fibroblast interferon has been purified to homogeneity
[75]. The purified interferon was capable of inhibiting cell multiplication.
This is probably the most convincing evidence that virus-type interferon
possesses biological activities in addition to being antiviral. It would be
interesting to determine the relationship of virus-type interferon to various
lymphokines that are capable of inhibiting DNA synthesis [15].

VIII. A MODEL

In Section I we discussed the cooperation that occurs between lymphocytes
and between lymphocytes and macrophages to help or suppress the immune
response. The question is how do interferons, with their immunosuppressive properties, fit into the suppressor cell picture of immunoregulation?
The answer is that we do not know; but if we focus on the B cells and antibody production and helper and suppressor T-cell effects, it might help
glue together the interferon data. Antigen contact induces the helper or
suppressor T cell. It is assumed that the presence of a receptor for the
antigen on both the B and T cell will bring the two cells into close proximity
when they bind to the same antigen so that a mediator, after release from
the T cell, is in sufficient concentration in the microenvironment of the
B cell to exert its effect.
     This model can be applied directly to explain how antigen-induced
mediators (such as immune interferon) may exert their suppressor effects.
Assuming similar interactions of T and B cells and antigen, the suppressor
substance (possibly interferon) could be released from the appropriate
antigen-stimulated T cell in the microenvironment of the B cell and inhibit
the B-cell antibody response to the same antigen (Figure 11). Thus, the
kinetics of the antibody response could be the reflection of a dynamic interaction of "helper" and "suppressor" activities with the responding B cell.

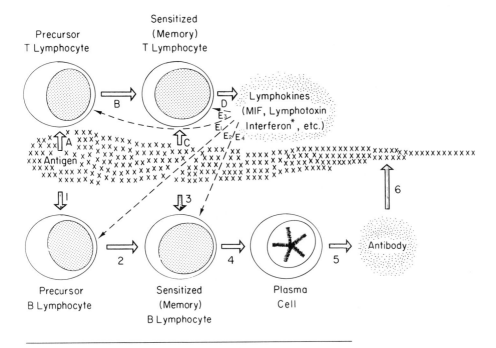

Time →

FIGURE 11. Cellular events in the induction and immunosuppressive action of interferons. Antigen comes into contact with a precursor T lymphocyte (A), which undergoes differentiation to a sensitized T lymphocyte (B). This cell, driven by antigen (C), may become a memory cell or it may release mediators known as lymphokines (D). Among the mediators produced by the T lymphocyte is immune interferon*. Antigen also reacts with a precursor B lymphocyte (1), which undergoes differentiation to a sensitized B lymphocyte (and memory B cell) (2). The sensitized B cell is further driven by antigen (3) to become a plasma cell (4), which is responsible for most of the antibody (5) that is produced. This antibody reacts with the specific antigen (6). Both antigen-induced (immune) and virus-induced interferons are capable of reacting with precursor T (E_1) and B (E_2) lymphocytes as well as sensitized T (E_3) and B (E_4) lymphocytes. As differentiation progresses, in part as a result of continued antigen presence, it becomes progressively more difficult to inhibit lymphocyte function by interferons. Plasma cell production of antibody is resistant to inhibition by interferon. The macrophage is not included in the figure, but interferons may exert their immunosuppressive effects via a required macrophage function in the immune response. The diagrammatic scheme does not necessarily imply, therefore, a direct effect of the interferons on the lymphocytes. From Ref. 1a. [Reprinted with permission from H. M. Johnson and S. Baron, Pharmacol. Ther. 1 (1977), Pergamon Press, Ltd.]

The model requires modification for postulating how cells interact in suppressor effects involving virus–type interferon. Virus–type interferon is produced by virtually every cell type in the body [1]. An agent (virus, for example) that is capable of stimulating the production of virus–type interferon can theoretically shut down the immune response, provided that the interferon–producing cell produces an effective concentration of interferon in the microenvironment of the responding B cell. Viruses with infectivities that are intimately associated with the lymphoid tissues may have, in general, a greater suppressive effect on the immune response than viruses not associated with lymphoid tissue [76]. Because of the intimate association of macrophages and T cells with the responding B cells, these cell types would be expected to play a prominent role in suppressing the immune response through virus–type interferon. As mentioned above, it has been shown that T cells are required for the virus–type interferon inducers poly rA: poly rU and poly rI: poly rC to inhibit the in vitro PFC response to E. coli 0127 LPS [48]. We have shown that this inhibition is blocked by antiserum to virus–type interferon [14].

Given this broadly outlined model, more work still needs to be done in order to precisely determine the role of various types of interferons in the regulation of the immune response. It remains to be determined whether other reported suppressions are related to interferon. This working model provides a guide for determining the role of interferon in the mechanism of regulation of the immune response. The cyclic AMP data can be incorporated into this working hypothesis without significant modification.

REFERENCES

1. N. B. Finter (ed.), in Interferon and Interferon Inducers, American Elsevier, New York, 1973.
1a. H. M. Johnson and S. Baron, Pharmacol. Ther. 1: 349 (1977).
2. A. Isaacs, Advan. Virus Res. 10: 1 (1963).
3. A. K. Field, A. A. Tytell, G. P. Lampson, and M. R. Hilleman, Proc. Nat. Acad. Sci. U.S. 58: 1004 (1967).
4. K. Paucker, Texas Repts. Biol. Med. in press (1978).
5. E. F. Wheelock, Science 149: 310 (1965).
6. J. A. Green, S. R. Cooperband, and S. Kibrick, Science 164: 1415 (1969).
7. S. B. Salvin, J. S. Youngner, and W. H. Lederer, Infec. Immun. 7: 68 (1973).
8. J. Stobo, I. Green, L. Jackson, and S. Baron, J. Immunol. 112: 1589 (1974).
9. L. B. Epstein, Texas Repts. Biol. Med. in press (1978).
10. H. M. Johnson, G. J. Stanton, and S. Baron, Proc. Soc. Exp. Biol. Med. 154: 138 (1977).

11. E. A. Havell, B. Berman, C. A. Ogburn, K. Berg, K. Paucker, and J. Vilček, Proc. Nat. Acad. Sci. U.S. 72:2185 (1975).

12. N. Maehara, M. Ho, and J. A. Armstrong, Infec. Immun. 17:572 (1977).

13. J. A. Youngner and S. B. Salvin, J. Immunol. 111:1914 (1973).

14. H. M. Johnson and S. Baron, Cell. Immunol. 25:106 (1976).

14a. L. C. Osborne, J. A. Georgiades, and H. M. Johnson, Cell. Immunol. in press (1980).

15. B. H. Waksman and Y. Namba, Cell. Immunol. 21:161 (1976).

16. W. Braun and H. B. Levy, Proc. Soc. Exp. Biol. Med. 141:769 (1972).

17. T. J. Chester, K. Paucker, and T. C. Merigan, Nature 246:92 (1973).

18. B. R. Brodeur and T. C. Merigan, J. Immunol. 113:1319 (1975).

19. B. R. Brodeur and T. C. Merigan, J. Immunol. 114:1323 (1975).

20. J. Ngan, S. H. S. Lee, and L. S. Kind, J. Immunol. 117:1063 (1976).

21. S. Ida, J. J. Hooks, R. P. Siraganian, and A. L. Notkins, J. Exp. Med. 145:892 (1977).

22. G. Sonnenfeld, A. D. Mandel, and T. C. Merigan, Cell. Immunol. 34:193 (1977).

23. R. H. Gisler, P. Lindahl, and I. Gresser, J. Immunol. 113:438 (1974).

24. H. M. Johnson, B. G. Smith, and S. Baron, IRCS Med. Sci. 2:1616 (1974).

25. H. M. Johnson, B. G. Smith, and S. Baron, J. Immunol. 114:403 (1975).

26. H. M. Johnson, J. A. Bukovic, and S. Baron, Cell. Immunol. 20:104 (1975).

27. R. J. Booth, J. M. Booth, and J. Marbrook, Eur. J. Immunol. 6:769 (1976).

28. C. W. Pierce, J. Exp. Med. 130:345 (1969).

29. R. J. Booth, J. M. Rostrick, A. R. Bellamy, and J. Marbrook, Aust. J. Exp. Biol. Med. Sci. 54:11 (1976).

30. B. A. Clinton, T. J. Mogoc, R. L. Aspinoll, and N. P. Rapoza, Cell. Immunol. 27:60 (1976).

31. T. Tadokuma, A. L. Kuhner, R. R. Rich, J. R. David, and C. W. Pierce, J. Immunol. 117:323 (1976).

32. G. Trivers, D. Braungart, and E. J. Leonard, J. Immunol. 117:130 (1976).

33. J. A. Georgiades, L. C. Osborne, R. Moulton, and H. M. Johnson, Proc. Soc. Exp. Biol. Med. 161:167 (1979).

34. H. M. Johnson, Cell. Immunol. 36:220 (1978).

35. R. M. Schultz, J. D. Papamatheakis, and M. A. Chirigos, Science 197:674 (1977).

36. R. M. Schultz, M. A. Chirigos, and U. I. Heine, Cell. Immunol. 35:84 (1978).

37. D. S. Nelson, in Immunobiology of the Macrophage (D. S. Nelson, ed.), Academic Press, New York, 1976, p. 235.

38. W. Braun, M. Nakano, L. Jaraskova, Y. Yajima, and L. Jimenez, in Nucleic Acids in Immunology (O. J. Plescia and W. Braun, eds.), Springer-Verlag, New York, 1968, p. 347.

39. A. G. Johnson, J. Schmidtke, K. Merritt, and T. Han, in Nucleic Acids in Immunology (O. J. Plescia and W. Braun, eds.), Springer-Verlag, New York, 1968, p. 379.

40. J. R. Schmidtke and A. G. Johnson, J. Immunol. 106:1191 (1971).

41. A. G. Johnson, in Immune RNA (E. P. Cohen, ed.), CRC Press, Cleveland, 1976.

42. H. Markowitz, D. A. Person, F. L. Gitnick, and R. E. Ritts, Science 163:476 (1969).

43. H. S. Egan, W. J. Reeder, and R. D. Ekstedt, J. Immunol. 112:63 (1974).

44. C. G. Romball and W. O. Weigle, J. Immunol. 11:556 (1975).

45. W. Braun and M. Ishizuka, Proc. Nat. Acad. Sci. U.S. 68:1114 (1971).

46. M. Ishizuka, W. Braun, and T. Matsumoto, J. Immunol. 107:1027 (1971).

47. R. E. Cone and J. J. Marchalonis, Aust. J. Exp. Biol. Med. 50:69 (1972).

48. H. M. Johnson, J. A. Bukovic, and B. G. Smith, Proc. Soc. Exp. Biol. Med. 149:599 (1975).

49. T. M. Chused, S. S. Kassan, and D. E. Mosier, J. Immunol. 116: 1579 (1976).

50. R. W. Dutton, J. Exp. Med. 136:1445 (1972).

51. R. R. Rich, and C. W. Pierce, J. Exp. Med. 137:205 (1973).

52. J. Watson, R. Epstein, I. Nakoinz, and P. Ralph, J. Immunol. 110: 43 (1973).

53. B. G. Smith and H. M. Johnson, J. Immunol. 115:575 (1975).

54. B. R. Brodeur, Y. Weinstein, K. L. Melmon, and T. C. Merigan, Cell. Immunol. 29:363 (1977).

54a. M. P. Langford, G. J. Stanton, and H. M. Johnson, Infec. Immun. 22:62 (1978).

55. P. Lindahl-Magnusson, P. Leary, and I. Gresser, Nature [New Biol.] 237:120 (1972).

56. K. R. Rozee, S. H. S. Lee, and J. Ngan, Nature [New Biol.] 245:16 (1973).

57. L. E. Mobraaten, E. De Maeyer, and J. De Maeyer-Guignard, Transplant. 16:415 (1973).

58. J. C. Cerottini, K. T. Brunner, P. Lindahl, and I. Gresser, Nature [New Biol.] 242:152 (1973).

59. M. S. Hirsch, D. A. Ellis, P. H. Black, A. P. Monaco, and M. L. Wood, Transplantation 17:234 (1974).

60. E. De Mayer, J. De Maeyer-Guignard, and M. Vandeputte, Proc. Nat. Acad. Sci. U.S. 72:1753 (1975).

61. J. De Maeyer-Guignard, A. Cochard, and E. De Maeyer, Science 190: 574 (1975).
62. I. Heron, K. Berg, and K. Cantell, J. Immunol. 117: 1370 (1976).
63. D. Killander, P. Lindahl, L. Lundin, P. Leary, and I. Gresser, Eur. J. Immunol. 6: 56 (1976).
64. H. Miörer, L. E. Landström, E. Larner, I. Larsson, E. Lundgren, and Ö. Strannegard, Cell. Immunol. 35: 15 (1978).
65. H. Cantor, R. Asofsky, and H. B. Levy, J. Immunol. 104: 1035 (1970).
66. M. L. Tyan, Proc. Soc. Exp. Biol. Med. 150: 628 (1975).
67. M. S. Hirsch, D. A. Ellis, M. R. Proffitt, P. H. Black, and M. A. Chirigos, Nature [New Biol.] 244: 102 (1973).
68. H. R. Bourne, L. M. Lichtenstein, K. L. Melmon, C. A. Henney, Y. Weinstein, and G. M. Shearer, Science 184: 19 (1974).
69. H. M. Johnson, Nature 265: 154 (1977).
70. H. M. Johnson, J. E. Blalock, and S. Baron, Cell. Immunol. 33: 170 (1977).
71. L. B. Epstein and H. R. Bourne, in Mitogens in Immunobiology (J. J. Oppenheim and D. L. Rosenstreich, eds.), Academic Press, New York, 1976, p. 453.
72. F. Dianzani, P. Neri, and M. Zucca, Proc. Soc. Exp. Biol. Med. 140: 1375 (1972).
73. R. R. Rich and C. W. Pierce, J. Immunol. 112: 1360 (1974).
74. D. W. Thomas, W. K. Roberts, and D. W. Talmage, J. Immunol. 114: 1616 (1975).
75. J. De Maeyer-Guignard, M. G. Tovey, I. Gresser, and E. De Maeyer, Nature 271: 622 (1978).
76. J.-L. Virelizier, A.-M. Virelizier, and A. C. Allison, J. Immunol. 117: 748 (1976).

AUTHOR INDEX

Numbers in brackets are reference numbers and indicate that an author's work is referred to although his name is not cited in the text. Underlined numbers give the page on which the complete reference is listed.

SUBJECT INDEX

A

ABMP (2-amino-5-bromo-6-methyl-4-pyrimidinol), 149, 157

Acenaphthene, 191

Actinomycin D, 8, 100, 103

Adenovirus, 121

Adenylate cyclase, 12

Albumin-sepharose columns, interferon purification, 36

Amnion, human, 150

Amphotericin B, effect on interferon response, 6

Amyotrophic lateral sclerosis, tilorone therapy, 212

Animal models, antiviral chemotherapy, 116-120

Anthraquinones, 147, 191

Antibody
  production affected by interferon, 263-290
  production enhanced by polynucleotides, 179
  production enhanced by pyran, 246

Antibody affinity chromatography
  of interferons, 28, 37
  qualitative data, 30

Antibody columns, stability of, 28

Antibody response, effect of interferon on, 269-275

Antigenic properties
  human interferons, 46
  masking of, 29

Anti-interferon antibody, 277-279
  absorption of, 29

Antiproliferation, by interferons, 89, 90, 91, 93, 94

Antitumor
  chemotherapy, 90
  polyanions, 249

Antiviral
  chemotherapy, 8-11, 114-140, 151
  polyanions, 251

Antiviral protein, 8

C

Carboxylic polyanions, interferon inducers, 245

Catecholamines, effect on interferon induction, 156

Cell growth, inhibition by interferon, 89

Chemotherapy, combination with interferon, 104

Chikungunya virus, 158

Cholera toxin
  effect on interferon, 10
  immune response, 285-287

Chromatography
  hydrophobic, 27
  of interferons, 22-50

Chromosome 21, 92

Chronic relapsing neuropathy, treatment with poly ICLC, 180

Ciba-cron blue F3Ga-Sepharose, purification of interferons, 36

Clinical trials, interferons, 96-99

Clinical use, interferons, 114-137